Foodborne Illness: Latest Threats and Emerging Issues

Editors

DAVID ACHESON
JENNIFER MCENTIRE
CHELESTE M. THORPE

INFECTIOUS DISEASE CLINICS OF NORTH AMERICA

www.id.theclinics.com

Consulting Editor
HELEN W. BOUCHER

September 2013 • Volume 27 • Number 3

ELSEVIER

1600 John F. Kennedy Boulevard • Suite 1800 • Philadelphia, Pennsylvania, 19103-2899.
http://www.theclinics.com

INFECTIOUS DISEASE CLINICS OF NORTH AMERICA Volume 27, Number 3
September 2013 ISSN 0891–5520, ISBN-13: 978-0-323-18858-6

Editor: Stephanie Donley

Infectious Disease Clinics of North America (ISSN 0891–5520) is published in March, June, September, and December by Elsevier Inc., 360 Park Avenue South, New York, NY 10010-1710. Periodicals postage paid at New York, NY and additional mailing offices. Subscription prices are $282.00 per year for US individuals, $482.00 per year for US institutions, $139.00 per year for US students, $334.00 per year for Canadian individuals, $596.00 per year for Canadian institutions, $398.00 per year for international individuals, $596.00 per year for international institutions, and $192.00 per year for Canadian and international students. To receive student rate, orders must be accompanied by name of affiliated institution, date of term, and the *signature* of program/residency coordinator on institution letterhead. Orders will be billed at individual rate until proof of status is received. Foreign air speed delivery is included in all *Clinics* subscription prices. All prices are subject to change without notice. **POSTMASTER**: Send address changes to *Infectious Disease Clinics of North America*, Elsevier Health Sciences Division, Subcription Customer Service, 3251 Riverport Lane, Maryland Heights, MO 63043. **Customer Service: 1-800-654-2452 (US). From outside of the US and Canada, call 1-314-447-8871. Fax: 1-314-447-8029. E-mail: JournalsCustomerService-usa@elsevier.com (print support) or JournalsOnlineSupport-usa@elsevier.com (online support).**

Infectious Disease Clinics of North America is also published in Spanish by Editorial Inter-MÅdica, Junin 917, 1er A 1113, Buenos Aires, Argentina.

Reprints. For copies of 100 or more, of articles in this publication, please contact the Commercial Reprints Department, Elsevier Inc., 360 Park Avenue South, New York, New York 10010-1710. Tel. 212-633-3874, Fax: 212-633-3820, E-mail: reprints@elsevier.com.

Infectious Disease Clinics of North America is covered in *MEDLINE/PubMed (Index Medicus), Current Contents/ Clinical Medicine, Science Citation Alert, SCISEARCH,* and *Research Alert.*

Printed and bound by CPI Group (UK) Ltd, Croydon, CR0 4YY

Transferred to digital print 2012

Contributors

CONSULTING EDITOR

HELEN W. BOUCHER, MD, FIDSA, FACP
Director, Infectious Diseases Fellowship Program; Associate Professor of Medicine, Division of Geographic Medicine and Infectious Diseases, Tufts Medical Center, Boston, Massachusetts

EDITORS

DAVID ACHESON, MD, FRCP
CEO, The Acheson Group, Frankfort, Illinois

JENNIFER McENTIRE, PhD
Vice President and Chief Science Officer, The Acheson Group, Frankfort, Illinois

CHELESTE M. THORPE, MD
Associate Professor, Tufts University School of Medicine; Staff Physician, Tufts Medical Center, Boston, Massachusetts

AUTHORS

DAVID ACHESON, MD, FRCP
CEO, The Acheson Group, Frankfort, Illinois

MICHAEL B. BATZ, MSc
Head, Food Safety Programs, Emerging Pathogens Institute, University of Florida, Gainesville, Florida

ERIK J. BOLL, PhD
Department of Microbiology and Physiological Systems, University of Massachusetts Medical School, Worcester, Massachusetts

CHRISTOPHER R. BRADEN, MD
Director, Division of Foodborne, Waterborne and Environmental Diseases, National Center for Emerging and Zoonotic Infectious Diseases, Centers for Disease Control and Prevention, Atlanta, Georgia

T. KEEFE DAVIS, MD
Division of Nephrology, Department of Pediatrics, Washington University School of Medicine, St Louis, Missouri

ERIN DiCAPRIO, MS
Department of Food Science and Technology, College of Food, Agricultural, and Environmental Sciences, The Ohio State University, Columbus, Ohio

MICHAEL S. DONNENBERG, MD
Professor, Department of Medicine, Department of Microbiology and Immunology;
Director, Medical Scientist Training Program, University of Maryland School of Medicine,
Baltimore, Maryland

EVAN HENKE, PhD
Professional Service Account Representative, 3M, St. Paul, Minnesota

DALLAS G. HOOVER, PhD
Professor, Department of Animal and Food Sciences, University of Delaware, Newark,
Delaware

JOHN HUGHES, PhD
Department of Molecular Virology, Immunology, and Molecular Genetics, College of
Medicine, The Ohio State University, Columbus, Ohio

DAKSHINA M. JANDHYALA, PhD
Division of Geographic Medicine and Infectious Diseases, Tufts Medical Center, Boston,
Massachusetts

GERALD T. KEUSCH, MD
Professor of Medicine and International Health, Boston University School of Medicine,
Boston, Massachusetts

BARBARA KOWALCYK, PhD
Assistant Research Professor, Department of Food, Bioprocessing and Nutrition
Sciences; CEO and Director of Research and Public Policy, Center for Foodborne Illness
Research and Prevention, North Carolina State University, Raleigh, North Carolina

YUSHUAN LAI
Department of Microbiology and Physiological Systems, University of Massachusetts
Medical School, Worcester, Massachusetts

JOHN M. LEONG, MD, PhD
Department of Molecular Biology and Microbiology, Tufts University School of Medicine,
Boston, Massachusetts

JIANRONG LI, PhD, DVM
Department of Food Science and Technology, College of Food, Agricultural, and
Environmental Sciences; Division of Environmental Health Sciences, College of Public
Health, The Ohio State University, Columbus, Ohio

YUANMEI MA, PhD
Department of Food Science and Technology, College of Food, Agricultural, and
Environmental Sciences, The Ohio State University, Columbus, Ohio

BETH A. McCORMICK, PhD
Department of Microbiology and Physiological Systems, University of Massachusetts
Medical School, Worcester, Massachusetts

JENNIFER McENTIRE, PhD
Vice President and Chief Science Officer, The Acheson Group, Frankfort, Illinois

RYAN McKEE, MD
Division of Emergency Medicine, Department of Pediatrics, Washington University School
of Medicine, St Louis, Missouri

SHIVAKUMAR NARAYANAN, MD
Clinical Fellow, Division of Infectious Diseases, Department of Medicine, Institute of Human Virology, University of Maryland Medical Center, Baltimore, Maryland

ALEXANDER RODRIGUEZ-PALACIOS, DVM, DVSc, PhD, Diplomate ACVIM, Diplomate ACVM
Division of Gastroenterology and Liver Disease, Digestive Health Research Center, Case Western Reserve University School of Medicine, Cleveland, Ohio

DAVID SCHNADOWER, MD, MPH
Division of Emergency Medicine, Department of Pediatrics, Washington University School of Medicine, St Louis, Missouri

THEODORE STEINER, MD
Associate Professor, Infectious Diseases, University of British Columbia, Vancouver, British Columbia, Canada

PHILLIP I. TARR, MD
Division of Gastroenterology, Hepatology, and Nutrition, Department of Pediatrics, Washington University School of Medicine, St Louis, Missouri

ROBERT V. TAUXE, MD, MPH
Deputy Director, Division of Foodborne, Waterborne and Environmental Diseases, National Center for Emerging and Zoonotic Infectious Diseases, Centers for Disease Control and Prevention, Atlanta, Georgia

VIJAY VANGURI, MD
Department of Pathology, University of Massachusetts Medical School, Worcester, Massachusetts

Contents

Immune-compromised hosts are at increased risk of life-threatening complications. This article reviews recommendations for the treatment of the most common and important foodborne illnesses, focusing on those caused by infections or toxins of microbial origin. The cornerstone of life-saving treatment remains oral rehydration therapy, although the use of other supportive measures as well as antibiotics for certain infections is also recommended.

T. Keefe Davis, Ryan McKee, David Schnadower, and Phillip I. Tarr

The management of Shiga toxin-producing *Escherichia coli* (STEC) infections is reviewed. Certain management practices optimize the likelihood of good outcomes, such as avoidance of antibiotics during the prehemolytic uremic syndrome phase, admission to hospital, and vigorous intravenous volume expansion using isotonic fluids. The successful management of STEC infections is based on recognition that a patient might have an STEC infection, and appropriate use of the microbiology laboratory. The timeliness of STEC identification cannot be overemphasized, because it avoids therapies prompted by inappropriate additional testing and directs the clinician to focus on effective management strategies. The opportunities during STEC infections to avert the worst outcomes are brief, and this article emphasizes practical matters relevant to making a diagnosis, anticipating the trajectory of illness, and optimizing care.

Michael B. Batz, Evan Henke, and Barbara Kowalcyk

Foodborne infections with *Campylobacter*, *E. coli* O157:H7, *Listeria monocytogenes*, *Salmonella*, *Shigella*, *Toxoplasma gondii*, and other pathogens can result in long-term sequelae to numerous organ systems. These include irritable bowel syndrome, inflammatory bowel disease, reactive arthritis, hemolytic uremic syndrome, chronic kidney disease, Guillain-Barré Syndrome, neurological disorders from acquired and congenital listeriosis and toxoplasmosis, and cognitive and developmental deficits due to diarrheal malnutrition or severe acute illness. A full understanding of the long-term sequelae of foodborne infection is important both for individual patient management by clinicians, as well as to inform food safety and public health decision making.

David Acheson

Certain subsets of the population are at a greater risk of acquiring foodborne infections and have a greater propensity to develop serious complications. Susceptibility to foodborne infection is dependent on numerous factors that largely relate to the status of an individual's defense systems in regard to both preventing and mitigating foodborne illness. Key examples include the increased susceptibility of pregnant women to listeriosis and increased severity of enteric bacterial infections in patients with AIDS. Clinicians must communicate with higher-risk patients about the risks of foodborne illness, and provide patients with information regarding safe food-handling practices.

regions of the world. In a global economy, both people and food travel the world. With this travel comes the potential for patients to acquire unexpected diseases. Clinicians need to consider foreign travel as well as the consumption of food from other parts of the world when determining the cause of foodborne disease.

INFECTIOUS DISEASE CLINICS
OF NORTH AMERICA

FORTHCOMING ISSUES

December 2013
Sexually Transmitted Diseases
Jeanne Marrazzo, MD, *Editor*

March 2014
Urinary Tract Infections
Kalpana Gupta, MD, *Editor*

June 2014
Antimicrobial Stewardship and Infection Prevention
Sara Cosgrove, MD, Pranita Tamma, MD, and Arjun Srinvasan, MD, *Editors*

RECENT ISSUES

June 2013
Infectious Disease Challenges in Solid Organ Transplant Recipients
Joseph G. Timpone Jr, MD, and Princy N. Kumar, MD, *Editors*

March 2013
Community-Acquired Pneumonia: Controversies and Questions
Thomas M. File Jr, MD, *Editor*

December 2012
Hepatitis C Virus Infection
Barbara McGovern, MD, *Editor*

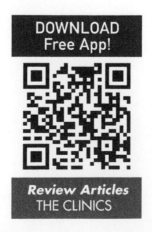

Preface

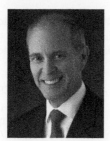 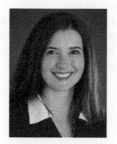 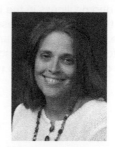

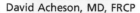

David Acheson, MD, FRCP   Jennifer McEntire, PhD   Cheleste M. Thorpe, MD

Editors

Foodborne illness in the United States continues to be a dynamic and, to us, fascinating field. Dr Keusch's introductory article provides an absorbing global perspective on the history of food and foodborne illness throughout the centuries. His contribution is a perfect launching point for a series of articles that highlight the state of foodborne illness in the United States in the early 21st century, and some of the emerging trends.

We know that much has changed in the past 15 years. In 1996, the US Food Safety and Inspection Service established requirements of the meat and poultry industry, to reduce the incidence of foodborne illness. This program has resulted in an overall decline in bacterial foodborne illness, but some bacterial foodborne illnesses, such as *Campylobacter* and *Vibrio*, continue to increase in incidence.

Drs Braden and Tauxe's article discusses these current epidemiologic trends. For diagnostic methodology and treatment updates, articles by Drs Donnenberg and Narayanan, and Dr Steiner are comprehensive resources for the infectious diseases physician faced with a patient suffering from a foodborne illness. An impact on foodborne illness is the fact that vulnerable populations in the United States continue to increase. There are more Americans age 65 and older now than at any other time in US history, and the United Network for Organ Sharing (UNOS) data show over the past 5 years (2008-2012) a steady number of approximately 28,000 solid organ transplants per annum. Dr Acheson discusses foodborne illness in these, and other, populations at risk, and reviews measures to prevent foodborne illness. Although the vast majority of cases of foodborne illness remain self-limited, Dr Batz's article describes the long-term sequelae of foodborne illness, and who is at higher risk for these sequelae.

We chose several organisms for special focus. Our understanding of treatment of Shiga toxin-producing *Escherichia coli* continues to be refined, and Dr Tarr's article provides a comprehensive review of treatment. The emergence of a novel Shiga toxin-producing enteroaggregative *E coli* is discussed in an article by Drs Leong and Jandhyala. As norovirus continues to be the most important foodborne illness in the United States hands down, with recent strides being made in vaccine development, an article by Dr Li is dedicated to this important pathogen. To round out the focus on emerging infections, Drs Hoover and Rodriguez-Palacios provides an extensive and highly intriguing review of the data supporting the concept that *Clostridium difficile*

Infect Dis Clin N Am 27 (2013) xiii–xiv
http://dx.doi.org/10.1016/j.idc.2013.06.002
0891-5520/13/$ – see front matter © 2013 Elsevier Inc. All rights reserved.

id.theclinics.com

may be a foodborne pathogen. Last but not least, just as Dr Keusch's article provides a historical global view of foodborne illness, Dr McEntire reviews present global impacts on foodborne illness in the United States.

We hope that infectious diseases physicians and others find this volume helpful to their practice. We also hope to transmit some of our interest in this field to others, as it is clear that foodborne illness is not a new problem, but continues, chameleon-like, to provide new challenges and has not yet been conquered.

David Acheson, MD, FRCP
The Acheson Group
1 Old Frankfort Way
Frankfort, IL 60423, USA

Jennifer McEntire, PhD
The Acheson Group
1 Old Frankfort Way
Frankfort, IL 60423, USA

Cheleste M. Thorpe, MD
Tufts Medical Center
800 Washington Street Box 041
Boston, MA 02111, USA

E-mail addresses:
david@achesongroup.com (D. Acheson)
jennifer@achesongroup.com (J. McEntire)
cthorpe@tuftsmedicalcenter.org (C.M. Thorpe)

Perspectives in Foodborne Illness

Gerald T. Keusch, MD

KEYWORDS

- Food safety • Contamination • Technology • Trade • Travel

KEY POINTS

- Foodborne illness has undoubtedly plagued humans from the beginning, as long as we have existed.
- The transition from hunter-gathering societies to settlements with agriculture and domesticated animals improved food security but increased the need for food safety and the opportunities for foodborne illnesses.
- Technology, from simple systems for sanitary disposal of human and animal waste, protection of water from fecal contamination, refrigeration, freezing, and other methods to inhibit microbial growth in food, for example pasteurization of milk, has contributed to the safety of the food supply chain and the reduction in foodborne illness.
- The globalization and increased magnitude of transport of food across the world, partly in response to the growth in population and in part to changes in the way that people obtain, prepare, and consume food, provides new ways for pathogens to be transported and transmitted.
- In addition to travel of the food supply, travel of people may expose them to foodborne illness to which they would not otherwise be exposed.
- Factory farming, the large-scale growth and processing especially of food animals, can easily promote unhygienic conditions and contamination in unprecedented scale of food products with pathogens, toxins, antibiotics, and other potentially dangerous substances.
- The scale of these factors has diminished the ability of regulatory agencies to monitor the safety of the products being consumed on a daily basis.
- Nonetheless, there are many opportunities to improve both technology and practice and, in turn, help to prevent or reduce future disease incidence.

INTRODUCTION

To many people in affluent nations, mere mention of the word food conjures up visions of heaped-up and sometimes well-presented piles of carbohydrate-laden and fat-laden items on a plate, daring to be consumed in 1 sitting. Thoughts may drift to nutritional value and health, or perhaps to weight control, but these thoughts usually do not linger. Rarely is there a concern for the safety of the food in front of the consumer.

Boston University School of Medicine, Boston, MA 02118, USA
E-mail address: Keusch@bu.edu

Infect Dis Clin N Am 27 (2013) 501–515
http://dx.doi.org/10.1016/j.idc.2013.05.005
0891-5520/13/$ – see front matter © 2013 Elsevier Inc. All rights reserved.

When this safety is considered, myths, superstitions, and urban legends abound. In contrast, to the poor, hungry, and destitute, food is a luxury in whatever form it takes (myths, superstitions, or urban legends notwithstanding). Therefore, perhaps it is best to start this perspective on foodborne illness with a fundamental and undeniable truth: to live we must eat, for that is where it all begins. What we eat, and whether or not it sustains and promotes our growth and our health, or if it might just kill us (whether that be sooner or later), is not on the table. Where food is scarce, or famines prevail, safety is definitely not an issue, for to live one must eat.

In the articles in this issue, the causes and consequences, the diagnosis and disposition, tracking and transmission, and treatment and travel aspects of foodborne illness are presented in depth. This introductory article has a different purpose; it is intended to provide a framework for the contemporary details to rest on, a perspective over the past 100 years or so (with a touch of ancient history) as particular issues that affect the safety of the food we eat have been appreciated, have evolved or at times been successfully dealt with, or have newly emerged or reemerged, in large part because of the impact of 3 critical and rapidly changing T words: technology, trade, and travel. The intent is to provide context for the details to follow in other articles, to avoid the possibility that the forest is missed because attention is entirely focused on the individual trees within it.

PREHISTORY

Without written records, it is difficult to reconstruct what life was really like for early prehumans, except that the search for food must surely have been central to daily life and survival. What impact climate change had on the environment and the availability of things to eat, and how this affected the evolution of early hominids into *Homo sapiens*, dropping from the trees to the ground and over time becoming bipedal, developing functional hands capable of crafting and using tools, including those for more efficient hunting and for cultivation, can only be inferred from the anthropologic, archeological, and paleontologic evidence that has accumulated in the recent past. This evidence includes hard evidence, based on the study of fossils and the use of new biochemical and isotopic methods (for example, carbon and nitrogen stable isotope concentrations in collagen),[1] about the prehistoric diet, which consisted primarily of terrestrial animal meat, predominantly deer and to a lesser extent a few other animals. By the time *Homo erectus* appeared about half a million years ago, this basic diet was supplemented by edible plants, initially seeds,[2] and in coastal areas by marine life as well.[3] We can only imagine how many times decayed meat contaminated with microbial pathogens or plants that contained rapidly lethal poisons, such as the ricin in castor plant seeds or the alkaloid coniine in hemlock leaves, or the more gradually lethal constituents such as heavy metals in plants grown in soil or water containing high levels of these natural elements, were consumed, and how many times the safe practice lessons had to be learned and at what cost in health or life. The dramatic events related to consuming toxic foods were the stuff to build myths on, without the science or the ability to preserve experience in writing, as occurred later in human development. As a consequence, also as a result of nutritional deficits related to limited dietary options, unsafe food, injury, and disease, life was short[4]: for men, who also risked injury or death in hunting, and for women, who had the added burden of mortality during pregnancy and childbirth to contend with.

Food historians, such as Reay Tannahill,[5] describe the discovery of cooking and preservation methods as a way of making some inedible food stuffs edible, enhancing taste (is this just a relatively modern imperative, the result of greater choice?), improving nutritive value, and preserving quality and safety. These innovations no doubt helped hunters of large animals to kill, butcher, cook, and haul the meat back to their camp or village, making it more efficient for those groups to settle down, rather than constantly moving to follow the animal herds on which they depended between winter caves in the lowlands and summer camps at the higher altitude pastures. Somewhere along the way, the discovery was made that plants could be cultivated, given the right soil and growing conditions, which further encouraged settlement rather than a migratory lifestyle. Tannahill comments on the likelihood that at some point it was known that animals regularly visited salt licks, which suggests that early human communities could have used salt to lure animals closer to their homes, especially in winter, making hunting even more efficient. With the domestication of the dog, herding of cattle and sheep undoubtedly became easier as well, and dogs proved to be more valuable alive than as a source of food. So, although populations could grow, other challenges awaited them.

The story of pigbel, the name in Papua New Guinea (PNG) Pidgin English for a necrotizing enteritis associated with traditional PNG pig feasts, and similar diseases in other societies elsewhere in the world,[6] is illustrative of some of the foodborne hazards for early humans. In PNG, common rituals and festivals involve pig feasts, in which pigs are slaughtered in a manner that often results in spillage of intestinal contents over the carcasses. These carcasses are slow cooked at low temperature using heated stones in earthen pits between layers of fruits and leaves to enhance flavor and aroma. Water is also added and the oven is then further sealed with large leaves and dirt so that the meat and offal are steamed anaerobically, essentially in the juices of the pig tissues. These events are sometimes followed after several days by acute intestinal syndromes in participants, varying from mild diarrheas to acute fulminating lethal diseases.[7] However, it is the fulminant lethal ones that really demand attention. Sharing of remnants of the pig feast over a few days to a few weeks with other clans and other villages, often the payback for previous debts or as part of celebrations like weddings, results in the geographic spread of these illnesses. The lack of consistency between feast and disease would have affected the appreciation of the relationship between the 2. From this description, it is not so surprising that soon after its clinical "discovery" in 1963 microbiological studies demonstrated the presence of β-toxin–producing *Clostridium perfringens* type C in bowel contents and stool of patients. This finding helped to make the etiologic connection with *Darmbrand* (gangrene of the bowel), a similar acute disease that appeared in Germany at the end of World War II, also associated with β-toxin–producing *C perfringens*.[8] Some have suggested that the effects of the toxin are enhanced by diets containing foods with large amounts of trypsin inhibitors, such as sweet potatoes, which limit the breakdown of the microbial toxin protein and increase the likelihood that it remain enzymatically active in those consuming the tainted feast, especially children, who are most at risk of the consequences. This syndrome is to be distinguished from food poisoning caused by type A *C perfringens*, which produces α-toxin, often associated with meat stews allowed to remain warm for hours or reheated after some time, although that too might have been a risk for these early human populations. Because societies in which food scarcity prevails are likely to be cultures in which all parts of an animal that can be eaten are eaten, contemporary examples of foodborne diseases suggest that primitive societies would also be subject to similar outbreaks. Given the barriers to good hygiene in primitive conditions, fecal-oral transmission of enteric pathogens introduced into foods would have been a frequent consequence of daily life.

THE AGRICULTURAL REVOLUTION

Although Tannahill cautions that food history is no better than informed speculation, the prevailing understanding is that the climate change associated with the end of the ice age some 10,000 to 12,000 years ago, as the Paleolithic period gave way to the Neolithic period, enhanced the growth of grains such as wheat and barley across more areas across the globe. Slowly, the gathering of wild grains morphed into the deliberate spreading of seeds to cultivate those same plants, and so modern agriculture had its beginnings. With this development, it became feasible to harvest and store grains in sufficient quantities to provide for families during lean times, serving as an additional factor in population increase. This population increase, in turn, was necessary to rapidly harvest the mature plants before the grains exploded and spread to reseed the earth. Although this event would reseed the fields, it would also waste the food that the same seeds could provide. Which came first, planting or population growth, is difficult to know for certain. Learning how to plant and harvest meant that the food supply could more effectively be moved adjacent to human habitats rather than requiring humans to go to where the food could be found. Clusters of individuals could now become fixed communities adjacent to the fields of grain, and the conditions under which they lived meant sharing not only chores and the resulting food supply but also hazards to health, including microbial pathogens. As gathering food slowly gave way to cultivating food, and gatherers became farmers, building fixed dwellings where the food was growing, the intimacies with pathogens also deepened, and toxins affecting some harvested bounty (ie, heavy metals accumulated during growth or aflatoxins during storage) became equal-opportunity poisons for the whole community. Community, let alone individual sanitation, is a recent advance.

The change to an agricultural society also meant that lessons were learned regarding the ill effects of eating raw grain, with its high and poorly digestible content of starch, along with methods for cooking the inner nutritionally valuable germ, or allowing for the sprouting of the seeds, which converted the starches into digestible sugars, increasing the content of vitamins, and partially digesting the proteins for better utilization. Cultivating and harvesting also required the creation of methods of threshing and winnowing in preparation for cooking, or otherwise preparing and storing edible foods. Along the way, the development of pottery allowed greater variation in preparation of food, because this made cooking and roasting in fires possible.

As fields were developed surrounding clusters of households, these settlements would have attracted wild ruminants also looking for food for survival. Tannahill posits that it was more effective to domesticate sheep and goats (and later on, cattle) than to constantly have to fend them off. Herding would also have allowed the addition of milk and products derived from milk into the diet, the use of animal fat for cooking (and as medicinal salves), as well as tallow for preparation of primitive candles (rush lights), the fabrication of containers from the skins for storage of solids and liquids, and the wool as well as clothing, and even the use of dried dung for fuel. Humans and animals must have lived in proximity, as they do in many rural societies to this day, sharing microbial flora and sometimes the resulting illnesses caused by commensals in one were or became pathogens in the other. As time passed, the variety of foods increased, sometimes locally depending on specific conditions, sometimes more universally, and sometimes moving with migrating people: other grains such as corn, rye, and oats, honey, pulses, olives, figs, dates, grapes, pomegranates, tomatoes, potatoes, and more. Technology improved yields, for example irrigation, the use of bulls and oxen as beasts of burden to help to till fields, thresh grain, and, with the development of the wheel, also to serve as the engines for transporting goods and materials. So, recognizable civilizations came into being, and with advances came adversities and new threats. Insects and parasites affecting plants and animals could become vectors for disease as well as direct threats to humans and domesticated animals. Ground waters used for irrigation could become contaminated with microbes and ova from the feces of infected individuals, both human and animal in origin, and so threaten the health and vitality of the whole of a village population.

EARLY CIVILIZATIONS

Records in art and texts, in addition to archeological finds, attest to the growth of civilizations in different parts of the world. As technology improved, diets became more varied, breads, and ale produced from the same grains, became staples, and fruits with high sugar content, such as dates or figs in the Middle East and North African countries where they originated, became popular. Drying and salting (another way to dry food, in addition to the salinity per se) for preservation were introduced. Awareness of medicinal plants grew. With increased yields of grains, storage in silos began, perhaps as early as the fifth millennium BC in the fertile crescent of the Middle East.[9]

In some settings, dietary laws were formulated, for example as codified in Deuteronomy, the fifth book of the Old Testament, defining what may and what may not be consumed. Although the latter are often thought of as principles in an early public health textbook, for example the separation of animals for food into clean and unclean categories, which certainly suggests a health rationale, the translation of the original terms and the context used may be misleading. Other interpretations at least as logical for prohibiting the consumption of certain items as food, even although in the case of pork, it may have been true with respect to transmission of trichinosis or the tapeworm *Taenia solium*, or the proscriptions against eating the flesh of animals found injured or dead of natural causes may have prevented some cases of intestinal anthrax or, from a modern perspective, the spillover of an animal infection to a human host. Specifically, social and cultural imperatives may also have played a major and perhaps even more important role in the development of Mosaic law, as the Hebrew tribes worked at creating an identity for themselves distinct from the Egyptians in as many ways as possible, including their food habits. For example, in Deuteronomy 14:21, we find the following: "You are not to eat any animal that dies naturally; although you may let a stranger staying with you eat it, or sell it to a foreigner; because you are a holy people for *Adonai* your God."[10] It is difficult to believe that it would have been considered holy to provide something known to be potentially harmful to a stranger or foreigner, suggesting that something other than health concerns must have underlain this, and potentially other dietary laws.

The rationale for the Mosaic rules about avoiding the consumption of fish without scales or fins is more difficult to interpret in terms of health consequences, with the exception of known toxin-producing fish of the order Tetraodontiformes, such as pufferfish (also known as blowfish, or in Japan, *fugu*). These creatures produce a potent neurotoxin (tetrodotoxin), which acts by blocking sodium channels in nerve cell membranes, interrupting the propagation of impulses along the axon and resulting in various dramatic neurologic manifestations, essentially causing progressive muscle paralysis, which interferes with breathing, often leading to respiratory death. Where these fish are consumed, for example Japan, preparation of the flesh for eating is highly regulated, only permitted at special restaurants by chefs specifically trained for the task. As a consequence, instances of *fugu* poisoning have become uncommon in Japan, especially in licensed restaurants, although cases continue to occur, especially among fishermen. However, this subject is not relevant to Egypt and The Levant.

The Mosaic dietary laws also preclude consumption of bottom feeders, such as catfish and eels, filter-feeding shellfish, shrimp, even swordfish. These creatures have become increasingly unhealthy to humans because they live in pesticide-polluted river beds, or bodies of water contaminated by heavy metals released into the air from coal-burning power plants and certain other industries, or concentrate the bacterial cause of cholera to an infectious dose. Such considerations would not have been so compelling when these laws were laid down, and their apparent prescient warning for our contemporary society, when several health hazards have been identified with these otherwise tasty seafoods, was at best serendipitous.

On the other hand, specific instructions to improve sanitation among inhabitants living in a community are also presented in the Old Testament, and these could be an attempt to implement practices that reduce disease incidence. In Deuteronomy 23:12–13, for example, the sanitary disposition of human feces is succinctly described: "You shall also have a place outside the camp and go out there, and you shall have a spade among your tools, and it shall be when you sit down outside, you shall dig with it and shall turn to cover up your excrement."[10] Because a major source of foodborne illness is contamination of food by pathogens excreted in human feces, any means to reduce the introduction of feces into foods by improving sanitation practices reduces the incidence of such infections. However, the early Israelites did not know about microorganisms, and the relationship between illness and deposits of feces close to where food was prepared or eaten, or where water was stored in cisterns, may not have been obvious to them. However, the associated smells would have been strong and perhaps unpleasant enough to make it worth the extra effort to deposit and bury fecal material in designated spots away from the home. For the system be effective, everybody would need to follow the same practice, hence codification as a rule would have made great sense. Later on, during the Roman Empire, elaborate systems for water supply and sewage disposal were implemented, but these did not last after the Empire fell, being replaced by a simpler method: chamber pots, which were simply emptied into the streets outside the closely clustered homes of the people, to be carried away in the gutters (or more widely dispersed) by the rains, because water was too precious to use.

Technology

Let us fast forward to London in the middle of the nineteenth century: a major urban center, a rapidly growing population hub, and a thriving center of the economic and industrial revolution. It was also a city of filth, covered with a veneer of human and animal feces, fetid, and lacking even a minimally effective system to remove human waste (usually just tossed out of the windows of the homes on to the streets below, and anybody unfortunate enough to be in the wrong place). Charles Dickens describes London as follows.

A dirtier or more wretched place he had never seen. The street was very narrow and muddy, and the air was impregnated with filthy odors...Covered ways and yards, which here and there diverged from the main street, disclosed little knots of houses, where drunken men and women were positively wallowing in filth.[11]

It was not atypical of the major cities around the world. The cholera epidemic of 1831 and 1832 drew new "attention to the deplorable lack of sanitation in the industrial cities. It was obvious that cholera was concentrated in the poorest districts, where sanitation was most neglected and the slum housing most befouled by excremental filth and other dirt. The relationship between disease, dirt and destitution clarified the need for sanitary reform as, in the crowded and congested cities, disease could fairly readily spread from the homes of the poor to the homes of the wealthy."[12]

In part, the realization that disease, dirt, and destitution were fellow travelers, all contributing to the pungent smells of filth and decay, supported and promoted the miasmic theory of disease, which really remained in vogue to the beginning of the twentieth century, well beyond the discovery of the microbial world as the cause of many diseases. Cholera also stimulated the movement to improve sanitation, exemplified by laws promulgated in London in 1848. During the cholera epidemic in London in 1854, Dr John Snow unraveled the role of contaminated water in cholera transmission, but it was the Great London Stink of 1858, when the polluted Thames was so foul that Parliament was forced into recess, that finally galvanized action, led by the Chief Engineer of the newly created Metropolitan Board of Works, Sir Joseph Bazalgette, to build an adequate sewage system, completed in 1875. Additional laws were put in to effect that prevented companies supplying drinking water from using the most contaminated Thames waters as a source, and requiring as well the use of some type of filtration. In conjunction with advances in the mechanics and uptake in the use of flush toilets, promoted by John Crapper, a nineteenth-century English plumbing entrepreneur and businessman who is immortalized in its common name,[13] significant improvements in environmental sanitation ultimately followed. Ultimately is the operative word, for an unintended consequence of the water closet was an initial increase in the amount of human excreta reaching the river,[14] until other reforms and administrative improvements in implementation finally had an impact and the incidence of foodborne infections could begin to diminish. This is an important point, for it is rarely the rule that single public health interventions have major impacts; more often than not, it is a combination of approaches, technical, legal, and administrative, that finally achieves the desired result.

Another technological advance affecting food safety was the development of reliable refrigeration for the storage of food (fresh or cooked) for consumption at a later date. Although earlier societies recognized the use of snow and ice as winter season refrigerants, this evolved later on (relatively recently) into the harvesting and long-term storage of ice obtained from lakes and rivers for use in domestic ice boxes year round and for shipment of goods around the globe.[15] Root cellars, as a reverse geothermal approach, became common in rural settings to safely store certain fruits, vegetables, and cooked preserves at a cool constant temperature below ground, and were especially accessible in rural settings. However, the major advance came with the identification of the microbial causes of foodborne illness and the effect of low temperature on their growth on the one hand, and on the other hand, the science behind evaporation and the development of mechanical refrigeration systems that could be used in commercial settings to produce ice. By 1882, a system to refrigerate a ship was developed by William Soltau Davidson, a Canadian entrepreneur working in Australia, leading to a global trade in refrigerated meat and dairy products, which has escalated to the present time.[16] With further innovation of the technology, home refrigerators became available around the time of World War I, but they were expensive and often used toxic chemicals as a refrigerant.[17] The development of Freon as a safer refrigerant (albeit subsequently identified as harmful to the atmospheric ozone layer and abandoned in favor of newer less harmful chemicals) and the economic boom after World War II led to a dramatic increase in the use of home refrigerators, with freezer compartments as a standard as well, after Clarence Birdseye's flash-freezing methods developed in the 1920s to preserve fish (and subsequently, a whole variety of foods) became a commercial enterprise, preserving food for later cooking and consumption that resembled the fresh item in texture and taste.[18] Refrigeration allowed longer shelf life for a variety of foods without spoilage, although freezing kept foods safe for a long time, although the desirable fresh quality was lost after variable periods of storage, depending on the food involved.

The Food Safety and Inspection Service of the US Department of Agriculture regularly publishes recommendations for the duration of safe storage of refrigerated foods kept at temperatures between 2.7°C (37°F) and 4.4°C (40°F).[19] However, it is likely that most households keep food considerably longer than recommended (for example, how many toss out cooked meat, poultry, or fish after the recommended 3–4 days is reached?); for some, the refrigerator temperature exceeds 4.4°C (40°F), and in some cases, food is kept until mold is obvious, foods smell off, or there is liquefaction or other evidence of spoilage. This situation sometimes but does not necessarily lead to intestinal illness of 1 sort or another. In addition, some organisms, such as *Listeria monocytogenes*, grow at refrigerator temperature, and can reach a level high enough to cause illness, particularly in highly susceptible individuals such as pregnant women, the immunocompromised, and the elderly.[20] There are no practical devices, such as the temperature indicators to monitor cold chain storage of vaccines, in use to indicate the safety of refrigerated foods. Without refrigeration, especially in warm and tropical climates, food spoilage occurs rapidly and the practical rule in such settings, but not necessarily followed, should be eat it or toss it.

Pasteurization, a process involving heating followed by rapid cooling to reduce microbial populations to levels that do not cause illness and delay spoilage, was developed by Louis Pasteur and subsequently has been highly successfully applied to milk and milk products, and has virtually eliminated milk transmission of infections. Implementation of pasteurization, and other initiatives to improve milk safety from "1870 to 1940 [launched] a vigorous public health movement to prevent the bacterial contamination of milk…In this period, the market milk supply gradually became safer, with improved sanitary conditions in dairy farms, pasteurization of milk, keeping milk at low temperatures during shipping and delivery, and prohibition of the sale of loose milk (unpackaged bulk milk stored in a large canister and sold using a dipper) in grocery stores."[21] There are now several methods to improve milk safety. The classic method, referred to as high-temperature, short-time (HTST), involves heating to 71.7°C (161°F) for 15 to 20 seconds, and extends the refrigerated shelf life to 2 to 3 weeks. The introduction of ultrapasteurized milk, which involves heating milk to a temperature of 135°C (275°F) for a minimum of 1 second, has increased refrigerated stored life to 2 to 3 months. When ultrapasteurization is coupled with sterile handling and container technology, a shelf life of 6 to 9 months can be achieved, even without refrigeration. A third technology, referred to as extended shelf life (ESL), processes HTST milk through a microbial filtration step that further increases the useful shelf life of the product, although a lack of established standards for its production results in variable shelf life among products labeled as ESL.

Another technology, tube wells, aimed at providing clean water for developing countries, has been extensively applied since the 1970s, especially in Bangladesh and India. By obtaining water from underground rather than surface sources, microbial contamination from human or animal feces deposited in the environment and present in ground water is precluded. This development has had a major impact on the incidence of cholera and dysentery in areas where it has been used. By the early 1990s, nearly all rural populations in Bangladesh and India had access to tube well water. However, in many locales, tube well water drawn from shallow sources, 10 to 70 m below ground, contained high concentrations of arsenic, leached from sediments via biogeochemical processes that promote reducing environments.[22] An unanticipated consequence, widespread evidence of chronic arsenic poisoning, had become evident. Presenting initially with nonspecific abdominal pain, diarrhea, weight loss, and skin changes consisting of hyperpigmented areas with diffuse or nodular keratotic thickening of the palms and soles, and hepatomegaly, over time involvement of the intestinal, cardiac, respiratory, genitourinary, neurologic, endocrine, and hematologic systems became evident. A significant increase in cancers of the skin, lung, liver, kidney, and bladder has since been documented,[23] with an excess in mortality compared with populations not affected by arsenic.[24] It has been difficult to mitigate this problem, although attempts have been made to test individual tube wells, taking those with high levels of arsenic out of service, and creating shared water resources using clean wells. To find a simple, cheap, readily maintained system, the US National Academy of Engineering offered a prize, supported by the Grainger Foundation, to develop a method to remove arsenic from contaminated tube well water, allowing its continued and safe use. A winning team was identified in 2007,[25] and by 2012, the investigators reported its successful field testing in more than 200 localities in West Bengal, India, with each unit serving around 150 families, who were able to monitor and maintain the system once trained.[26] Technology may solve 1 problem and in so doing create another, as is the case with tube wells, but when the secondary problem is recognized and addressed, it is often possible to identify technological fixes to solve it.

Trade

The technological revolution not only provided options for the safe storage of perishable foods for increasing periods, but coupled with the emergence of economically viable rapid air freight systems and the development of genetic food variants that reduced damage in shipping (often at the cost of flavor and taste), has allowed a global food transportation system to develop, with an unprecedented increase in volume in the past 2 decades. The food markets, at least in affluent countries, are no longer seasonal; you can more or less consume the foods you want when you want them. Raspberries in December? Done! All sorts of tropical fruits can be obtained, at a price of course, in the dead of winter in New York, London, Paris, and most developed world centers. Bananas in January? Done! Although some warm weather fruits and vegetables can be grown in hot-house conditions in the northern hemisphere, the ability to transport them from the southern hemisphere and tropical agricultural regions to the north is now big business. The value of this global trade escalated from an estimated $50 billion in 1960, to $438 billion in 1998, to nearly $1060 billion in 2008.[27] The North American Free Trade Agreement area, the European Union, and Asia (much of it representing food exported from China to Japan) are the major destinations. All 3 regions depend on southern hemisphere countries for imports of juices and off-season fresh fruits, and on equatorial regions for bananas, the leading global fresh fruit import.[28] In the United States, in the first 10 months of 2012 alone, nearly 32 million metric tonnes of food and agricultural products were imported, legally, exclusive of wine and beer.[29] To conceptualize this statistic, to deliver a load of that magnitude would require nearly 800 Boeing 747–400 cargo planes landing every day. Now think of conducting comprehensive food safety inspections on that number of aircraft. Of course, foods are moved by every means of transportation, from ships, to railroads, to trucks, making it even more complicated as the entry points and routes of transport are so numerous and diverse; if only it were confined to the airports! Moreover, it is not just fresh foods that are involved, because increasingly, frozen and processed or at least partially processed foods are being imported. The US Food and Drug Administration (FDA) estimates that 10% to 15% of all food consumed in the United States is produced elsewhere, and that 75% of processed foods in the United States contain ingredients that originated in other countries, almost impossible to fully trace.[30] The FDA recognizes that in the future "(p)roducts entering the U.S. will come from new and different markets and will flow through long, multi-step processes to convert globally sourced materials into finished goods. As global product flows change, many individuals will encounter the growing dangers of fraud and economic or other intentional adulteration of both foods and medical products."[30] It is not without reason that the international food trade network has been characterized as "a perfect platform to spread potential contaminants with practically untraceable origins."[27]

As we move forward in a period of climate change, which will have a variety of impacts on food production, at the same time that growth in populations will require an increasing volume of food trade, there may be additional impacts on food safety. Among the more likely of these impacts are an increase in contamination of food products by mycotoxins in a variety of crops, a likely increase in the use of pesticides at higher concentrations, and variable effects on the transfer of trace elements (some necessary and some potentially toxic).[31] On top of these effects, the deliberate adulteration of foods for animals and humans for economic gain (eg, the recent scandals in China in which melamine has been added to milk in order to boost the measurement of protein content) has resulted in an international outbreak of severe kidney disease in young children consuming the tainted products.[32] As food becomes more precious with population growth, the likelihood of adulteration of foods for economic gain will undoubtedly increase. Regulatory and inspection services will be stressed in technology, resources, and human capacity, which can only partially be ameliorated by point-of-use technology to identify pathogens or toxins in foodstuff, or drugs, pesticides, or adulterants, which, of course, is still to be developed.

Another aspect of this problem is the trade in wildlife intended for consumption.[33] The magnitude of this trade and its relationship to food safety is uncertain, especially because a considerable proportion is illicit, and some of it relates to trade in ivory, skins, hair, or parts reputed to have medicinal or aphrodisiac properties, that is, not for food. However, all the indications are that the volume is big, and potentially dangerous.[34] In an era when we recognize the global problem of emerging and reemerging infectious diseases of humans, most of which originate in animals that infect humans[35] and, in the nightmarish scenario, can successfully transmit from human to human, there is great concern about the potential of this trade to introduce new diseases, particularly when it is illicit, underground, and difficult to monitor. Given the likely origins of human immunodeficiency virus/AIDS in nonhuman primates consumed as food in the bush in Africa,[36] an agent that only subsequently became capable of transmitting from human to human, it can be thought about as an originally foodborne disease, and a dead-end infection as well. How many more like it are out there? How many can make the species jump to humans and to efficient transmission between humans? Can these possibly be monitored? And if they can, will it be possible to intervene in time to prevent the next global pandemic? The increasing global trade in bush meat for consumption suggests the virtual impossibility of accomplishing that goal, and (very) creative thinking will be essential. Another issue, generally overlooked, is the role of wildlife in the transmission of disease at the wildlife-livestock interface.[37] Because the agents that may be found are often capable of being transmitted to humans, this relationship is of potential importance. It may not be simply transmission of organisms from wildlife to livestock. In 1 study conducted in Spain, cattle were identified as the source of transmission of serovars of *Salmonella* to wildlife, in this case, wild boars.[38] In environments in which wildlife, livestock, and humans interact frequently and closely, disease transmission among them must be considered in developing models for disease control. The concept of One Health, the interrelated health of animals and humans, is even broader than is generally considered, and these more complex relationships will need to be considered as an appropriate and effective One Health research, surveillance, and response policy is developed.[39] As this development happens, and wildlife are increasingly seen as contributing to the risk of human disease, the message needs to be carefully crafted in order to avoid serious effects on wildlife conservation programs.[40]

Two other brief comments: first, although we are paying attention to viruses and bacteria, we should not forget about parasitic infections of humans. It has recently been noted that "(c)hanging eating habits, population growth and movements, global trade of foodstuff, changes in food production systems, climate change, increased awareness and better diagnostic tools are some of the main drivers affecting the emergence or reemergence of many foodborne parasitic diseases in recent years. In particular, the increasing demand for exotic and raw food is one of the reasons why reports of foodborne infections, and especially water-borne parasitosis, have increased in the last years."[41] This concern demands greater attention. Second, considered as a domestic US issue, the twin movements toward huge commercial farms and, for livestock, the crowded and often filthy conditions in which the animals are sometimes kept on the one hand, and the desire for small, local, organic, and not necessarily well-run farms on the other, may each in their own way increase the risk of marketing unsafe foods. The risks in factory farming are already known, including runoff of pathogen-containing waste, which can contaminate nearby fields of vegetables, not to mention the effect of the use of antimicrobials to promote animal growth and earlier marketing on the selection of antibiotic-resistant human pathogens, and the large-scale processing that goes along with it, which may put many people at risk when 1 contaminated carcass is processed with many clean carcasses, resulting in a lot of contaminated meat. The potential risks in small farms, struggling to compete and perhaps leading to cutting corners, is a still poorly assessed risk.[42] Proposed legislation to tighten up regulatory and inspection oversight for large farms is meeting resistance from small farmers, who fear that the costs of implementation may make them uncompetitive.[43]

Travel

If the discussion on trade is seen as moving potentially unsafe foods across the globe and within countries to the consumer, travel of people, especially to low-income and middle-income countries, can move them to risky foods, an equally problematic situation made potentially more risky where the regulatory environment is worse than in their home country, and access to good medical care, if necessary, may be problematic. Although not all travel-related illness is foodborne, many disease episodes, in particular diarrhea, result from eating food contaminated with bacterial, protozoal, and viral pathogens.[44] Younger travelers, on limited budgets, extended trips, and more likely to engage in risky behavior, experience frequent episodes of diarrhea and other foodborne infections.[45] Cruise ships have been the scene and source of outbreaks of diarrheal disease affecting the more affluent, often older traveler, frequently caused by norovirus but also associated with a variety of bacterial and other enteric pathogens.[46]

It has been known for a long time that disease may spread along travel and trade routes. The movement of cholera is an excellent example of this. Even before the cause was identified, evidence emerged in New York in 1832 that cholera spread with human movement along the newly constructed Erie Canal.[47] It is ironic that the author of the report did not believe in his own data, succumbing to the lure of the miasmic theory of disease. Contemporary proof of this theory is provided by the origins of the cholera epidemic in Haiti, after the devastating earthquake of January 2010, introduced by Nepalese soldiers who had joined the UN Peacekeeping Force to deal with security aspects of the response to the earthquake.[48] Transport of pathogens by travelers can be an efficient way to distribute an agent widely across the globe. Albeit not foodborne, the severe acute respiratory syndrome outbreak of 2003 shows the rapid dissemination of an agent carried by airline passengers, which in this instance led to a pandemic within a few days of the transmission of the infection from the index case to secondary cases.[49]

SUMMARY

Foodborne illnesses have been a part of the human experience from the beginning. Over time, keen observation and deduction have identified particular illnesses associated with particular foods or food-related behavior. Such observations have stimulated attempts to mitigate these risks, often with significant success when generally applied. However, such lessons are hard won, and many have suffered and many have succumbed over time until, in a Darwinian fashion, lessons learned with positive survival value have been incorporated into cultural practices.

With the growth of science, and the ability to identify specific causes of foodborne illnesses, several technological solutions have been developed that have significantly reduced the burden of disease. Not only are they technological (eg, pasteurization), but sometimes, they are in the form of regulatory oversight to ensure good practice. However, in the real world, technology and optimal practice can break down from time to time, resulting in periodic outbreaks of illnesses that could have been avoided. The scale of contemporary food production, preservation, trade, and storage in the modern era not only makes these incidents more likely but has also introduced many new ways for foodborne disease to be transmitted, sometimes in outbreak or epidemic form. These new opportunities for transmission of illness must be identified, unraveled, and addressed, often in a manner unique to each setting. The future presents us with opportunities to improve both technology and practice and, in turn, to help to reduce disease incidence. The magnitude of the food trade, partly in response to the growth in population and in part to changes in the way that people obtain, prepare, and consume food, provides new ways for pathogens to be transported and transmitted. The emergence of new agents, and the economic incentives for some to put others at risk through poor practice or adulteration of food, ensures that the incidence of foodborne diseases will continue to be high.

In the articles that follow in this issue, the agents, the epidemiology, the clinical aspects and treatment, and the prevention of foodborne illnesses are more thoroughly examined. Although it remains a significant problem even in the United States and in all other developed countries, it also results in a major burden of disease and death in low-income and middle-income countries as well. Although some of the potential approaches to reduce these burdens are common across all environments, many will need to be targeted to the specific conditions that create the risk. For this goal, we need a continued vigorous research agenda, attention to improving practices in the food industry and culturally sensitive customs in different populations, and sensible and affordable regulation in individual nations and in the international setting. There is the need to understand how human health, animal health, and wildlife health are linked together in order to develop policies that address systemic issues that can only be, or are best, tackled together. This approach is termed One Health, and although taken in the abstract, it makes great sense, until the scientific and political leadership truly buy in, and until the general public is engaged, based on knowledge and fact, progress will be slow and avoidable illnesses will, all too often, continue to occur. This issue of Infectious Diseases Clinics of North America is a timely presentation of the most contemporary information, and is of use to all interested in the issue, regardless of their background.

REFERENCES

1. Boutton TW, Lynott MJ, Bumsted MP. Stable carbon isotopes and the study of prehistoric human diet. Crit Rev Food Sci Nutr 1991;30:373–85.
2. Chaney RW. Food of Peking man. Nature 1935;136:577.
3. Walker PL, DeNiro MJ. Stable nitrogen and carbon isotope ratios in bone collagen as indices of prehistoric dietary dependence on marine and terrestrial resources in southern California. Am J Phys Anthropol 1986;71:51–61.
4. Eshed V, Gopher A, Gage TB, et al. Has the transition to agriculture reshaped the demographic structure of prehistoric populations? New evidence from the Levant. Am J Phys Anthropol 2004;124:315–29.
5. Tannahill R. Food in history. New York: Stein and Day; 1973.
6. Murrell TG. Pigbel in Papua New Guinea: an ancient disease rediscovered. Int J Epidemiol 1983;12:211–4.
7. Murrell TG, Roth L. Necrotising jejunitis: a newly discovered disease in the Highlands of New Guinea. Med J Aust 1963;50:61–9.
8. Egerton JR, Walker PD. The isolation of *Clostridium perfringens* type C from necrotic enteritis man in Papua New Guinea. J Pathol Bacteriol 1964;88:275–8.
9. Available at: http://en.wikipedia.org/wiki/Silo#History. Accessed June 21, 2013.
10. New American Standard Bible. Available at: http://www.biblegateway.com/passage/?search=Deuteronomy+23%3A12-13&version=NASB. Accessed June 21, 2013.
11. Dickens C. Oliver Twist [1837]. 3rd edition. New York: Washington Square Press; 1962. p. 62.
12. Fee E, Brown TM. The Public Health Act of 1848. Bull World Health Organ 2005; 83:866–7.
13. DuPont HL, Bean WB. Sir John Harington, Thomas Crapper, and the flush toilet. South Med J 1978;71:1145–7.
14. The city in history. London in the 19th century. University of North Carolina at Pembroke. Available at: http://www.uncp.edu/home/rwb/london_19c.html. Accessed June 21, 2013.
15. Available at: http://en.wikipedia.org/wiki/Frederic_Tudor. Accessed June 21, 2013.
16. Available at: http://en.wikipedia.org/wiki/William_Soltau_Davidson. Accessed June 21, 2013.
17. Available at: http://en.wikipedia.org/wiki/Refrigerator. Accessed June 21, 2013.
18. Available at: http://en.wikipedia.org/wiki/Clarence_Birdseye. Accessed June 21, 2013.
19. Available at: http://www.fsis.usda.gov/FACTSheets/Refrigeration_&_Food_Safety/index.asp. Accessed June 21, 2013.
20. Gandhi M, Chikindas ML. *Listeria*: a foodborne pathogen that knows how to survive. Int J Food Microbiol 2007;113:1–15.
21. Lee KS. Infant mortality decline in the late 19th and early 20th centuries: the role of market milk. Perspect Biol Med 2007;50:585–602.
22. Flanagan SV, Johnston RB, Zheng Y. Arsenic in tube well water in Bangladesh: health and economic impacts and implications for arsenic mitigation. Bull World Health Organ 2012;90:839–46.
23. Ratnaike RN. Acute and chronic arsenic toxicity. Postgrad Med J 2003;79:391–6.
24. Argos M, Kalra T, Rathouz PJ, et al. Arsenic exposure from drinking water, and all-cause and chronic-disease mortalities in Bangladesh (HEALS): a prospective cohort study. Lancet 2010;376:252–8.

25. Available at: http://www.nae.edu/Projects/48083/page2007PrizeWinners.aspx. Accessed June 21, 2013.
26. Sarkar S, Greenleaf JE, Gupta A, et al. Sustainable engineered processes to mitigate the global arsenic crisis in drinking water: challenges and progress. Annu Rev Chem Biomol Eng 2012;3:497–517.
27. Ercsey-Ravasz M, Toroczkai Z, Lakner Z, et al. Complexity of the international agro-food trade network and its impact on food safety. PLoS One 2012;7(5):e37810.
28. Huang SW. Global trade patterns in fruits and vegetables. USDA Agriculture and Trade Report WRS 04–06, 2004. Available at: http://www.ers.usda.gov/media/320504/wrs0406_1_.pdf. Accessed June 21, 2013.
29. US Agricultural Trade Data Update. USDA Economic Research Service. Updated January 14, 2013. Available at: http://www.ers.usda.gov/data-products/foreign-agricultural-trade-of-the-united-states-%28fatus%29/#.UcULspxtwoE. Accessed June 21, 2013.
30. US Food and Drug Administration. Pathway to global product safety and quality 2011. Available at: http://www.fda.gov/downloads/AboutFDA/CentersOffices/OfficeofGlobalRegulatoryOperationsandPolicy/GlobalProductPathway/UCM262528.pdf. Accessed June 21, 2013.
31. Miraglia M, Marvin HJ, Kleter GA, et al. Climate change and food safety: an emerging issue with special focus on Europe. Food Chem Toxicol 2009;47:1009–21.
32. Bhalla V, Grimm PC, Chertow GM, et al. Melamine nephrotoxicity: an emerging epidemic in an era of globalization. Kidney Int 2009;75:774–9.
33. Karesh WB, Cook RA, Bennett EL, et al. Wildlife trade and global disease emergence. Emerg Infect Dis 2005;11:1000–2.
34. Sonricker Hansen AL, Li A, Joly D, et al. Digital surveillance: a novel approach to monitoring the illegal wildlife trade. PLoS One 2012;7(12):e51156.
35. Woolhouse M, Gaunt E. Ecological origins of novel human pathogens. Crit Rev Microbiol 2007;33:231–42.
36. Hemelaar J. The origin and diversity of the HIV-1 pandemic. Trends Mol Med 2012;18:182–92.
37. Siembieda JL, Kock RA, McCracken TA, et al. The role of wildlife in transboundary animal diseases. Anim Health Res Rev 2011;12:95–111.
38. Mentaberre G, Porrero MC, Navarro-Gonzalez N, et al. Cattle drive *Salmonella* infection in the wildlife-livestock interface. Zoonoses Public Health 2012. [Epub ahead of print]. http://dx.doi.org/10.1111/zph.12028.
39. Coker R, Rushton J, Mounier-Jack S, et al. Towards a conceptual framework to support one-health research for policy on emerging zoonoses. Lancet Infect Dis 2011;11:326–31.
40. Decker DJ, Evensen DT, Siemer WF, et al. Understanding risk perceptions to enhance communication about human-wildlife interactions and the impacts of zoonotic disease. ILAR J 2010;51:255–61.
41. Broglia A, Kapel C. Changing dietary habits in a changing world: emerging drivers for the transmission of foodborne parasitic zoonoses. Vet Parasitol 2011;182:2–13.
42. Van Loo EJ, Alali W, Ricke SC. Food safety and organic meats. Annu Rev Food Sci Technol 2012;3:203–25.
43. Luntz T. Will new food safety rules hurt organic farmers? Sci Am April 3, 2009. Available at: http://www.scientificamerican.com/article.cfm?id=food-rules-hurt-organic. Accessed June 21, 2013.
44. Kollaritsch H, Paulke-Korinek M, Wiedermann U. Traveler's diarrhea. Infect Dis Clin North Am 2012;26:691–706.

45. Fhogartaigh CN, Sanford C, Behrens RH. Preparing young travellers for low resource destinations. BMJ 2012;345:e7179.
46. Lawrence DN. Outbreaks of gastrointestinal diseases on cruise ships: lessons from three decades of progress. Curr Infect Dis Rep 2004;6:115–23.
47. Tuite AR, Chan CH, Fisman DN. Cholera, canals, and contagion: rediscovering Dr. Beck's report. J Public Health Policy 2011;32:320–33.
48. Frerichs RR, Boncy J, Barrais R, et al. Source attribution of 2010 cholera epidemic in Haiti. Proc Natl Acad Sci U S A 2012;109(47):E3208 [author reply: E3209].
49. Christian MD, Poutanen SM, Loutfy MR, et al. Severe acute respiratory syndrome. Clin Infect Dis 2004;38:1420–7.

Emerging Trends in Foodborne Diseases

Christopher R. Braden, MD*, Robert V. Tauxe, MD, MPH

KEYWORDS

- Foodborne infections • Outbreak investigations • Laboratory diagnosis
- Molecular subtyping • Trends • Imports • Burden of illness • Food poisoning

KEY POINTS

- About 1 in 6 (or 48 million) Americans become ill with a foodborne illness each year.
- Successful food safety interventions significantly decreased rates of some foodborne illnesses before 2005.
- Progress in decreasing rates of foodborne illness has stalled; *Salmonella* infection rates are the same as in 1998.
- Public health surveillance, outbreak detection, and investigation serve to focus prevention efforts.
- Clinicians play a critical role in linking clinical observations and findings with public health action.

WAS IT SOMETHING I ATE?

Infections transmitted through foods are common. Presenting with a variety of symptoms and syndromes, these infections complicate school, work, and travel and can lead to hospitalization and even death, particularly in high-risk patients. The spectrum of infections and the food sources that transmit them has changed as new pathogens have emerged or are better detected, the number of high-risk persons in the population has increased, previously idiopathic syndromes have been linked to foodborne infection, and as the nature and sources of the foods we eat has changed. Since the 1990s, some infections have been reduced by intensive and focused control efforts in some parts of the food chain, whereas others remain as common or are increasing.

Disclosure: No commercial relationships to disclose.
Division of Foodborne, Waterborne and Environmental Diseases, National Center for Emerging and Zoonotic Infectious Diseases, Centers for Disease Control and Prevention, Mailstop C-09, 1600 Clifton Road Northeast, Atlanta, GA 30333, USA
* Corresponding author.
E-mail address: crb5@cdc.gov

Infect Dis Clin N Am 27 (2013) 517–533
http://dx.doi.org/10.1016/j.idc.2013.06.001
0891-5520/13/$ – see front matter Published by Elsevier Inc.

Some foodborne pathogens, like *Campylobacter,* Shiga toxin–producing *Escherichia coli* (STEC), nontyphoidal *Salmonella*, and *Listeria* have animal or environmental reservoirs, and humans are most often incidental hosts, after foods or ingredients are contaminated from those reservoirs somewhere along the chain of production, slaughter and processing. Secondary spread, particularly of *Salmonella* from food handlers and of STEC among young children can also be important. Other pathogens, like norovirus, hepatitis A, or *Shigella* have a primary human reservoir and cause foodborne illness when an infected human contaminates foods. Some of these pathogens also spread via water or animal contact, so the source of an infection is not necessarily food.

Our food supply is changing as more food is imported from distant lands, food processing becomes more centralized and industrial, and consumer tastes and cooking practices evolve. Food animals are raised in close quarters and are slaughtered and processed with ever-greater efficiency. Fresh fruits and vegetables are available year round, often shipped from warmer countries. Processed foods like peanut butter and raw cookie dough have caused large outbreaks when food safety measures were insufficient to prevent microbial contamination. In the kitchen, microwaving is replacing traditional cooking, which means that the heating that kills microbes is less thorough and more difficult to monitor. Consumers may desire local foods and foods eaten with minimal cooking as well as convenience. In 25 states, the sale of raw unpasteurized milk is now permitted, despite the raw milk–associated outbreaks that occur more frequently in those states.[1]

Diagnosing these infections is important for individual patients, who may be helped by specific treatment, and also for the general public health. Diagnosis and reporting is the foundation of public health surveillance, which makes it possible to detect and investigate outbreaks, to halt ongoing transmission, to better prevent similar outbreaks in the future, and to track progress in making the food supply safer.

PUBLIC HEALTH BURDEN OF FOODBORNE INFECTIONS

In 2011, the Centers for Disease Control and Prevention (CDC) estimated that each year approximately 48 million illnesses, 320 000 hospitalizations, and 3000 deaths caused by foodborne diseases occur in the United States.[2,3] The 31 known foodborne pathogens with sufficient data to make estimates account for an estimated 9.4 million illnesses, 56 000 hospitalizations, and 1400 deaths annually. These estimates are based on population surveys of acute gastroenteritis and pathogen-specific surveillance data. Eight pathogens account for most of the health burden caused by known pathogens (**Table 1**), accounting for 91% of illnesses, 88% of hospitalizations, and 88% of deaths. Norovirus accounts for most foodborne illnesses (58%), whereas nontyphoidal *Salmonella* accounts for the most hospitalizations (35%) and deaths (28%). Beyond the 31 defined pathogens, unspecified agents account for the balance of the total estimated burden. These unspecified agents represent those with insufficient data to estimate agent-specific burden (eg, *Plesiomonas* spp); known agents not yet identified as causing foodborne illness; marine and mycotic biotoxins; microbes, chemicals, or other substances known to be in food whose ability to cause illness is unproven or unknown; and agents yet to be identified.

The 2011 estimates update the previous 1999 estimate of 76 million cases with improved methods and data.[4] Because the analyses and data differed, direct comparison is not possible between the two sets of estimates. Additional population survey data used for the 2011 estimates revealed a more precise rate of acute gastroenteritis (0.6 per person per year) compared with data used for the 1999

Table 1
Reported incidence of culture-confirmed cases (from FoodNet in 2011) and estimated actual incidence of principal foodborne pathogens tracked in the United States

Pathogen	Culture-confirmed Cases per 100 000 Population	Estimated Actual Cases per 100 000 Population	Percent Foodborne (%)
Norovirus	n/a*	7000	26
Campylobacter spp	14.3	442	80
Salmonella	16.7	411	94
Cryptosporidium spp	2.8	408	8
Clostridium perfringens	n/a*	324	100
Shigella	3.2	165	31
STEC	2.1	88.7	77[a]
Staphylococcus aureus (foodborne)	n/a*	80.9	100
Yersinia enterocolitica	0.3	39	90
Toxoplasma gondii	n/a*	58	50
Vibrio	0.3	27	74[a]

* Surveillance data not available for all pathogens.
[a] Weighted mean for category.
Adapted from Scallan E, Hoekstra RM, Angulo FJ, et al. Foodborne illness acquired in the United States–major pathogens. Emerg Infect Dis 2011;17(1):7–15; and CDC. FoodNet 2011, final report; 2012. Available at: http://www.cdc.gov/foodnet/PDFs/2011_annual_report_508c.pdf. Accessed January 28, 2013.

estimates (0.8 episodes per person per year), and new study data revealed a smaller proportion of norovirus illnesses to be foodborne (26%) compared with previous estimates (40%). The 2011 estimates also excluded travel- related illnesses associated with international travel and included uncertainty estimates (90% credibility limits).

NEW ANALYSES THAT ATTRIBUTE FOODBORNE ILLNESS TO SPECIFIC FOODS

The estimates of foodborne illnesses, hospitalizations, and deaths form the foundation for policy and research activities in foodborne diseases and food safety, akin to the US census data used for population-based policies and research. Because food safety policies and research are often focused on specific foods, analyses are needed that attribute foodborne illnesses to specific food commodities, called *foodborne illness source attribution*. These analyses can draw on a variety of data and can use several methods. The issue is challenging because most pathogens are transmitted through a variety of foods, the food source of individual illnesses is rarely known, and because there are so many types of foods. To help make attribution more systematic, the CDC proposed 17 categories of foods (or commodities), such as leafy greens, eggs, and shellfish, and suggested that *simple* foods could be defined as those whose major ingredients were a single commodity, whereas *complex* foods were those made with more than one commodity.[5]

One important source of data on food sources for a broad range of pathogens comes from outbreak investigations in which the source of illnesses is determined. Approximately 1000 foodborne outbreak investigations conducted at the local (ie, county or city), state, and national levels are reported each year to the CDC in the National Foodborne Outbreak Surveillance System.[6] Based on an analysis of illness in 1565 outbreaks that were linked to a single food commodity in 2003 to 2008, poultry, leafy greens, beef, and dairy commodities were together responsible for more than half of the outbreak-associated illnesses (**Fig. 1**).

In 2013, a deeper analysis of outbreak data included outbreaks linked to complex foods (ie, foods that contain ingredients from more than one food commodity).[7] These foods have previously been excluded from such analyses. Using foodborne outbreak surveillance data from 1998 to 2008, the analysis included 4589 outbreaks with an implicated food vehicle and a single etiologic agent, accounting for 120 233 outbreak-associated illnesses caused by 37 agents. The percentage of outbreak-associated illnesses attributed to each of the 17 food commodities were applied to the pathogen-specific illnesses, hospitalizations, and deaths from the 2011 CDC estimates of public health burden to derive the annual disease burden by food commodity. Forty-six percent of the illnesses were attributed to the produce commodities, for which infections caused by norovirus were the major driver, and 29% of deaths were attributed to meat and poultry, largely caused by *Salmonella* and *Listeria* infections. This analysis combines information over 11 years into a single number and relies on the assumption that food vehicles for infection are similar for outbreak-related and sporadic cases. This assumption may be truer for some pathogens than for others, and it is important to remember that outbreak-associated cases account for only 3% of foodborne illnesses reported in active case-based surveillance.[8]

A different approach combined foodborne outbreak surveillance data from 1999 to 2008 with the opinions solicited from a panel of experts.[9] This analysis matched 14 major pathogens with 12 broad categories of foods resulting in 168 pathogen-food combinations and ranked them by quality-adjusted life-years (QALY) and cost of illness. The top 10 pairs accounted for more than $8 billion and 36 000 QALY (more than 50% of total). The top 5 were *Campylobacter* from poultry ($1257 million, 9541 QALY), *Toxoplasma gondii* from pork ($1219 million, 4495 QALY), *Listeria monocytogenes* in deli meats ($902 million, 3281 QALY), *Salmonella* from poultry ($693 million, 3513 QALY), and *L monocytogenes* from dairy products ($773 million, 2812 QALY). This analysis differs from the 2013 CDC report in that produce items are not included

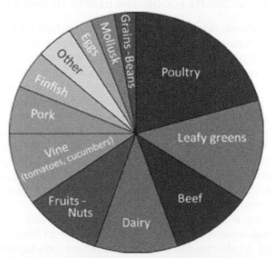

Fig. 1. Distribution of outbreak-associated illnesses in 1565 outbreaks caused by single food commodity and reported to CDC (2003–2008), National Foodborne Outbreak Surveillance System.

among the top 5 pathogen-commodity pairs, likely as a result of lower cost and QALY burden for illnesses caused by norovirus compared with the other pathogens and because complex food vehicles were not included in the analysis.

These estimates are being further refined using more methods and data sources in an interagency work group including the CDC, the Food and Drug Administration (FDA), and the US Department of Agriculture-Food Safety and Inspection Service (USDA-FSIS) called the *Interagency Food Safety Analytics Collaboration*.

RECENT SURVEILLANCE TRENDS

To reliably track some infections regularly transmitted through foods, the FoodNet active surveillance program was launched in 1996. FoodNet gathers systematic information on all laboratory-diagnosed infections with 8 different bacterial pathogens and 2 parasites often transmitted through foods, as well as hemolytic uremic syndrome (HUS), in 10 sites encompassing 15% of the US population.[10] In 2011, salmonellosis was the most common of the infections (16.4 cases per 100 000 population), followed by campylobacteriosis (14.3 per 100 000), shigellosis (3.2 per 100 000) and infection with Shiga toxin-producing *E coli* (2.1 per 100 000) (see **Table 1**). Diagnosed infections may represent only 1 in 20 to 1 in 30 of the actual infections.[2,8] Norovirus infection is the most frequent of all but is not captured in FoodNet because the clinical laboratory diagnosis of this infection is not routine at this time. FoodNet surveillance tracks changes in incidence for specific infections over time (**Fig. 2**). Compared with the baseline period from 1996 to 1998, infection with *Campylobacter, E coli* O157, *Listeria*, *Shigella*, and *Yersinia enterocolitica* have decreased significantly, although most of that occurred before 2003, with little recent progress. In fact, *Campylobacter* has increased slightly in the last 5 years. Importantly, *Salmonella* infections have not decreased over this 16-year span, although the incidence of individual serotypes has changed. The most common serotype, Typhimurium, declined significantly and the serotype Enteritidis first declined and then increased again (**Fig. 3**).

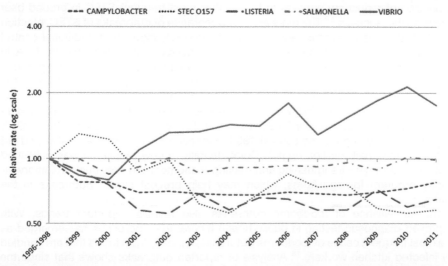

Fig. 2. FoodNet trends in relative incidence of 5 pathogens often transmitted by food from baseline in 1996–1998 to 2011 (http://www.cdc.gov/foodnet/data/trends/index.html).

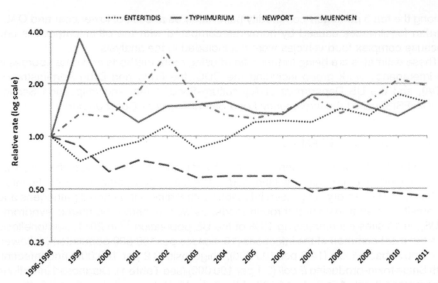

Fig. 3. FoodNet trends in top 4 serotypes of *Salmonella* from baseline in 1996–1998 to 2011 (http://www.cdc.gov/foodnet/data/trends/index.html).

Decreases in infections with *E coli* O157, *Listeria*, and *Campylobacter* likely reflect the impact of efforts by industry and regulatory authorities to address specific problems as well as a greater level of concern on the part of consumers. For example, changes in ground-beef processing and the designation of *E coli* O157 as an adulterant in ground beef by the USDA-FSIS (thus requiring immediate regulatory action if detected) were followed by a major decline in the frequency of contamination of ground beef with this organism by 2003.[11] More systematic and thorough cooking of ground beef in commercial and private kitchens also likely helped. The recent expansion of regulatory concern to the 6 other most frequent STEC in ground beef builds on this success.[12] The more recent appearance of outbreaks of STEC infection due to leafy greens, sprouts and other fresh produce shows that additional control measures are needed such as the produce regulations proposed by the FDA in 2013 to address the quality of agricultural water, wild animal incursions into produce fields and seed treatment of sprouts.[13] Beginning in the 1990s, voluntary efforts by the egg industry to reduce contamination with *Salmonella* Enteritidis and the growing use of pasteurized eggs were followed by decreases in the number of outbreaks and illnesses caused by *Salmonella* Enteritidis.[14,15] This success was incomplete; in 2010, eggs from 2 Iowa egg farms caused 1900 diagnosed infections in 47 states and led to the recall of half a billion eggs.[16] Coincidentally, a new regulation was published that same summer strengthening and making mandatory the previously voluntary industry program for egg farms, which may help prevent similar outbreaks in the future.[17]

The surveillance of foodborne outbreaks also reveals important trends. With improved diagnostic testing in public health laboratories, norovirus has emerged as the most frequent cause of foodborne outbreaks, typically from foods that are handled by infected kitchen workers.[18] Analysis of reported outbreaks shows that since the 1970s, fresh produce food vehicles account for a growing part of the overall problem. In the 1970s, fresh-produce food vehicles accounted for 1% of the outbreaks for which a vehicle was determined and 1% of the illnesses associated with those out-breaks.[19] By the 1990s, these had increased to 6% of the outbreaks and 12% of the outbreak-associated illnesses. The importance of produce as a source of out-breaks has continued to increase. In 2009 to 2010, 10% of the outbreaks with a known food vehicle and 14% of the outbreak-associated illnesses were attributed to one of several produce categories.[6] The 2013 CDC attribution analysis that included the complex food vehicles estimated that 46% of foodborne illnesses were related to pro-duce.[7] Some produce outbreaks may reflect a specific biologic association that *Salmonella*, *E coli* O157:H7, and other pathogens have with plants.[20] Recent observa-tions of microbial adaptations that facilitate internalization and persistence inside plant hosts suggest that for some bacteria, colonizing a plant may be a strategy for reaching the next herbivorous host.

Progress in food safety proceeds in a cycle linking surveillance, investigation, and prevention. As recurrent problems are identified by repeated outbreaks or careful monitoring, specific points of intervention are identified and targeted measures applied. If prevention is improved by those measures, the incidence of illness de-creases. For example, a series of outbreaks linked to raw fruit juice and cider in the 1990s led to new requirements for pasteurizing juices, and such outbreaks are now less frequent.[21] When surveillance improves, such as when pathogen subtyping is introduced routinely, more outbreaks are detected. Prevention can improve further by showing which infections are caused by precisely the same pathogen subtype and, thus, may have the same source; subtyping can find clusters of related cases that would otherwise be unapparent. Thus, improved subtype–based surveillance can have the seemingly paradoxic effect of both increasing the number of outbreaks detected and decreasing the incidence of disease. For example, outbreaks of listeri-osis used to be rarely detected in the United States. Then in 1996, PulseNet subtyping of *Listeria* began nationwide, which increased the number of outbreaks detected by an order of magnitude, including large multistate foodborne outbreaks (**Fig. 4**). Many of those outbreaks were caused by processed meats, like hot dogs and sliced deli turkey. Changes in the processed-meat industry and its regulation made contamina-tion with *Listeria* less likely, and listeriostatic compounds added to many meat

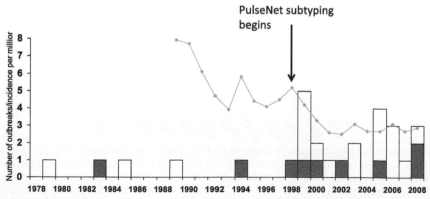

Fig. 4. Incidence of *Listeria* infections per million and outbreaks of listeriosis (1978–2008). White bars indicate single-state outbreaks, gray bars indicate multistate outbreaks, and solid line indicates incidence. (*Data from* Cartwright EJ, Jackson KA, Johnson SD, et al. Liste-riosis outbreaks and associated food vehicles, United States, 1998–2008. Emerg Infect Dis 2013;19(1):1–9.)

products now inhibit *Listeria* growth even if contamination occurs. Outbreaks from processed meats became less frequent, and the incidence of listeriosis declined.[22]

TRENDS IN ANTIMICROBIAL RESISTANCE

Antimicrobial resistance can complicate clinical treatment and can also increase the number of illnesses that occur because resistant strains may cause illness at lower doses when the exposed person is also taking an antibiotic to which the organism is resistant.[23] Antimicrobial resistance in clinical isolates of enteric bacteria has been tracked systematically at the CDC since 1996 for *Salmonella* and 1997 for *Campylobacter*. In the late 1990s, multidrug-resistant strains of *Salmonella* Typhimurium and of *Salmonella* Newport emerged and spread.[24] Multidrug-resistant Typhimurium and Newport strains continue to circulate at lower frequencies, and the plasmid that encoded the Newport resistance has moved into other *Salmonella* serotypes. Currently 11% of clinical nontyphoidal *Salmonella* infections are caused by multidrug-resistant strains, that is, by strains resistant to 2 or more classes of agents, substantially lower than in the 1990s (**Fig. 5**).[25] Strains of serotype Heidelberg that are resistant to ceftriaxone have recently emerged; in 2010, 24% of Heidelberg strains were resistant.[25] Fluoroquinolone resistance in *Campylobacter* from humans increased rapidly after this class of drug was approved for use in poultry. Fluoroquinolone-resistant campylobacter infections were related to eating poultry in the United States and to international travel.[26] In 2005, the FDA withdrew approval to use fluoroquinolones in poultry. Fluoroquinolone resistance in isolates from humans peaked at 25.8% of *Campylobacter jejuni* strains in 2007, declining to 21.8% as of 2010 (see **Fig. 5**). Macrolide resistance in *Campylobacter* remains rare.

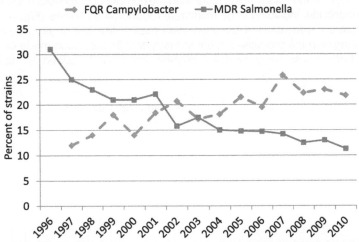

Fig. 5. Proportion of *Salmonella* resistant to 2 of more antimicrobial agents and of *Campylobacter jejuni* resistant to fluoroquinolones from 1996–1997 to 2010, National Antimicrobial Resistance Monitoring System for isolates from humans. FQR, Fluoroquinolone resistant; MDR, multidrug resistant. (*Data from* CDC. National Antimicrobial Resistance Monitoring System for Enteric Bacteria - annual report for 2000. Available at: http://www.cdc.gov/ncidod/dbmd/narms/. Accessed January 31, 2013; and CDC. National Antimicrobial Resistance Monitoring System for Enteric Bacteria (NARMS): human isolates final report, 2010. In: Centers for Disease Control and Prevention. Atlanta (GA): 2011. Available at: http://www.cdc.gov/narms/pdf/2010-annual-report-narms.pdf. Accessed January 31, 2013.)

THE SIGNIFICANCE OF MULTISTATE FOODBORNE OUTBREAKS

Most foodborne outbreaks occur at the county level and have local solutions. Of the almost 5000 foodborne outbreaks that were reported from 2006 to 2010, 94% were confined to a single county (CDC, 2012, unpublished data). Typically these local outbreaks are investigated by local public health officials who identify specific food preparation and handling problems, leading to corrections to food handling in retail, institutional, or catering kitchens.

Two percent of the approximately 5000 reported outbreaks involved patients who were exposed in multiple states. These multistate outbreaks accounted for 7% of all outbreak-associated illnesses, 31% of hospitalizations, and 34% of deaths. Thus, multistate foodborne outbreaks tend to be larger and more severe than local outbreaks. Investigating multistate outbreaks typically requires national coordination, and they often garner national press attention. Multistate outbreaks are the result of food contamination occurring during production, slaughter, processing, or distribution of foods that are widely distributed before the foods reach the kitchen. These investigations often reveal important gaps in food safety regulation and industry processes, with major implications for food safety policy in government and industry.

Outbreak investigations can be complicated if the contaminated food is an ingredient in multiple other foods (eg, spices) or is a minor component of dishes that is not likely to be remembered, (eg, sprouts). Therefore, thorough public health investigations are critical to stop the outbreak by removing contaminated food from the marketplace and also to prevent similar ones from occurring in the future. Multistate outbreaks serve to identify new and previously unknown risks that develop as the nation's food production and supply systems continuously change. Two recent examples illustrate this impact.

MULTIDRUG-RESISTANT *SALMONELLA* AND GROUND TURKEY

In May of 2011, the CDC detected a cluster of illnesses caused by a particular strain of *Salmonella* serotype Heidelberg infections; the outbreak strain was resistant to multiple antimicrobial agents, including ampicillin, streptomycin, tetracycline, and gentamicin. A total of 136 cases from 34 states were eventually associated with the outbreak.[27] Multiple lines of investigative evidence implicated ground turkey as the food vehicle. Most ill people reported ground turkey consumption. The outbreak strain of *Salmonella* Heidelberg was isolated from ground turkey remaining in a patient's home and from 5 ground-turkey samples purchased at retail stores, and source tracing of the ground turkey consumed by patients from retail store purchase sites led to a single large turkey-processing facility. As a result, the implicated company recalled approximately 36 million pounds of ground-turkey products that may have been contaminated with the multidrug-resistant strain of *Salmonella* Heidelberg. This large and severe outbreak led to the recall of a raw poultry product caused by contamination with *Salmonella*. The company has implemented additional measures to reduce the prevalence of *Salmonella* among its source turkey flocks and turkey-meat products, reducing the risk of future illnesses and outbreaks. That same spring, the USDA-FSIS finalized tighter standards for permissible levels of *Salmonella* in raw poultry.[28]

SALMONELLA AND PEANUT BUTTER

Thirteen cases in 12 states detected by national molecular subtype surveillance heralded an historic outbreak of *Salmonella* serotype Typhimurium infections in November 2008, linked to peanut butter and peanut paste that was used as an ingredient in thousands of food products.[29] More than 700 cases were eventually reported from 46 states, although many more were likely affected but not captured by national public health surveillance systems; 9 case-patients died. This outbreak exemplified the difficult epidemiologic task of implicating contaminated ingredients used in multiple foods. Many of the early illnesses were related to an institutional peanut butter rather than peanut butter available in retail stores. The connection with peanut butter was only identified because of an investigator's suspicion that the same food might be served at different institutions with cases (including schools and nursing homes). Then, even after that peanut butter was recalled, persons with no institutional connections continued to become ill, and it was learned that the same peanut butter factory also provided peanut paste to other companies to make a range of peanut butter–flavored foods from peanut butter crackers to dog biscuits. The resulting recall of peanut-containing products was one of the largest in the United States; more than 2100 different products from more than 200 companies were recalled.

This outbreak was the second largest outbreak of salmonellosis from peanut butter in the United States, following closely after the first one that occurred in 2006.[30] Before these outbreaks, low water activity foods, such as peanut butter, were not considered foods at risk for significant *Salmonella* contamination. That perception has changed as a result of these large outbreaks, and the need for specific food safety measures for such foods is now evident.[31] These outbreaks helped to propel the development of new legislation in 2011, the Food Safety Modernization Act, which is changing the approach to regulation and oversight of many parts of the food industry.[32]

CRITICAL ROLE OF PATHOGEN SUBTYPING

Traditional case surveillance activities, and citizen reports of illnesses, often serve to identify local foodborne outbreaks when illnesses are clustered within a community over a short period of time. However, national scale outbreaks caused by widely distributed foods often cannot be recognized early in their onset by local clustering of cases. In these circumstances, only one or a few cases may occur in any one state, defying identification by traditional surveillance, unless they become extremely large. In most circumstances, national-scale outbreaks would not be detected at all.

For this reason, surveillance based on subtyping the pathogens from patients in public health laboratories has been established for several foodborne pathogens. Subtype-based surveillance started with *Salmonella* serotyping, which has been done in state and large city health department laboratories in all 50 states since 1967.[33] Serotyping all *Salmonella* isolates provided a new means of finding dispersed outbreaks, which has been central to *Salmonella* surveillance ever since. Starting in 1996, the PulseNet molecular subtyping system has provided enhanced strain discrimination for surveillance.[34] PulseNet is a national network coordinated by the CDC that links 87 public health and food regulatory laboratories, including all state health department laboratories, some large city health department laboratories, and laboratories at the CDC, USDA, and FDA. PulseNet-participating laboratories perform routine molecular subtyping of bacterial foodborne pathogens including *Salmonella*, STEC, *Listeria*, and *Shigella*. State health departments require or request clinical laboratories to send in isolates of these pathogens to serotype *Salmonella* and *E coli* and to conduct molecular analyses. The principle method of molecular analysis is pulsed-field gel electrophoresis, although other complementary methods, such as multivariable tandem repeat analysis, may also be used. The subtype data are submitted to a national database at the CDC in real time, and the data are reviewed to identify clusters of molecular subtypes that may represent outbreaks. The overarching presumption is that persons infected with the same genetic strain of a pathogen likely acquired their infection from the same source. PulseNet now gathers approximately 50 000 patient isolate subtype submissions each year (**Fig. 6**). Each participating laboratory can view the data, and local and state health departments regularly use Pulse-Net to help detect clusters and define cases for investigation at their level. Approximately 200 multistate clusters are assessed epidemiologically each year leading to 15 to 20 large multistate outbreak investigations, most of which would not be detected without PulseNet. PulseNet does not replace traditional epidemiologic investigation but rather enhances it, focusing detailed interviews on those patients most likely to have an exposure in common and assessing the similarity of isolates from food or other sources to those from patients. The success of the PulseNet system is being replicated for other pathogens, including molecular subtype surveillance for norovirus, *Cryptosporidium*, and *Mycobacterium tuberculosis*.

LOOKING FORWARD
New Culture-Independent Diagnostic Tests

New diagnostic tests for enteric infections that do not depend on bacterial culture and isolation are changing the landscape of foodborne disease diagnosis and outbreak detection. These culture-independent diagnostic tests are 2-edged tools. A positive consequence is that diagnosis can be improved. For example, tests that detect Shiga toxin make it simpler to find infections with non-O157 STEC, and new *Campylobacter* diagnostic assays based on enzyme immunoassay make it possible to more rapidly start treatment. Public health surveillance currently depends on definitive identification by culture and on characterizing bacterial isolates by serotype, subtype, and resistance pattern. If new tests are more likely to yield a positive signal or are used more broadly than current diagnostics, the number of reported cases could increase because of the change in diagnostic testing rather than because the actual frequency of infection has increased.[35] Most importantly, unless bacterial isolates are still available for characterization in public health laboratories, the ability to detect widespread outbreaks will disappear, returning us to the limited capacity of the 1960s whereby clusters of related infections disappear into the background incidence of infections.[36] Thus, the CDC has recommended that when a specimen has evidence of Shiga toxin

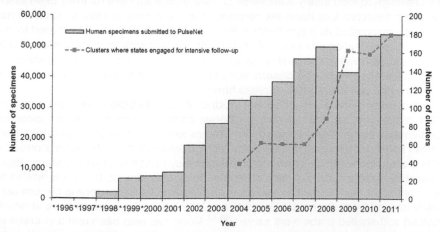

Fig. 6. Number of isolates from humans uploaded to PulseNet and clusters with intensive epidemiologic follow-up by year, 1996 to 2011 (CDC, 2012, unpublished data). *Data are incomplete for 1996 to 2000.

by a rapid test, it is important to culture that specimen for STEC, either in the clinical laboratory or by sending the positive broth to the state public health laboratory for culture there.[37,38] Similarly, if rapid *Salmonella* diagnostics are used, reflex bacterial culture of positive specimens will be critically important to preserve the ability to detect and investigate outbreaks, at least for the near term. In the future, new diagnostic surveillance platforms based on DNA sequencing that include specific gene markers for serotype, molecular subtype, virulence markers, and antimicrobial resistance could offer even better detection and characterization capacity than currently exists, but these methods urgently need to be developed. Public health laboratory-based surveillance of the future may be based on rapid transfer of selected DNA sequences to public health databases rather than referral of the actual strain itself.

New Pathogens and New Food Vehicles

New or unusual pathogens are identified, usually in the course of investigating outbreaks, and new food hazards can be characterized. In 2011, an outbreak of sprout-associated illnesses in Germany drew attention to a highly pathogenic combination of virulence factors in *E coli* rarely seen before, a strain of *E coli* O104:H4 that was both enteroaggregative and Shiga toxin producing.[39,40] In Germany, 3816 cases were reported, 22% (845) of which developed HUS and 54 died, whereas a related outbreak occurred in France a month later.[41] The remarkably severe illness may have been caused by the combination of adherence factors and Shiga toxin 2a, a particularly virulent toxin subtype. In 2008, an outbreak of gastroenteritis associated with consumption of chicken following a wedding reception in Wisconsin seems to have been caused by *Arcobacter butzleri,* a pathogen similar to *Campylobacter* that is also frequently found on poultry.[42] This outbreak is the first foodborne outbreak to be identified with this pathogen, which is difficult to isolate with traditional microbiological approaches but can be detected through gene probes. The calicivirus Sapovirus is emerging as the likely cause of oyster-associated foodborne outbreaks in Japan.[43]

New and unsuspected food vehicles are also identified in these investigations. Since 2006, at least 15 foods have been the source of outbreaks that had not previously been recognized as problems in the United States (**Box 1**). Of these 15, 11 (73%) were derived from plants and 7 (14%) were imported. Each of these represents a new challenge to food safety authorities. *Listeria* outbreaks have recently been associated with fresh produce items like sprouts, celery, and cantaloupes, which were not previously recognized as major hazards for that pathogen.[22] Outbreaks traced to imported foods, including produce, spices like pepper, and scraped tuna, have recently been associated with major outbreaks of *Salmonella* infection, highlighting the ease with which pathogens can be disseminated around the world through trade and travel (See www.cdc.gov/salmonella/outreaks.html).

In other parts of the world, important foodborne-disease challenges have emerged in the last decade. In South America, Chagas disease is emerging as a foodborne infection even as traditional vector-borne Chagas wanes. Outbreaks have been linked to fresh unpasteurized acai juice and to fresh guava juice.[44,45] Infected triatomid insects present in the fruits as they are processed may be the source of contamination. Fortunately, pasteurization of juice eliminates trypanosomes, so the risk is limited to consumption of fresh unpasteurized juice. In Western China, foodborne cholera outbreaks caused by toxigenic *Vibrio cholerae* O139 have followed banquets at which steamed soft-shelled crabs were served.[46,47] *Vibrio* has also been found in crabs at retail locations and may be present in the waters where the crabs are raised to meet the banquet market.[48] In Taiwan, multidrug-resistant *Salmonella* Choleraesuis infections, often presenting as aortitis, have been difficult to treat and have been

Box 1
Fifteen new food vehicles identified in outbreaks affecting the United States since 2006 (CDC unpublished data)

- Bagged spinach
- Carrot juice
- Peanut butter
- Broccoli powder on a snack food
- Dry dog food
- Frozen potpies
- Canned chili sauce
- Hot peppers
- White and black pepper
- Raw cookie dough (likely the flour)
- Hazelnuts
- Fenugreek sprouts
- Papayas
- Pine nuts
- Raw scraped tuna

resistant to fluoroquinolones and more recently to ceftriaxone.[49,50] It has been suggested that this is a consequence of a simultaneous epizootic of these infections in pigs and that at least some of this resistance is a consequence of the use of antimicrobials to treat pigs.[51] In Bangladesh, outbreaks of lethal Nipah virus encephalitis have been linked to drinking sugar palm sap, a sweet beverage like maple sap that is harvested from trees in pots overnight.[52] Giant fruit bats harbor the Nipah virus without signs and shed it in their urine. The palm sap becomes contaminated when fruit bats visit the trees to harvest sap from pots themselves. In some outbreaks, respiratory symptoms and limited person-to person transmission has occurred, a scenario that was amplified and dramatized in the 2011 movie *Contagion*.

More syndromes may prove to be foodborne in the future, just as HUS has been linked to STEC infection and Guillain-Barre syndrome to *Campylobacter* infection. It has been suggested that urinary *E coli* infections may follow transient gut colonization with uropathogenic strains after food exposure.[53,54] There is growing evidence that irritable bowel syndrome may be associated with *Campylobacter* and other enteric infections.[55] *Toxoplasma gondii* is known to induce important behavior changes in the mice they infect, making them curious about cats rather than fearful and, thus, more likely to be caught and eaten, perpetuating the predator-prey cycle to the benefit of the parasite.[56] Many humans have long-term infection with *Toxoplasma*, as a result of foodborne exposures and contact with kittens.[57] It has been suggested that the presence of encysted *Toxoplasma* encysted in human brains may also have neuropsychiatric consequences.[58] Other hypotheses link illness to the state of the gut flora considered as a community, which is modulated by the microbes and nutrients in food. This rapidly evolving arena includes the demonstration that in mice, the efficiency of energy extraction from foods is affected by gut flora, thereby perhaps affecting obesity.[59] It also includes the hygiene hypothesis that suggests the immune system is more likely to react to autogenous antigens because of reduced exposure to antigenic diversity in childhood.[60] The health benefit of consuming specific probiotic organisms or beneficial communities of organisms is a target for further research.

Critical Role of the Specialist in Infectious Diseases

Public health surveillance and outbreak detection for foodborne diseases depends to a great degree on the actions of astute clinicians. Knowledge of the clinical syndromes of foodborne diseases guides appropriate diagnostic testing to identify significant pathogens and the treatment of infections. In many instances, the standard stool culture panel available at the local clinical laboratory is either unnecessary (eg, for illness very likely caused by norovirus infection) or insufficient (eg, for illness consistent with STEC infection or *Vibrio*). Some of the new nonculture diagnostic tests currently or soon to be available can have variable sensitivity or specificity and may require culture to confirm and characterize the pathogen to guide treatment (ie, Shiga toxin profile, antimicrobial sensitivity testing). Appropriate testing also serves the public's health through national surveillance systems, and a cultured isolate may also be critical to linking ill patients involved in an outbreak.

Infectious diseases physicians should develop relationships with local public health officials to share information about patients or groups of patients with illnesses, which may portend a public health issue requiring public health investigation and intervention. Infectious diseases specialists have a critical role to play within their professional communities to guide and teach primary care and other providers of the importance of appropriate testing and diagnosis of patients with significant foodborne illness and to provide direct communication with public health officials.

REFERENCES

1. Langer AJ, Ayers T, Grass J, et al. Nonpasteurized dairy products, disease outbreaks, and state laws-United States, 1993–2006. Emerg Infect Dis 2012;18(3): 385–91.
2. Scallan E, Hoekstra RM, Angulo FJ, et al. Foodborne illness acquired in the United States–major pathogens. Emerg Infect Dis 2011;17(1):7–15.
3. Scallan E, Griffin PM, Angulo FJ, et al. Foodborne illness acquired in the United States–unspecified agents. Emerg Infect Dis 2011;17(1):16–22.
4. Mead P, Slutsker L, Dietz V, et al. Food-related illness and death in the United States. Emerg Infect Dis 1999;5(5):607–25.
5. Painter J, Ayers T, Woodruff R, et al. Recipes for foodborne outbreaks: a scheme for categorizing and grouping implicated foods. Foodborne Pathog Dis 2009; 6(10):1259–64.
6. CDC. Surveillance for foodborne disease outbreaks - United States, 2009–2010. MMWR Morb Mortal Wkly Rep 2013;62:41–7.
7. Painter J, Hoekstra R, Ayers T, et al. Attribution of foodborne illnesses, hospitalizations, and deaths to food commodities by using outbreak data, United States, 1998–2008. Emerg Infect Dis 2013;19(3):407–15. http://dx.doi.org/10.3201/eid1903.111866.
8. CDC. FoodNet 2011-final report. 2012. Available at: http://www.cdc.gov/foodnet/PDFs/2011_annual_report_508c.pdf. Accessed January 28, 2013.
9. Batz MB, Hoffmann S, Morris JG Jr. Ranking the disease burden of 14 pathogens in food sources in the United States using attribution data from outbreak investigations and expert elicitation. J Food Prot 2012;75(7):1278–91.

10. Scallan E, Mahon BE. Foodborne Diseases Active Surveillance Network (Food-Net) in 2012: a foundation for food safety in the United States. Clin Infect Dis 2012;54(Suppl 5):S381–4.

11. Naugle AL, Holt KG, Levine P, et al. Sustained decrease in the rate of *Escherichia coli* O157:H7-positive raw ground beef samples tested by the Food Safety and Inspection Service. J Food Prot 2005;68(12):2504–5.

12. FSIS. Proposed rule: Shiga toxin-producing *Escherichia coli* in certain raw beef products. Fed Regist 2012;76(182):58157–65.

13. FDA. Produce safety Standards; 2013. Available at: http://www.fda.gov/Food/FoodSafety/FSMA/ucm304045.htm. Accessed January 30, 2013.

14. Mumma GA, Griffin PM, Meltzer MI, et al. Egg quality assurance programs and egg-associated *Salmonella* Enteritidis infections, United States. Emerg Infect Dis 2004;10(10):1782–9.

15. Braden CR. *Salmonella enterica* serotype Enteritidis and eggs: a national epidemic in the United States. Clin Infect Dis 2006;43(4):512–7.

16. CDC. Investigation update: multistate outbreak of human *Salmonella* Enteritidis infections associated with shell eggs. 2010. Available at: http://www.cdc.gov/salmonella/enteritidis/index.html. Accessed March 27, 2011.

17. FDA. Final rule: prevention of *Salmonella* enteritidis in shell eggs during production, storage, and transportation, 21 CFR Parts 16 and 118. Fed Regist 2009; 74(130):33029–101. Available at: http://wwwgpogov/fdsys/pkg/FR-2009-07-09/pdf/E9-16119pdf. Accessed April 8, 2012.

18. Hall AJ, Eisenbart VG, Etingue AL, et al. Epidemiology of foodborne norovirus outbreaks, United States, 2001–2008. Emerg Infect Dis 2012;18(10):1566–73.

19. Sivapalasingam S, Friedman C, Cohen L, et al. Fresh produce: a growing cause of outbreaks of foodborne illness in the United States; 1973 through 1997. J Food Prot 2004;67(10):2342–53.

20. Fletcher J, Leach J, Eversole K, et al. Human pathogens on plants: designing a multidisciplinary strategy for research. Phytopathology 2013;103:306–15.

21. Vojdani JD, Beuchat LR, Tauxe RV. Juice-associated outbreaks of human illness in the United States, 1995 through 2005. J Food Prot 2008;71:356–64.

22. Cartwright EJ, Jackson KA, Johnson SD, et al. Listeriosis outbreaks and associated food vehicles, United States, 1998–2008. Emerg Infect Dis 2013;19(1):1–9.

23. Barza M, Travers K. Excess infections due to antimicrobial resistance: the "attributable fraction". Clin Infect Dis 2002;34(Suppl 3):S126–30.

24. Tauxe R. *Salmonella* Enteritidis and *Salmonella* Typhimurium DT104: successful subtypes in the modern world. In: Shield WM, Craig WA, Hughes JM, editors. Emerging infections 3, vol. 3. Washington, DC: ASM Press; 1999. p. 37–52.

25. CDC. National Antimicrobial Resistance Monitoring System: Enteric bacteria - 2010-human isolates final report. 2012. Available at: http://www.cdc.gov/narms/pdf/2010-annual-report-narms.pdf. Accessed July 6, 2012.

26. Nelson J, Chiller T, Powers J, et al. Fluoroquinolone-resistant *Campylobacter* species and the withdrawal of fluoroquinolones from use in poultry; a public health success story. Clin Infect Dis 2007;44:977–80.

27. CDC. Multistate outbreak of human *Salmonella* Heidelberg infections linked to ground turkey; 2011. Available at: http://www.cdc.gov/salmonella/heidelberg/index.html. Accessed January 30, 2012.

28. FSIS. New performance standards for *Salmonella* and *Campylobacter* in young chicken and turkey slaughter establishments: response to comments and announcement of implementation schedule. Fed Regist 2011;76(54): 15282–90.

29. Cavallaro E, Date K, Medus C, et al. *Salmonella* Typhimurium infections associated with peanut products. N Engl J Med 2011;365(7):601–10.
30. Sheth AN, Hoekstra M, Patel N, et al. A national outbreak of *Salmonella* serotype Tennessee infections from contaminated peanut butter: a new food vehicle for salmonellosis in the United States. Clin Infect Dis 2011;53(4):356–62.
31. Beuchat LR, Komitopoulou E, Beckers H, et al. Low-water activity foods: increased concern as vehicles of foodborne pathogens. J Food Prot 2013; 76(1):150–72.
32. FDA. The New FDA Food Safety Modernization Act; 2011. Available at: http://www.fda.gov/food/foodsafety/fsma/default.htm. Accessed January 31, 2013.
33. CDC. *Salmonella* surveillance - report number 10, January, 1963-First nationwide surveillance, February 28, 1963. In: Public Health Service. Atlanta (GA): Communicable Diseases Center; 1963.
34. Gerner-Smidt P, Hise K, Kincaid J, et al. PulseNet USA – A 5-year update. Foodborne Pathog Dis 2006;3(1):9–19.
35. Cronquist AB, Mody RK, Atkinson R, et al. Impacts of culture-independent diagnostic practices on public health surveillance for bacterial enteric pathogens. Clin Infect Dis 2012;54(Suppl 5):S432–9.
36. Jones TF, Gerner-Smidt P. Nonculture diagnostic tests for enteric diseases. Emerg Infect Dis 2012;18(3):513–4.
37. Gould LH, Bopp C, Strockbine N, et al. Recommendations for diagnosis of Shiga toxin–producing *Escherichia coli* infections by clinical laboratories. MMWR Morb Mortal Wkly Rep 2009;58(RR-12):1–14.
38. Atkinson R, Besser J, Bopp C, et al. Guidance for public health laboratories on the isolation and characterization of Shiga toxin-producing *Escherichia coli* (STEC) from clinical specimens. Silver Spring (MD): Association of Public Health Laboratories; 2012.
39. Buchholz U, Bernard H, Werber D, et al. German outbreak of *Escherichia coli* O104:H4 associated with sprouts. N Engl J Med 2011;365(19):1763–70.
40. Frank C, Werber D, Cramer JP, et al. Epidemic profile of Shiga-toxin-producing *Escherichia coli* O104:H4 outbreak in Germany. N Engl J Med 2011;365(19): 1771–80.
41. King LA, Nogareda F, Weill FX, et al. Outbreak of Shiga toxin-producing *Escherichia coli* O104:H4 associated with organic fenugreek sprouts, France, June 2011. Clin Infect Dis 2012;54(11):1588–94.
42. Lappi V, Archer J, Cebelinski E, et al. An outbreak of foodborne illness among attendees of a wedding reception in Wisconsin likely caused by *Arcobacter butzleri*. Foodborne Pathog Dis 2013;9:250–5.
43. Nakagawa-Okamoto R, Arita-Nishida T, Toda S, et al. Detection of multiple sapovirus genotypes and genogroups in oyster-associated outbreaks. Jpn J Infect Dis 2009;62(1):63–6.
44. Nobrega AA, Garcia MH, Tatto E, et al. Oral transmission of Chagas disease by consumption of açai palm fruit, Brazil. Emerg Infect Dis 2009;15(4):653–5.
45. Alarcon de Noya B, Diaz-Bello Z, Colmenares C, et al. Large urban outbreak of orally acquired acute Chagas disease at a school in Caracas, Venezuela. J Infect Dis 2010;201(9):1308–15.
46. Xia B-Z, Li Q, Long J, et al. Analysis of a foodborne outbreak of cholera. J Tropical Medicine 2010;10(1):88–9 [in Chinese].
47. Tang X-F, Liu L-G, Ma H-L, et al. Outbreak of cholera associated with consumption of soft-shelled turtles, Sichuan Province, China, 2009. Zhonghua Liu Xing Bing Xue Za Zhi 2010;31(9):1050–2 [in Chinese].

48. Xie Q, Zeng X-J, Zheng W. Survey of *Vibrio cholerae* -carrying rate of short-shelled turtles sold in markets of Chenzou City. China Tropical Medicine 2009; 9(1):135–6 [in Chinese].
49. Chiu C, Wu T, Su L, et al. The emergence in Taiwan of fluoroquinolone resistance in *Salmonella enterica* serotype choleraesuis. N Engl J Med 2002;346(6): 413–9.
50. Su L, Teng W, Chen C, et al. Increasing ceftriaxone resistance in *Salmonellae*, Taiwan. Emerg Infect Dis 2011;17(6):1086–90.
51. Hsueh P, Teng L, Tseng S, et al. Ciprofloxacin-resistant *Salmonella enterica* and Choleraesuis from pigs to humans, Taiwan. Emerg Infect Dis 2004;10(1):60–8.
52. Luby SP, Hossain MJ, Gurley ES, et al. Recurrent zoonotic transmission of Nipah virus into humans, Bangladesh, 2001–2007. Emerg Infect Dis 2009;15(8): 1229–35.
53. Manges AR, Johnson JR, Foxman B, et al. Widespread distribution of urinary tract infections caused by a multidrug-resistant *Escherichia coli* clonal group. N Engl J Med 2001;345(14):1007–13.
54. Manges AR, Johnson JR. Food-borne origins of *Escherichia coli* causing extra-intestinal infections. Clin Infect Dis 2012;55(5):712–9.
55. Spiller R, Garsed K. Postinfectious irritable bowel syndrome. Gastroenterology 2009;136(6):1979–88.
56. Vyas A, Kim SK, Giacomini N, et al. Behavioral changes induced by *Toxoplasma* infection of rodents are highly specific to aversion of cat odors. Proc Natl Acad Sci U S A 2007;104(15):6442–7.
57. Jones JL, Dargelas V, Roberts J, et al. Risk factors for *Toxoplasma gondii* infection in the United States. Clin Infect Dis 2009;49(6):878–84.
58. Yolken RH, Dickerson FB, Fuller Torrey E. Toxoplasma and schizophrenia. Parasite Immunol 2009;31(11):706–15.
59. DiBaise JK, Zhang H, Crowell MD, et al. Gut microbiota and its possible relationship with obesity. Mayo Clin Proc 2008;83(4):460–9.
60. Bisgaard H, Li N, Bonnelykke K, et al. Reduced diversity of the intestinal microbiota during infancy is associated with increased risk of allergic disease at school age. J Allergy Clin Immunol 2011;128(3):646–652.e1–5.

How to Diagnose a Foodborne Illness

Michael S. Donnenberg, MD[a,b,c],*, Shivakumar Narayanan, MD[d]

KEYWORDS

- Outbreaks • Diagnosis • Foodborne illness • Food poisoning • Microbiology
- Stool culture • Pulsed-field gel electrophoresis • Stool antigen detection

KEY POINTS

- Foodborne infections are of major public health importance, owing to their potential to cause widespread illness.
- The timely recognition of foodborne origin of a gastrointestinal illness, appropriate testing, and reporting to public health authorities can help curtail further spread of an outbreak.
- Identification of common food-vehicle exposures and knowledge of incubation periods of common foodborne pathogens can provide epidemiologic clues to diagnosing a pathogen in an outbreak.
- Stool cultures can be ordered when signs of inflammatory diarrhea are observed. The "3-day rule" is a useful guide to selective ordering of cultures in hospitalized patients.
- Culture-independent methods of stool identification of pathogens present their own advantages and disadvantages.
- Molecular subtyping and surveillance by pulsed-field gel electrophoresis has greatly aided investigation and confirmation of foodborne outbreaks.

Funding: Public Health Service awards R01 AI 32074, U19 AI 090873, R03 AI 097953 from the National Institute of Allergy and Infectious Diseases (M.S. Donnenberg); None (S. Narayanan).
Conflict of Interest: None.

[a] Department of Medicine, University of Maryland School of Medicine, 20 Penn Street, S243, Baltimore, MD 21201, USA; [b] Department of Microbiology and Immunology, University of Maryland School of Medicine, 20 Penn Street, S243, Baltimore, MD 21201, USA; [c] Medical Scientist Training Program, University of Maryland School of Medicine, 20 Penn Street, S243, Baltimore, MD 21201, USA; [d] Division of Infectious Diseases, Department of Medicine, Institute of Human Virology, University of Maryland Medical Center, 725 West Lombard Street, Room N149, Baltimore, MD 21201, USA
* Corresponding author. Health Sciences Facility II, University of Maryland School of Medicine, 20 Penn Street, S243, Baltimore, MD 21201.
E-mail address: mdonnenb@umaryland.edu

Infect Dis Clin N Am 27 (2013) 535–554
http://dx.doi.org/10.1016/j.idc.2013.05.001
0891-5520/13/$ – see front matter © 2013 Elsevier Inc. All rights reserved.

id.theclinics.com

INTRODUCTION

Acute diarrheal illnesses are a significant cause of global morbidity and mortality, especially among those at the extremes of ages and those who are malnourished. On a global scale, diarrhea is estimated to account for 18% of all deaths in children younger than 5 years.[1] Foodborne diseases are challenges in both developing and developed countries, owing to changes in our food production and supply chains, changes in our environment leading to contamination, new and emerging pathogens, antibiotic resistance among pathogens, and the propensity of the known pathogen vehicles to cause multistate outbreaks. The Centers for Disease Control and Prevention (CDC) estimate that each year roughly 48 million people in the United States become ill, 128,000 are hospitalized, and 3000 die from infections from foodborne pathogens.[2] In addition to the acute morbidity and mortality, some of these infections can cause significant long-term sequelae, for example, hemolytic-uremic syndrome causing renal failure following infection with Shiga toxin–producing Escherichia coli, and Guillain-Barré syndrome following Campylobacter jejuni infection.[3] An estimated $6 billion is spent each year in the United States on medical care and lost productivity attributable to foodborne illnesses.[4]

The Foodborne Diseases Active Surveillance Network (FoodNet) is a system of active population-based surveillance of laboratory-confirmed cases of infection in 10 geographic regions in the United States caused by 9 common foodborne pathogens of public health importance. FoodNet estimates that, during 2011, 18,964 cases of foodborne illness were documented, which resulted in 4398 hospitalizations and 82 deaths.[5] Advances in pathogen detection and discrimination in identification by molecular methods have enabled early and effective surveillance for specific foodborne pathogens and the detection and control of outbreaks.[6]

More than 30 pathogens cause the major burden of foodborne illnesses in the United States (**Table 1**). Of these, Norovirus accounted for 58% of all illness followed by nontyphoidal Salmonella spp (11%), Clostridium perfringens (10%), and Campylobacter spp (9%). Salmonella was also the leading cause of hospitalization and death.[7]

ASSESSMENT

The health care provider's initial approach to patients with a suspected foodborne illness is to conduct a careful history and physical examination, and to evaluate and treat for dehydration if present. The provider often assumes responsibility not just to the individual patient but to the community as a whole if an outbreak is suspected. A clinician should be alert to the possibility that any patient with foodborne illness may represent the sentinel case of a more widespread outbreak. A foodborne disease outbreak (FBDO) is defined as an incident whereby 2 or more persons experience a similar illness resulting from the ingestion of a common food.[12] The CDC's Outbreak net Web site (http://www.cdc.gov/outbreaknet/report_healthcare.html) can be accessed for descriptive criteria, incubation periods, descriptions of clinical syndromes, and guidelines for confirmation, as well as contact information of the CDC.

The provider should ascertain how and when the illness began, stool characteristics (frequency, consistency, and quantity), signs or symptoms of dehydration, and previous significant medical conditions. The history should include symptoms suggesting severity (ie, fever, blood in stool, weight loss, lethargy, voluminous diarrhea, proctalgia, tenesmus, or abdominal pain). A clinician should also be aware that not all foodborne illnesses have gastrointestinal manifestations.

An epidemiologic history requires asking about specific foods consumed in the period leading up to the symptoms, the onset of symptoms in relation to the time of consumption of food, and whether others are ill. Some foodborne agents may cause symptoms in minutes (chemical agents) to hours (preformed toxins) to days (most viral/bacterial pathogens), whereas some may not cause symptoms until weeks after exposure (hepatitis A or listeria). One should ask about high-risk foods (raw or under-cooked meat and seafood, unpasteurized dairy products, uncooked vegetables), or food that has been left outside unrefrigerated for many hours, in the period of up to 72 hours before onset of symptoms. In the FoodNet data, the top commodities to which outbreaks were attributed were poultry (15%) and beef (14%). In most cases of foodborne outbreaks, foods were served in a single establishment or at a single event (eg, restaurant, wedding, party, or conference), and were attributed to contamination that occurred before final preparation or serving.[13]

Each pathogen has a characteristic incubation period between ingestion of contaminated food and manifestation of symptoms (**Table 2**). Based on this period, and to some extent the symptoms, a differential diagnosis can be built and further diagnostic testing can be ordered.

The provider should ask about other illnesses in the family or in other contacts; day-care exposure; travel outside the United States, to the sea coast, or to rural or mountainous areas; and attendance at group picnics or similar outings. Around 13% of cases under the FoodNet surveillance for enteric pathogens are associated with international travel.[14] A history of recent antibiotic use or hospitalization should be elicited. Alerting public health officials when a foodborne illness outbreak is suspected is critical in identifying the source, aiding detection of potentially more wide-scale outbreaks, and curtailing further spread.

An analysis of FBDO investigations in the period 2003 to 2008 indicated that the overwhelming majority of viral outbreaks and approximately one-third of bacterial outbreaks were first reported by private citizens.[13]

Although deliberate contamination of food is a rare event, it has occurred.[15,16] The following red flags may be suggestive of intentional contamination: an unusual pathogen in a common food; or a common agent, either affecting an unusually large number of people or that is not usually seen in clinical practice (eg, pesticide poisoning).[17]

The extent of diagnostic evaluation depends on the clinical picture, the differential diagnosis considered, and clinical judgment. Physical signs that demand greater attention and should be evaluated in detail include bloody diarrhea, dehydration, fever, prolonged diarrhea, severe abdominal pain, dehydration, weight loss, and neurologic changes such as motor weakness and paresthesiae. These features are particularly important in the very young, the very old, and the immunocompromised.[18]

REPORTING AND SURVEILLANCE

Reporting should take place in parallel with diagnosis and treatment. Reporting is of critical importance, as it helps public health officials to assess the burden of disease and to curtail spread by:

- Aiding in detection of the implicated food and, thus, early removal from commercial supply
- Correction of food-preparation practices, if necessary
- Public education about proper food handling
- Identification of hitherto unknown agents
- Identification and appropriate management of human carriers in high-risk jobs

State or local health agencies establish criteria for voluntary or mandatory reporting of specific diseases that are foodborne and are on the CDC list for pathogen-specific

Table 1
Major pathogens causing foodborne illnesses, their clinical syndromes, implicated foods, and environmental factors

Etiology	Clinical Syndrome	Foods Commonly Linked	Season	Geographic Predilection
Bacterial				
Staphylococcus aureus	Nausea, vomiting within 6 h	Cream-filled pastries, ham, beef, poultry, potato and egg salads	Summer	None
Clostridium botulinum	Nausea, vomiting, in 6 h, paralysis in 18–36 h	Home-canned vegetables, fruits, preserved fish, honey (infants)	Summer, fall	None
Bacillus cereus	Emetic: nausea, vomiting in 6 h; Diarrheal: abdominal cramps and diarrhea within 8–16 h	Fried rice (short incubation period), meats, vegetables (long incubation period)	Year-round	None
Clostridium perfringens	Abdominal cramps and diarrhea within 8–16 h	Beef, poultry, gravy. Stored between 15°C and 50°C[8]	Fall, winter, spring	None
Salmonella	Fever, abdominal cramps and diarrhea within 6–48 h	Beef, poultry, eggs (raw, undercooked or unpasteurized), dairy products, produce	Summer, fall	None
Campylobacter jejuni	Fever, abdominal cramps, and diarrhea within 6–48 h	Poultry, raw milk	Spring, summer	None
Shigella	Fever, abdominal cramps, and diarrhea within 6–48 h	Egg salad, lettuce (cool, moist foods)	Summer	None
Vibrio parahaemolyticus	Fever, abdominal cramps, and diarrhea within 6–48 h	Bivalve mollusks and crustaceans	Spring, summer, fall	Coastal states
Yersinia enterocolitica	Fever and abdominal cramps without diarrhea within 16–48 h	Milk, pork, chitterlings	Winter	Unknown

Organism	Symptoms / incubation	Food source	Season	Geography
Enterotoxigenic *Escherichia coli*	Abdominal cramps and diarrhea within 16–72 h	Salads, imported cheese, fresh produce[9]	Varies, summer	Cruise ship, Latin America
Vibrio cholerae O1	Abdominal cramps and diarrhea within 16–72 h	Shellfish	Variable	Tropical, Gulf Coast, Latin America
Vibrio cholerae non-O1	Abdominal cramps and diarrhea within 16–72 h	Shellfish	Unknown	Tropical, Gulf Coast
Shiga toxin–producing *Escherichia coli*	Bloody diarrhea, no fever within 72–120 h	Ground beef, leafy greens, sprouts, salami.[10] Person to person reported[11]	Summer, fall	Northern states
Viral				
Noroviruses	Vomiting, nonbloody diarrhea within 24–48 h	Salads, shellfish, sandwiches	Year-round	None
Parasitic				
Cyclospora	Diarrhea over 1–3 wk	Imported fresh produce: raspberries, basil, lettuce	Year-round	None
Chemical				
Ciguatera	Paresthesiae within 1–6 h	Barracuda, snapper, amberjack, grouper	Spring, summer (in Florida)	Tropical reefs
Histamine fish poisoning (scombroid)	Paresthesiae within 1 h	Tuna, mackerel, bonito, skipjack, mahi-mahi	Year-round	Coastal
Mushroom poisoning	Various	Mushrooms	Spring, fall	Temperate
Heavy metals	Nausea, vomiting, cramps within 1 h	Acidic beverages	Year-round	None
Monosodium-L-glutamate	Head, upper torso burning, flushing, diaphoresis, cramps, nausea, headache	Chinese food	Year-round	None
Paralytic shellfish poisoning	Paresthesiae of face, lips, extremities progressing to weakness, dysphagia, respiratory muscle weakness	Shellfish	Summer, fall	Temperate coastal zones
Neurotoxic shellfish poisoning	Somewhat similar features to above	Shellfish	Spring, fall	Subtropical

Table 2
Clinical syndromes of foodborne infections

Incubation Period	Vomiting	Abdominal Cramps and Pain	Voluminous, Less Frequent Bowel Movements	Small-Volume Multiple Bowel Movements	Proctalgia, Tenesmus, Fecal Urgency	Dysentery	Fever, Systemic Symptoms	Systemic Illness	Pathogenesis Correlate	Pathogens Likely	Comments
				Symptoms							
1–6 h	++	±	–	–	–	–	–	±	Preformed toxin	*Staphylococcus aureus, Bacillus cereus, Clostridium botulinum*	Descending paralysis with botulism
8–16 h	–	+	+	–	–	–	–	–	Toxin produced in vivo	*Clostridium perfringens, Bacillus cereus*	
6–48 h	± to +	+	–	++	+	++	++	±	Inflammatory diarrhea of lower small and large intestine	*Shigella, Salmonella, Campylobacter jejuni, Yersinia enterocolitica*	Reactive arthritis (15%) and erythema nodosum late complications of *Yersinia*. Guillain-Barré syndrome as a late complication of *Campylobacter*

Incubation period							Syndrome and representative agents
12–72 h	± to ++	+	++	++	−	±	+	Toxin-mediated diarrhea — *Enterotoxigenic E coli, Vibrio cholera* non-O1, *Vibrio parahaemolyticus,* Noro- and other caliciviruses
16–72 h	± to +	++	−	++	++	+	±	Renal failure with associated hemolytic-uremic syndrome — Shiga toxin–producing *E coli*; Toxin-mediated inflammation
2–28 d	− to ±	± to +	+ to ++	−	−	−	−	*Cryptosporidium, Cyclospora, Giardia,* Brainerd diarrhea
2–6 wk	+	±	±	±	±	+	++	*Listeria, Vibrio vulnificus,* trichinellosis

surveillance. Infections can be reported through electronic medical records directly or through laboratory information. Isolates or other clinical materials are forwarded to public health laboratories for confirmation and further characterization, as required by state laws or regulations. The CDC works with states to compile national surveillance data. The agent is identified and, after serotyping, molecular subtyping, and susceptibility assays to characterize the agent, reports are issued and specimen data are uploaded on national data systems such as PulseNet (discussed later) and the Public Health Laboratory Information System (PHLIS). Widespread clusters of presumably related cases can be identified by subtype-/serotype-based surveillance, or pulsed-field gel electrophoresis (PFGE) using PulseNet (see later discussion). Once a cluster is identified, a hypothesis-generating questionnaire may be used to implicate particular foods. Systematic interviews of ill persons can then be conducted with a matched healthy population of controls.

Through interviews with more than 1 ill person, a common food, brand, restaurant, or food commodity is identified as a vehicle. Both ill and well persons who were present must be questioned. Epidemiologists can calculate food-specific attack rates for all foods and beverages served at the meal. Food-specific attack rates are defined as the proportion of persons who consumed a food and who subsequently became ill. To be able to incriminate a specific food, people who ate the food should have a higher attack rate than those who did not. One should minimize recall bias by trying to interview people as near to exposure as possible.

An increase in the diagnosis of FBDOs may be due to improvement in detection using molecular typing data available on PulseNet. The number of FBDOs investigated by the CDC has increased from 50 in 2006 to 180 in 2011/2012.[19] Diagnosis is more efficient, and PulseNet data are accessed between partners at state health departments, local health departments, and federal agencies, enabling them to compare strains and communicate in real time to identify common sources of FBDOs.

In January 2011, Congress passed the Food Safety and Modernization Act (FSMA), with the goal of creating preventive control strategies for food facilities. Under the FSMA provisions, in September 2011 the Food and Drug Administration (FDA) established the Coordinated Outbreak Response and Evaluation (CORE) Network, which monitors potential foodborne disease clusters at an early stage. The CDC's Outbreak Response Team and the FDA's CORE Network monitor clusters of disease via PulseNet, and the 2 agencies meet weekly to exchange information.

When submitting specimens for microbiologic testing, it is important to realize that in identifying and testing pathogens, clinical microbiology laboratories differ in procedures and standards used. It is often important to be familiar with the merits and shortcomings of methodology used in the local laboratory.

WHOM TO TEST

A complete laboratory evaluation to determine the etiology of diarrhea is not appropriate for every patient, as this would squander valuable health care resources with little benefit. However, under the following circumstances efforts should be made to determine the cause of the illness:

High-Risk Personnel

Food preparers, handlers in food service establishments, health care workers involved in direct patient care, day-care attendees, day-care employees, or residents of an institutional facility should be tested for bacterial pathogens if they have diarrhea.[18]

These groups should ideally also have follow-up testing before returning to work, even if they are asymptomatic. Two consecutive negative stool samples taken 24 hours apart and at least 48 hours after resolution of symptoms are required. If the patient has received antimicrobial therapy, the first stool specimen should be obtained at least 48 hours after the last dose of medication.[18]

Some patients who may be at increased risk for developing severe illness from foodborne pathogens (eg, human immunodeficiency virus [HIV]-positive patients or transplant recipients) should also be considered high risk, and should be tested.

Average Risk

Although anyone with gastrointestinal symptoms who has had exposure to possibly incriminated food and can provide a specimen may be tested in an outbreak setting, a more selective approach is recommended in an individual clinical case.[18] Specifically, patients with bloody stool, systemic symptoms such as fever and abdominal pain, and those with severe dehydration must be sought and tested. A positive stool white blood cell count/fecal lactoferrin may help the clinician decide in this regard. The physician should take a culture for the most commonly recognized invasive pathogens: C jejuni Salmonella, Shigella, and E coli O157 (by growth on sorbitol–MacConkey agar) and for other Shiga-producing E coli (STEC) by a specific assay (immunoassay or polymerase chain reaction). Stool culture is also recommended in those with moderate to severe diarrhea failing empiric treatment, when diarrhea is persistent or day-care attendance is known.[18]

WHAT SPECIMENS TO TEST

Appropriate specimens for laboratory confirmation vary with the etiologic agents but include feces, vomitus, serum, plasma, and blood (**Table 3**). In addition, specimens from leftover food, the food-preparation environment, and food handlers may be examined. Appropriate stool-collection methods may need to be followed when requesting immunoelectron microscopy or other specialized tests on specimens forwarded to the CDC. The use of stool-collection kits delivered to patients can improve the frequency of specimen collection and confirmation of etiologic agents in FBDOs.[20]

An analysis of FBDOs conducted by FoodNet sites showed that although a food vehicle is implicated in only around 30% of cases, the odds of identifying a food vehicle were 4.9 times greater when food specimens were tested, compared with investigations whereby food specimens were not tested. In the absence of standard methods for identification of viral pathogens in food vehicles, food testing is applicable for only for bacterial pathogens and, in an appropriate setting, testing for bacterial pathogens must be encouraged.[13]

Swab or diaper specimens appear to be less sensitive than cup specimens for fecal leukocytes.[21] Careful specimen collection and transport are critical to successful diagnosis. Rectal or stool swabs for bacteriologic diagnosis should be inserted 1 to 1.5 inches into the rectum, and have visible fecal material on them. The swabs should be transported under refrigeration to the laboratory in a nonnutrient holding medium such as Cary-Blair or Stuart medium, and should be frozen if they cannot be plated within 48 hours. For identification of a virus, liquid stools should be collected in a clean dry container and transported under refrigeration without freezing. Parasitic diagnosis depends on collection of a stool sample and its transport in specialized parasitic transport media (1 part stool and 3 part preservative: 10% formalin and polyvinyl alcohol fixative refrigerated for up to 48 hours).[22]

Table 3
Specimens to be collected for investigating a foodborne illness outbreak

	Patient				Food Handler				Environment	
	Stools	Vomitus	Urine	Blood	Blood	Stools	Nose	Hands	Food	Food-Preparation Environment
Bacterial										
Staphylococcus aureus	C	C, P, T	—	—	—	—	C	C	C, P, T	—
Clostridium botulinum	C, T, P	C, T	T	T	—	—	—	—	C, T, P	—
Bacillus cereus	C	C, P	—	—	—	—	—	—	C, P, T	—
Clostridium perfringens	C, T	—	—	—	—	—	—	—	C, P, T	—
Salmonella	C, P	—	C	C, S	C, S	C, P	—	—	C	C, P
Campylobacter jejuni	Cª, P, A	—	—	C	—	C, P, A	—	—	C	C, P
Shigella	C, P	—	—	—	—	C, P	—	—	C	C, P
Vibrio parahaemolyticus	C	—	—	—	—	—	—	—	C	C
Yersinia enterocolitica	C, P	—	—	C	S	C, P	—	—	C	C
Vibrio cholerae O1 and non-O1	Cª, P, A	—	—	—	S	C, P	—	—	C	C
Shiga toxin–producing Escherichia coli	C, T, P	—	C, T, P	—	S	C, T, P	—	—	C, T, P	C, T, P
Listeria monocytogenes	C	—	—	C, S	—	—	—	—	C	C

Viral							
Norovirus	I, P, A	P	—	—	S	I, P, A	P
Parasitic							
Cryptosporidium	O, A	—	—	—	—	O	O
Cyclospora	O, P	—	—	—	—	O	O
Giardia	O, A	—	—	—	S	O, A	O, P
Trichinella	—	—	—	—	S, P	—	—
Chemical							
Ciguatera	—	—	—	—	—	—	T
Histamine fish poisoning (scombroid)	—	—	—	—	—	—	T
Mushroom	T	T	—	T	—	—	T
Paralytic shellfish poisoning	—	—	—	T	—	—	T
Neurotoxic shellfish poisoning	—	—	—	—	—	—	T

Abbreviations: A, antigen testing; C, culture; I, immunoelectron microscopy; O, other; P, polymerase chain reaction probe; S, serology; T, toxin testing.

[a] Direct examination of stool of utility.

Adapted from Sodha SV, Griffin PM, Hughes JM. Foodborne disease. In: Mandell D, editor. Bennett's Principles and practice of infectious diseases. vol. 1. 7th edition. Churchill Livingstone Elsevier; 2010. p. 1423; with permission.

WHAT TESTS TO ORDER

The specific tests to be ordered depend on the clinically suspected diagnosis. One can aid the clinical suspicion of inflammatory diarrhea by checking for evidence of a luminal inflammatory process, in the form of either inflammatory cells or inflammatory markers.

White Blood Cells in Stool

A fresh stool specimen is necessary to identify fecal leukocytes, as the morphology of white blood cells (WBCs) is altered by stored specimens. Mucus from stool is of high yield. The sample is mixed with a drop of Loeffler methylene blue on a slide and is examined under a microscope.[23,24] In most cases, no leukocytes are noted. Presence of 5 or more leukocytes per high-power field is considered positive and indicates the presence of colonic mucosal inflammation or proctitis, which could be inflammatory or infectious. Negative stool WBC is consistent with a small-bowel process, or viral/parasitic or toxigenic bacterial processes. In an analysis of the utility of stool WBC for the diagnosis of community-acquired diarrhea, the reported sensitivity was only 50%, with positive predictive value of 45%.[25] The sensitivity is higher for shigellosis, the prototype inflammatory diarrheal infection.[26]

Amebic colitis can often be distinguished from bacterial dysenteries by microscopic fecal examination. In addition to the amebic trophozoites or cysts, fecal neutrophils are usually pyknotic or absent with amebiasis, probably because of the cytopathic effect of virulent amoebae on mammalian cells, including neutrophils.[27]

Stool Lactoferrin

Lactoferrin is an iron-binding glycoprotein found in secondary granules in leukocytes. It is used as an inflammatory marker in a commercially available latex agglutination test.[28] Sensitivity of the lactoferrin assay in detecting disease caused by Salmonella, Campylobacter, and Shigella was 93% and its specificity was 83%, at a cutoff titer of 1:50. Compared with the fecal leukocyte test, the fecal lactoferrin assay is more sensitive but less specific.[29] In addition, it does not need fresh stool specimens and is not so observer dependent. It does have false positives, especially in breast-fed infants.

Stool Culture

Although the utility of stool cultures has been questioned in the care of an individual patient, they may provide valuable information in the epidemiologic investigation of an outbreak.[18,30]

The positivity of stool cultures for acute infectious diarrhea has been reported to be as low as 2.5% to 15%,[31,32] depending on the setting. The price per unit positive stool culture result has been estimated by Koplan and colleagues[31] in the 1980s to be in the region of $1000. While this relatively poor value could be due to low sensitivity for tested pathogens, it could also be due to poor selection of patients. Siegel and colleagues[33] found that up to 50% of ordered stool cultures were for patients who had been hospitalized for more than 3 days. The yield of stool cultures in these patients is exceedingly low (see "3-day rule"). Unfortunately the poor yield of stool cultures has encouraged empiric treatment of diarrheal illnesses without testing. In an analysis of 315,828 diarrheal episodes in a Tennessee Medicaid population, Carpenter and colleagues[34] found that stool cultures were performed for only 5% of diarrheal episodes, whereas antimicrobials were prescribed for around 10% to 25%, of which almost 90% did not have accompanying stool cultures. This practice of empirically treating without testing is dangerous, because inappropriate antimicrobial use can lead to adverse outcomes, increased costs, and antimicrobial resistance.[35] In addition, this issue becomes important in cases where appropriate antibiotics need to be chosen (eg, avoiding quinolones, which can prolong the carrier state in salmonellosis[36]), where the administration of antibiotics could worsen the course of the illness itself (hemolytic-uremic syndrome related to *E coli* O157:H7[37]), or in situations where drug-resistant pathogens could be causal, such as fluoroquinolone-resistant campylobacteriosis.

The practice of sending stool cultures also helps public health authorities take appropriate early steps to prevent the spread of the infection, such as identifying and treating the source food handler or providing appropriate follow-up information to the individual infected patient if an infection is identified. FBDO investigations are most often successful when 4 or more stool specimens are obtained and analytical studies are conducted.[13] The low yield of stool cultures could be overcome by more selective ordering of stool specimens if appropriate epidemiologic cues in the history are considered.[18] The "3-day rule" proposed by some researchers states that fecal specimens should not be submitted from patients who have been hospitalized for more than 3 days, unless they have a community onset of diarrhea, have non-diarrheal manifestations of an enteric infection, are older than 65 years, are neutropenic, or are HIV positive.[26,38] In most laboratories, routine stool cultures are limited to screening for *Salmonella* and *Shigella* spp, *E coli* O157:H7, and *C jejuni/C coli*.

The laboratory should be alerted to suspected causes, so that special techniques can be used for identification of *C perfringens*, *Vibrio* spp (selective thiosulfate citrate bile salt sucrose [TCBS] media), *C jejuni* (42°C requirement and media without cephalosporins), *E coli* O157:H7 (sorbitol-MacConkey), *Cyclospora* (phase-contrast microscopy with autofluorescence), and *Y enterocolitica*, and so that organisms that may appear similar to the normal flora (eg, other *E coli*, *Bacillus cereus*) are not overlooked.

Routine stool culture also includes a medium, such as MacConkey, that selects for aerobic gram-negative rods. In addition, more selective media (eg, Hektoen, *Salmonella-Shigella* agar) and enrichment broths (eg, selenite-F and tetrathionate broths) that inhibit most organisms except *Salmonella* and *Shigella* should be used. Routine techniques must include selective culture for *C jejuni* in a selective atmosphere of reduced oxygen (4%–6%) and increased carbon dioxide (6%–10%) at 42° C.

In the United States, STEC are the most common cause of bloody diarrhea, and should be suspected especially if fever is absent.[39] Around 90% of patients with *E coli* O157:H7 isolated in stool specimens reported bloody diarrhea.[40] Hence sorbitol–MacConkey agar should be used whenever bloody diarrhea is reported. On this medium the O157:H7 colonies appear white owing to their inability to ferment sorbitol, whereas the colonies of the usual sorbitol-fermenting serotypes of *E coli* appear red. Because this serotype is unusual in its inability to ferment sorbitol, other assays must be used to detect non-O157:H7 STEC (see later discussion). Enterotoxigenic *E coli* (ETEC) is detected by commercial latex agglutination assays for labile toxin (LT) and stable toxins (ST) in an outbreak setting.

Culture of *Vibrio* spp (eg, *V cholerae*, *V parahaemolyticus*), which should be suspected after exposure to coastal areas or seafood, requires the highly selective TCBS agar.

Culture of *Y enterocolitica* in stool is often hampered by slow growth and overgrowth by normal flora. Isolation may require cold enrichment on sheep blood agar or phosphate-buffered saline, alkaline medium, and isolation in CIN agar over weeks. *Y enterocolitica* may be suspected or ordered in patients receiving iron chelators or with a history of consumption of raw pork chitterlings, or in certain ethnic at-risk populations (Asian Americans in California and African American infants).[41]

Sometimes (in up to 40% of cases) fragile organisms such as *Shigella* fail to grow, even with very careful culture methods.[23]

Growth of *E coli* as purple lactose fermenting colonies on MacConkey agar would be considered as normal fecal flora unless one were investigating unexplained dysentery in a specific host, or in an outbreak setting.

Staphylococcus aureus as a cause of food poisoning is usually apparent from the hyperacute onset of symptoms, prominence of emesis, history of ingesting foods with high protein or meat content, and concomitant illness in those who shared the meal. Staphylococcal enterotoxin can be detected by enzyme immunoassay (EIA). Alternatively, primers are available to detect enterotoxin by PCR.[42] Either the isolation of more than 10^5 organisms per gram of suspected food or detection of enterotoxin by EIA or enterotoxin gene by PCR constitutes epidemiologic evidence of staphylococcal food poisoning.[22]

Because *C perfringens* organisms are part of the normal flora in many people, the number of organisms should be greater than 10^6 per gram of stool in 2 or more affected people, or 10^5 organisms per gram of epidemiologically implicated food in stool to implicate *C perfringens* in an outbreak. Other evidence may be provided by detection of enterotoxin in the stool by enzyme-linked immunosorbent assay (ELISA) or latex agglutination.[43]

B cereus outbreaks may be documented by isolating 10^5 or more *B cereus* organisms per gram of incriminated food. One must remember, however, that *B cereus* can be found in stool in some healthy persons. There are immunoassays for the diarrheagenic toxin that are relatively less sensitive, and a cell cytotoxicity assay for cereulide, the emetic toxin.[44] PCR probes are available for all 4 toxins.

Culture-Independent Methods

For decades, isolation by culture has been the mainstay of diagnostic testing for bacterial enteric pathogens. This paradigm is changing as clinical laboratories adopt culture-independent methods, such as antigen-based tests and nucleic acid–based assays.[45] Such tests provide quicker availability of results along with accuracy, reliability, ease of validation/standardization, ease of use, potential for automation, lower cost, and convenience.

These methods are based around detection of either the toxin or other antigen by EIA/ELISA or gene determinant of the antigen or toxin by nucleic acid amplification methods such as PCR. Traditional bioassays could also be included in culture-independent methods.

The FDA approved rapid test kits for the detection of *Campylobacter* antigen directly from stool in 2009. Several these are available in the form of EIA (Premier CAMPY EIA, the ImmunoCard STAT! CAMPY test [Meridian Diagnostics, Cincinnati, OH]) with sensitivities and specificities greater than 98%. PCR tests are also available for rapid and specific identification of *Campylobacter*.[46]

Compared with culture, the overall sensitivity and specificity of PCR detection of *Salmonella*, *Campylobacter*, and *Yersinia* species and of *Shigella* species/enteroinvasive *E coli* were 92% and 98%, respectively, from fresh or Cary-Blair stool. For individual genera, PCR was as sensitive as the culture method, with the exception of *Salmonella* culture using selenite enrichment, for which PCR was less sensitive than culture. Multiplex PCR assays yield results in 3 hours (or less) versus 2 to 5 days with conventional culture. This enhanced expediency may direct appropriate care, mitigate inappropriate antibiotic use, and aid epidemiologic investigations.[47] The FDA recently approved a new qualitative multiplex PCR assay to detect simultaneously 15 different pathogens in human stool samples. The xTAG GPP assay

(Luminex Corp, Austin, TX) is able to detect viruses (rotavirus A, norovirus GI/GII, and adenovirus 410/41), protozoa/parasites (*Cryptosporidium*, *Entamoeba*, *Giardia*), and bacteria (*Salmonella*, *Shigella*, *Campylobacter*, *Yersinia*, ETEC LT/ST, *E coli* O157:H7, STEC stx1/stx2, *Clostridium difficile* toxin A/B, *Vibrio cholerae*). Sensitivity is greater than 95% for most pathogens except *Salmonella* (85%). Clinical sensitivity was not assessed for ETEC, *Yersinia enterocolitica*, and *V cholerae*.[48] Culture-independent tests are usually less labor intensive, faster to perform, and hence less expensive. In some cases they can provide virulence information, such as detection of Stx, and provide for a wider range of pathogen detection (eg, non-O157 STEC). Specimen collection may be easier (dry swab specimens); however, they do not yield an isolate that can be checked for antimicrobial susceptibility or forwarded to public health laboratories for definite identification or linkage by PFGE (see later discussion), for accuracy of testing or comparison with other isolates to detect outbreaks.

A multisite validation of antigen-based and PCR methods of *Campylobacter* identification in stool showed that the positive predictive value varied from 55% (ProSpecT Ag based assay) to 80% (PCR) with negative predictive value in the region of 99%.[49] The variable positive predictive value (PPV) could reflect that in the studies done on the stool antigen and PCR methods, higher proportions of cultures were positive with *Campylobacter* than in practice, where the prevalence is around 3% to 5%. In the real world the expected PPV of *Campylobacter* antigen–based assay would be less than 50%. Preliminary results from a multisite, validation study of *Campylobacter* culture and culture-independent methods were similar.[49]

The ImmunoCard STAT! *E coli* O157:H7 tests are available for *E coli* O157 antigen in stool and enrichment-broth stool culture incubated overnight. Compared with culture for O157 STEC, the assay has an overall sensitivity of 81% and specificity of 97%.[50] However, the assay does suffer the disadvantage of not detecting non-O157 STEC serogroups. Moreover, if used for screening one must remember that not all *E coli* O157 produce Shiga toxin, resulting in at least some false positives.

TOXIN DETECTION

Traditionally toxins were detected by the effects of toxins on animal models, such as the rabbit ileal loop or Chinese hamster ovary cell, to demonstrate the activity of the toxins of ETEC.[51] The invasiveness of enteroinvasive *E coli* was identified by inoculation into the conjunctival sac of the guinea pigs (Sereny test).[52] The effect of the Shiga toxin was demonstrated by neutralization of cytopathic changes on Vero or HeLa cell lines using anti-Stx 1 and anti-Stx 2 antibodies. These tests are no longer routinely used, owing to the need for availability of and experience with the assays.[53] The mice lethality test is used for diagnosis of botulism, at the expense of sacrificing a laboratory animal.

Toxin detection can also be accomplished by immunoassays, which include EIAs, reverse passive latex agglutinations, and gel diffusion.[54] PCR primers are also available for detection of *B cereus* nonhemolytic enterotoxin/enterotoxin T/cytotoxin K, *Clostridium botulinum* toxin types A/B/E/F, *C perfringens* enterotoxin, *E coli* Stx1 and Stx2, *S aureus* enterotoxins A to E, and *V cholerae* toxin ctxA.[44]

The FDA has approved several immunoassays for the detection of Shiga toxin in human specimens. Free fecal Shiga toxin in stools is often low, so broth cultures incubated overnight should be tested.

Four FDA-approved immunoassays are available in the United States. The Premier EHEC (Meridian Diagnostics) and the ProSpecT Shiga Toxin *E coli* Microplate Assay (Remel, Lenexa, KS) are in a microplate EIA format; the Immunocard STAT! EHEC

(Meridian Diagnostics) and the Duopath Verotoxins Gold Labeled Immunosorbent Assay (Merck, Darmstadt, Germany) are lateral-flow immunoassays. Both the Immunocard STAT! EHEC and the Duopath Verotoxins assays differentiate between Stx1 and Stx2; the Premier EHEC and the ProSpecT assays do not differentiate between Stx1 and Stx2.

Shiga-toxin PCR assays on DNA extracted from whole stool specimens are not recommended because the sensitivity is low.[55]

Any patient with a history of recent antibiotic use or hospitalization should have a stool assay for *C difficile* toxins or a PCR for *C difficile* checked, regardless of the results of the microscopic stool examination.

THE ROLE OF PULSED-FIELD GEL ELECTROPHORESIS

The investigation and confirmation of foodborne outbreaks of bacterial origin have been aided greatly by the establishment of standardized PFGE methods used by public health laboratories in the United States and Canada in a molecular subtyping network called PulseNet.[56]

PFGE allows for the resolution of DNA fragments to up to 800 kb in size.[57] For PFGE, the bacterial suspension is prepared with an optimal concentration and is mixed with molten agarose, then cast into plug molds. After releasing DNA with enzymes such as sarcosine or proteinase K, which lyse the cells, the plug is thoroughly washed to remove cellular debris and is treated with a restriction endonuclease. The plugs are then inserted into an agarose gel and the restriction fragments separated under conditions of alternating polarity. Following electrophoresis, the pattern of DNA separation is visualized after staining with a fluorescent dye, such as ethidium bromide.[58] The banding pattern from one isolate can be compared with those of other isolates, and information about the relatedness of the strains can be detected and shared via the Internet.

Tenover and colleagues[59] developed standardized criteria comparing the number of PFGE fragment differences in a test strain with those in an outbreak strain, to determine the genetic relatedness of isolates. This standardization of technique has allowed PFGE to become a widely accepted method for comparison of the genetic identity of bacteria during a disease outbreak.[56] PFGE typing has demonstrated a high level of reproducibility for foodborne pathogens. In a later article, Barrett and colleagues[60] proposed a modified approach for PFGE analysis of heterogeneous foodborne pathogens.

OVA AND PARASITE EXAMINATION

Ova and parasite examination should be considered if diarrhea persists for more than 10 days, is unresponsive to antimicrobial therapy, or if there is a history of travel to endemic areas or mountainous regions, being in contact with children in day-care centers, HIV infection, or immune compromise.

A modified acid-fast stain on stool detects *Cryptosporidium* and *Cyclospora*. The latter shows autofluorescence under ultraviolet light, which helps to differentiate the two. On phase-contrast or bright-field microscopy the oocysts appear as 8- to 10-μm spherical structures.[61]

Giardia can be diagnosed by iodine or trichrome staining. Stool-antigen detection with immunofluorescence and ELISA are now available for *Cryptosporidium* and *Giardia*, and are more sensitive methods for detection.

Stool trichrome stain for cysts and trophozoites of *Entamoeba histolytica* can be diagnostic if erythrophagocytosis is seen. Otherwise the specificity is poor in distinguishing from commensal *Entamoeba dispar* and *Entamoeba moshkovskii*.[62] A microwell ELISA, which detects the Gal/GalNAc lectin of *E histolytica*, offers a rapid (<2 hours) and sensitive way of distinguishing the 3 species.[63] PCR techniques offer superior sensitivity and specificity.[64] Serologic testing may be useful in the diagnosis of extraintestinal amebiasis, but should be used in conjunction with antigen or PCR testing in early cases where sensitivity may be limited.

REFERENCES

1. Bryce J, Boschi-Pinto C, Shibuya K, et al. WHO estimates of the causes of death in children. Lancet 2005;365:1147–52.
2. CDC Web site. Available at: http://www.cdc.gov/foodborneburden/. Accessed January 27, 2013.
3. Nachamkin I, Allos BM, Ho T. *Campylobacter* species and Guillain-Barré syndrome. Clin Microbiol Rev 1998;11:555–67.
4. Buzby JC, Roberts T, Jordan Lin CT, et al. Bacterial foodborne disease: medical costs and productivity losses. Agricultural economic report. United States Department of Agriculture; 1996. p. 93. No. (AER-741).
5. CDC. Foodborne Diseases Active Surveillance Network (FoodNet): FoodNet surveillance report for 2011 (final report). Atlanta (GA): U.S. Department of Health and Human Services, CDC; 2012.
6. CDC update on *Salmonella typhimurium* outbreak related to peanut butter. Available at: http://www.cdc.gov/salmonella/typhimurium/update.html. Accessed January 27, 2012.
7. Scallan E, Hoekstra RM, Angulo FJ, et al. Foodborne illness acquired in the United States—major pathogens. Emerg Infect Dis 2011;1:7–15.
8. Brynestad S, Granum PE. *Clostridium perfringens* and foodborne infections. Int J Food Microbiol 2002;74:195–202.
9. Dalton CB, Mintz ED, Wells JG, et al. Outbreaks of enterotoxigenic *Escherichia coli* infection in American adults: a clinical and epidemiologic profile. Epidemiol Infect 1999;123:9–16.
10. Rangel JM, Sparling PH, Crowe C, et al. Epidemiology of *Escherichia coli* O157:H7 outbreaks, United States, 1982-2002. Emerg Infect Dis 2005;11:603–9.
11. Belongia EA, Osterholm MT, Soler JT, et al. Transmission of *Escherichia coli* O157:H7 infection in Minnesota child day-care facilities. Clin Microbiol Rev 1993;269:883–8.
12. CDC's outbreak net resource Web site. Available at: http://www.cdc.gov/outbreaknet/references_resources/guide_confirming_diagnosis.html. Accessed January 27, 2013.
13. Murphree R, Garman K, Phan Q, et al. Characteristics of foodborne disease outbreak investigations conducted by FoodNet sites, 2003-2008. Clin Infect Dis 2012;54(Suppl 5):S498–503.
14. Kendall ME, Crim S, Fullerton K, et al. Travel-associated enteric infections diagnosed after return to the United States, Foodborne Diseases Active Surveillance Network (FoodNet), 2004–2009. Clin Infect Dis 2012;54(Suppl 5):S480–7.
15. Torok T, Tauxe RV, Wise RP, et al. A large community outbreak of *Salmonella* caused by intentional contamination of restaurant salad bars. JAMA 1997;278: 389–95.
16. Kolavic SA, Kimura A, Simons SL, et al. An outbreak of *Shigella dysenteriae* type 2 among laboratory workers due to intentional food contamination. JAMA 1997; 278:396–8.

17. American Medical Association, American Nurses Association-American Nurses Foundation, Centers for Disease Control and Prevention, Center for Food Safety and Applied Nutrition, Food and Drug Administration, Food Safety and Inspection Service, US Department of Agriculture. Diagnosis and management of foodborne illnesses. A primer for physicians and other health care professionals. MMWR Recomm Rep 2004;53(RR04):1–33.
18. Guerrant RL, Van Gilder T, Steiner TS, et al. Practice guidelines for the management of infectious diarrhea. Clin Infect Dis 2001;32:331–51.
19. The CDC's National Outbreak Reporting System Web site. Available at: http://www.cdc.gov/nors/resources.html. Accessed January 27, 2013.
20. Jones TF, Bulens SN, Gettner S, et al. Use of stool collection kits delivered to patients can improve confirmation of etiology in foodborne disease outbreaks. Clin Infect Dis 2004;39:1454–9.
21. Korzeniowski OM, Basada FA, Rouse JD, et al. Value of examination for fecal leukocytes in the early diagnosis of shigellosis. Am J Trop Med Hyg 1979;28: 1031–5.
22. Lew JF, LeBaron CW, Glass RI, et al. Recommendations for collection of laboratory specimens associated with outbreaks of gastroenteritis. MMWR Recomm Rep 1990;39(RR-14):1–13.
23. Harris JC, DuPont HL, Hornick RB. Fecal leukocytes in diarrheal illness. Ann Intern Med 1972;76:697–703.
24. Guerrant RL, Shields DS, Thorson SM, et al. Evaluation and diagnosis of acute infectious diarrhea. Am J Med 1985;78(6B):91–8.
25. Chitkara YK, McCasland KA, Kenefic L. Development and implementation of cost-effective guidelines in the laboratory investigation of diarrhea in a community hospital. Arch Intern Med 1996;156(13):1445–8.
26. Hines J, Nachamkin I. Effective use of the clinical microbiology laboratory for diagnosing diarrheal diseases. Clin Infect Dis 1996;23:1292–301.
27. Guerrant RL, Brush JE, Ravdin JI, et al. The interaction between *Entamoeba histolytica* and human polymorphonuclear leukocytes. J Infect Dis 1981;143:83–93.
28. Choi SW, Park CH, Silva TM, et al. To culture or not to culture: fecal lactoferrin screening for inflammatory bacterial diarrhea. J Clin Microbiol 1996;34:928–32.
29. Silletti RP, Lee G, Ailey E. Role of stool screening tests in diagnosis of inflammatory bacterial enteritis and in selection of specimens likely to yield invasive enteric pathogens. J Clin Microbiol 1996;34(5):1161–5.
30. Morris AJ, Murray PR, Reller LB. Contemporary testing for enteric pathogens: the potential for cost, time, and health care savings. J Clin Microbiol 1996;34:1776–8.
31. Koplan JP, Fineberg HV, Ferraro MJ, et al. Value of stool cultures. Lancet 1980;2: 413–6.
32. DeWitt TG, Humphrey KF, McCarthy P. Clinical predictors of acute bacterial diarrhea in young children. Pediatrics 1985;76:551–6.
33. Siegel DL, Edelstein PH, Nachamkin I. Inappropriate testing for diarrheal diseases in the hospital. JAMA 1990;263(7):979–82.
34. Carpenter LR, Pont SJ, Cooper WO, et al. Stool cultures and antimicrobial prescriptions related to infectious diarrhea. J Infect Dis 2008;197:1709–12.
35. Devasia RA, Varma JK, Whichard J, et al. Antimicrobial use and outcomes in patients with multidrug-resistant and pansusceptible *Salmonella* Newport infections, 2002–2003. Microb Drug Resist 2005;11:371–7.
36. Neill MA, Opal SM, Heelan J, et al. Failure of ciprofloxacin to eradicate convalescent fecal excretion after acute salmonellosis: experience during and outbreak in health care workers. Ann Intern Med 1991;114:195–9.

37. Wong CS, Jelacic S, Habeeb RL, et al. The risk of the hemolytic-uremic syndrome after antibiotic treatment of *Escherichia coli* O157:H7 infections. N Engl J Med 2000;342:1930–6.
38. Bauer TM, Lalvani A, Fahrenbach J, et al. Derivation and validation of guidelines for stool cultures for enteropathogenic bacteria other than *Clostridium difficile* in hospitalized adults. JAMA 2001;285:313–9.
39. Slutsker L, Ries AA, Greene KD, et al. *Escherichia coli* O157:H7 diarrhea in the United States: clinical and epidemiologic features. Ann Intern Med 1997;126:505–13.
40. Mead PS, Griffin PM. *Escherichia coli* O157-H7. Lancet 1998;352:1207–12.
41. Lee LA, Taylor J, Carter GP, et al. *Yersinia enterocolitica* O:3: an emerging cause of pediatric gastroenteritis in the United States. The *Yersinia enterocolitica* Collaborative Study Group. J Infect Dis 1991;163:660–3.
42. Bennett RW. Staphylococcal enterotoxin and its rapid identification in foods by enzyme-linked immunosorbent assay-based methodology. J Food Prot 2005; 68(6):1264–70.
43. Birkhead G, Vogt RL, Heun EM, et al. Characterization of an outbreak of *Clostridium perfringens* food poisoning by quantitative fecal culture and fecal enterotoxin measurement. J Clin Microbiol 1988;26:471–4.
44. Foley SL, Grant K. Molecular techniques of detection and discrimination of foodborne pathogens and their toxins. In: Simjee S, editor. Foodborne diseases. Totowa (NJ): Humana Press; 2007. p. 485–510.
45. Cronquist AB, Mody RK, Atkinson R, et al. Impacts of culture independent diagnostic practices on public health surveillance for bacterial enteric pathogens. Clin Infect Dis 2012;54(Suppl 5):S432–9.
46. Bessede E, Delcamp A, Sifre E, et al. New methods for detection of campylobacters in stool samples in comparison to culture. J Clin Microbiol 2011;49:941–4.
47. Cunningham SA, Sloan LM, Nyre LM, et al. Three-hour molecular detection of *Campylobacter*, *Salmonella*, *Yersinia*, and *Shigella* species in feces with accuracy as high as that of culture. J Clin Microbiol 2010;48:2929–33.
48. Wessels E, Rushman L, van Bussel M. Prospective application of the Luminex xTAG-GPP multiplex PCR in diagnosing infectious gastroenteritis [abstract P1792]. In: Programs and Abstracts of the 22nd European Congress of Clinical Microbiology and Infectious Diseases. London, March 31–April 3, 2012. p. 503.
49. Fitzgerald C, Patrick M, Jerris R, et al. Multicenter study to evaluate diagnostic methods for detection and isolation of *Campylobacter* from stool In: Programs and Abstracts of the 111th General meeting of the American Society of Microbiology [abstract P2553]. May 21–24, New Orleans (LA), 2011.
50. Stapp JR, Jelacic S, Yea YL, et al. Comparison of *Escherichia coli* O157:H7 antigen detection in stool and broth cultures to that in sorbitol-MacConkey agar stool cultures. J Clin Microbiol 2000;38:3404–6.
51. Morris GK, Merson MH, Sack DA, et al. Laboratory investigation of diarrhea in travellers to Mexico: evaluation of methods for detecting enterotoxigenic *Escherichia coli*. J Clin Microbiol 1976;3:486–95.
52. Sereny B. Experimental *Shigella* keratoconjunctivitis: a preliminary report. Acta Microbiol Acad Sci Hung 1955;2:293–6.
53. Paton JC, Paton AW. Pathogenesis and diagnosis of Shiga toxin-producing *Escherichia coli* infections. Clin Microbiol Rev 1998;11:450–79.
54. Jay JM. Modern food microbiology. Gaithersburg (MD): Aspen; 2000.
55. Gould LH, Bopp C, Strockbine N, et al. Recommendations for diagnosis of shiga toxin-producing *Escherichia coli* infections by clinical laboratories. MMWR Recomm Rep 2009;58:1–14.

56. Swaminathan B, Barrett TJ, Hunter SB, et al. PulseNet: the molecular subtyping network for foodborne bacterial disease surveillance, United States. Emerg Infect Dis 2001;7:382–9.
57. Schwartz DC, Cantor CR. Separation of yeast chromosome-sized DNAs by pulsed field gradient gel electrophoresis. Cell 1984;37:67–75.
58. Gautom RK. Rapid pulsed-field gel electrophoresis protocol for typing of *Escherichia coli* O157:H7 and other gram-negative organisms in 1 day. J Clin Microbiol 1997;35:2977–80.
59. Tenover FC, Arbeit RD, Goering RV, et al. Interpreting chromosomal DNA restriction patterns produced by pulsed-field gel electrophoresis: criteria for bacterial strain typing. J Clin Microbiol 1995;33:2233–9.
60. Barrett TJ, Gerner-Smidt P, Swaminathan B. Interpretation of pulsed-field gel electrophoresis patterns in foodborne disease investigations and surveillance. Foodborne Pathog Dis 2006;3:20–31.
61. Eberhard ML, Pieniazek NJ, Arrowood MJ. Laboratory diagnosis of *Cyclospora* infections. Arch Pathol Laboratory Med 1997;121:792–7.
62. Pillai DR, Keystone JS, Sheppard DC, et al. *Entamoeba histolytica* and *Entamoeba dispar*: epidemiology and comparison of diagnostic methods in a setting of nonendemicity. Clin Infect Dis 1999;29:1315–8.
63. Haque H, Mollah NU, Ali IK, et al. Diagnosis of amebic liver abscess and intestinal infection with the TechLab *Entamoeba histolytica* II antigen detection and antibody tests. J Clin Microbiol 2000;38:3235–9.
64. Roy S, Kabir M, Mondal D, et al. Real-time PCR assay for the diagnosis of *Entamoeba histolytica* infection. J Clin Microbiol 2005;43:2168–72.

Treating Foodborne Illness

Theodore Steiner, MD

KEYWORDS

- Antiemetics • Antidiarrheals • Diarrhea • Antibiotics

KEY POINTS

- Most foodborne illnesses are self-limited without treatment, but may have important long-term consequences in immune-compromised hosts and children.
- Oral rehydration therapy and other supportive measures have a significant impact on morbidity and mortality caused by enteric infections.
- Randomized, controlled trials have shown that antibiotic treatment improves outcomes in selected foodborne infections and specific hosts, although in general the benefits are relatively mild.

INTRODUCTION

Foodborne illnesses are among the most frequent diseases experienced worldwide. Most cases in developed countries are mild and self-limited, but severe and life-threatening complications do occur, even in previously healthy people. However, the greatest burden of disease is in developing areas, where gastrointestinal infections are a leading cause of mortality in early childhood and in patients with human immunodeficiency virus (HIV)/AIDS. Although many of these infections are capable of being spread through person-to-person contact, contaminated food and particularly water remain important transmission vehicles.

In addition to infectious agents, food and water can be the vehicle for transmission of illness caused by toxins, including those that originate from microbes (eg, *Staphylococcus aureus* enterotoxins, botulinum toxin) and environmental sources (eg, heavy metals, pesticides, mushrooms). This review focuses on those foodborne illnesses of microbial origin, but treating physicians need to remain aware of the possibility of environmental toxin ingestion, because the therapeutic and epidemiologic implications can be different.

PATIENT EVALUATION OVERVIEW

As a general rule, it is difficult if not impossible to definitively identify the specific cause of a foodborne illness from the clinical presentation alone. However, a thorough history (including symptoms, exposure, and timing) can almost always allow the treating

Infectious Disease, University of British Columbia, Rm. D452 HP East, VGH, Vancouver, British Columbia V5Z 3J5, Canada
E-mail address: tsteiner@mail.ubc.ca

Infect Dis Clin N Am 27 (2013) 555–576
http://dx.doi.org/10.1016/j.idc.2013.05.006
0891-5520/13/$ – see front matter © 2013 Elsevier Inc. All rights reserved.

id.theclinics.com

clinician to identify the presenting syndrome, which guides the appropriate diagnostic and therapeutic algorithms. There are a few syndromes that are so characteristic that they can be diagnosed with high accuracy from the history alone (for example, ciguatera after consumption of barracuda, or norovirus infection during an institutional outbreak).

The major clinical syndromes of foodborne illness and some of the leading causes include:

- Acute bacterial toxin ingestion. The patient who ingests food that was improperly handled or stored, allowing for growth of toxigenic organisms, generally becomes ill 1 to 8 hours later with the abrupt onset of severe nausea and vomiting, sometimes followed by abdominal pain/cramps and watery diarrhea. Fever is usually absent and symptoms should resolve within 24 hours.[1] In some cases (such as with nonemetic *Bacillus cereus*), cramping and diarrhea are the predominant symptoms.[2] Many patients who present with this syndrome are already better by the time they are seen by a care provider. Often, there is a clear food exposure (such as a picnic or other informal gathering) and others attending the same event have a similar illness at the same time. The major causes are *Staphylococcus aureus*, *Bacillus cereus*, and *Clostridium perfringens*, and commonly implicated foods include prepared salads that are not kept cold enough during storage.
- Viral gastroenteritis. This category contains similar illnesses caused by a growing number of recognized viruses. Although most exposure is through direct contact, food can also be a source when it is handled by any person shedding virus.
  - Norovirus and related viruses. A patient exposed to norovirus generally presents after an incubation period of 12 to 48 hours with abrupt onset of nausea and vomiting followed by watery diarrhea.[3] Norovirus infections can easily be confused with acute bacterial toxin ingestion, but rather than resolving within a few hours, symptoms generally last for 1 to 3 days, and can be more prolonged in young children and the elderly. Many patients have an obvious exposure to a sick family member or coworker, but during annual winter outbreaks, there may be no clear source of the infection. Several more recently described enteric viruses can produce a similar syndrome.
  - Rotavirus syndrome. Rotavirus is most common and most dangerous in children, in whom it typically presents with diarrhea and fever, which can lead to fatal dehydration if not treated appropriately. Symptoms may be prolonged,[4] although the mean is about 6 days.[5] Immunity is not lifelong and rotavirus infection can present in healthy adults. An extended duration of symptoms and relative lack of vomiting can sometimes help to distinguish rotavirus from norovirus.[6]
- Microbial neurotoxin exposure. This term refers to ingestion of stable, preformed toxins produced by bacteria or protozoa that concentrate in foods and disseminate in the individual after ingestion. In a few of these cases, there is an acute gastrointestinal syndrome of nausea, vomiting, intestinal pain, or diarrhea immediately after ingestion, but generally the predominant symptoms occur after the toxin reaches its target cells. Some important examples include:
  - Botulism. *Clostridium botulinum* is a common environmental contaminant, and forms spores that are resistant to boiling. When canned products are not sterilized properly, the organism can germinate and produce the highly lethal botulinum toxins, which impair neurotransmitter function in motor neurons, leading to paralysis. The disease usually presents with descending paralysis,

beginning with the cranial nerves, and if not appropriately recognized and treated with antitoxin, can lead to diffuse paralysis, requiring respiratory support for a period of weeks.[7] The major item in the differential diagnosis is Guillain-Barré syndrome.

o Ciguatera. Ciguatoxins are a family of neurotoxins produced by ocean dinoflagellates that become concentrated as they move up the food chain, concentrating in tissues of large predator fish (particularly barracuda, red snapper, and other tropical and subtropical species). After an acute nonspecific gastrointestinal syndrome, ciguatera progresses to neurologic symptoms, which may include neuropathic pain, cold allodynia, headache, ataxia, and confusion.[8] Symptoms generally last for days to weeks (or occasionally years), and clinical relapses can occur after periods of well-being.

o Scombroid. Histidine in improperly stored fish can be converted to bioactive histamine, which is relatively heat stable. Patients who ingest large quantities of histamine can present with acute onset of headache, flushing, tachycardia, and occasionally diarrhea and nausea. These symptoms are self-limited to a few hours to days.

• Small intestinal infection. Infectious agents that colonize the small intestine can produce symptoms through toxin production or local tissue invasion.

o Nontoxigenic organisms (eg, Giardia, Cryptosporidium, Cyclospora) frequently lead to an inflammatory response that causes villous blunting, fluid hypersecretion, and impaired absorption. This response produces a syndrome of abdominal cramping, bloating, flatulence, and watery or loose stools, occasionally with a greasy appearance caused by fat malabsorption. Nausea may be present, but vomiting is generally less prominent. Symptoms may persist for days or weeks, depending on the organism. A history of consumption of untreated water (eg, from lakes or streams) or travel to a developing area is often present in these cases.

o Toxin-producing bacteria (such as Vibrio cholerae and enterotoxigenic Escherichia coli) also produce mild mucosal inflammation, but most symptoms are caused by effects of the toxins on the epithelium, leading to fluid hypersecretion. Patients typically present with acute onset of nausea, occasionally vomiting, and high-volume, watery diarrhea. Fever, if present, is low-grade. If untreated, the illness is short-lived (typically <3 days), but can be fatal if appropriate rehydration is not provided.

• Inflammatory diarrhea. Invasive infections can present with a nonspecific diffuse gastroenteritis or a more characteristic dysentery syndrome. The symptoms are not specific enough to provide a diagnosis without microbiological investigation.

o Inflammatory enterocolitis typically presents as diarrhea, significant abdominal pain, and fever. Nausea and vomiting may be present but are typically not the major symptoms. Patients may pass frequent, low-volume stools with blood or pus, or may have larger watery stools. The presence of a high fever and duration for more than 48 hours can usually help to distinguish this syndrome from viral gastroenteritis. Although foodborne bacteria such as Salmonella and Campylobacter are common causes, Clostridium difficile can present in an identical fashion and must be considered in any patient with recent hospitalization, antibiotic use, or gastrointestinal surgery.

o Dysentery refers to colonic infection presenting with tenesmus and bloody or mucusy, small-volume stools, typically with fever and considerable discomfort. Although this infection is classically associated with Shigella or Entamoeba histolytica infection, it is neither sensitive nor specific for these organisms, but clearly warrants evaluation and appropriate treatment. The differential diagnosis includes ulcerative colitis and sexually transmitted proctitis.

- Hemorrhagic colitis. This syndrome classically consists of acute onset of watery diarrhea and abdominal cramps and tenderness, progressing to frankly bloody diarrhea and severe abdominal pain, but with a conspicuous absence of fever in most cases.[9,10] Although intestinal symptoms are self-limited, the disease can progress to hemolytic-uremic syndrome (HUS) with potentially fatal consequences. There is no clear evidence for benefit, and some evidence for harm, with the use of antibiotics in this syndrome, which makes it important to recognize (discussed in detail later).
- Enteric fever. *Salmonella enterica* serovar Typhi and related strains can be transmitted through food and water after contamination by infected individuals. After ingestion, the bacteria invade the intestinal epithelium and take up residence in macrophages, which disseminate the organism. The typical presentation involves fever, abdominal discomfort, headache, and other nonspecific symptoms.[11] These symptoms often progress in a stepwise fashion, becoming more severe until either resolution or fatal complications result. Because the symptoms are so nonspecific, enteric fever should be considered in the differential diagnosis of fever in endemic areas or travelers to these areas, in whom it can be confused with malaria or dengue fever, particularly early in its course.
- Other pathogen-specific conditions. There are certain pathogens that are foodborne but do not fit easily into the other categories. Some examples are:
  - *Listeria monocytogenes.* This gram-positive bacillus grows well at refrigerator temperatures and is classically associated with ingestion of unpasteurized cheese or contaminated cold cuts. It frequently causes a nonspecific diarrheal illness, but this can be followed by bacteremia with meningitis or endocarditis, particularly in immune-compromised hosts, and fetal loss in pregnant women.
  - *Yersinia enterocolitica.* This organism can present as a nonspecific inflammatory enterocolitis, but has a propensity to cause mesenteric adenitis that can mimic acute appendicitis or ileal Crohn disease.
  - Helminthic infections. Various cestodes (tapeworms), trematodes (flukes), and nematodes (roundworms) are transmitted primarily through contaminated food or water. They are described in **Table 1**.
  - *Toxoplasma gondii.* This apicomplexan protozoon causes systemic infection after ingestion of infectious cysts. This infection can occur through 2 means. Food or water can be directly contaminated with oocysts excreted by cats, which are the definitive host for the organism. In addition, other animals that have ingested toxoplasma oocysts can develop infectious muscle cysts, allowing for transmission through contaminated meat. Although toxoplasmosis is benign in most people, immunocompromised hosts are at particular risk of serious consequences, and primary infection during pregnancy can lead to severe fetal anomalies.

NONPHARMACOLOGIC TREATMENT OPTIONS

Most foodborne illnesses are self-limited and require only symptomatic treatment, but there are certain diseases in which specific therapy is indicated by either randomized, controlled trial (RCT) data or expert opinion based on case series in the setting of severe illness. In the case of diarrheal foodborne infections, even in the absence of effective specific therapy, it is important to provide supportive treatment whenever possible to prevent potentially fatal complications, which include:

Table 1
Treatment of foodborne helminthic pathogens

Pathogen	Presentation of Infection	Complications if Untreated	Recommended Treatment
Nematodes			
Trichinella spp	Muscle cysts: intense pain, orbital edema	Rare cardiac or neurological involvement	Supportive care; albendazole ± corticosteroids
Ascaris lumbricoides	Usually asymptomatic	Obstruction with heavy worm burden, biliary sepsis	Single-dose pyrantel, levamisole, mebendazole, albendazole
Trichuris trichiura	Usually asymptomatic	Heavy infestation can lead to rectal prolapse	Mebendazole
Anisakis	Acute nausea, vomiting, abdominal pain	Self-limited	Worm may self-expel as a result of vomiting; can be extracted endoscopically
Cestodes			
Taenia solium	Adult phase: asymptomatic; cyst phase: seizures	Parenchymal brain calcifications leading to seizure foci	Adult worm: praziquantel Cysts: early phase: albendazole or praziquantel, often with steroids Late phase: treatment benefit unclear
Taenia saginata, Hymenolepis nana, Diphyllobothrium latum, and others	Generally asymptomatic	Rarely, vitamin deficiencies; growth impairment in children	Praziquantel or niclosamide
Echinococcus spp	Gradually expanding cyst	Compression of surrounding viscera; anaphylaxis caused by cyst rupture	Surgical removal, PAIR (percutaneous aspiration, injection, reaspiration). Treatment with albendazole or praziquantel alone occasionally successful
Trematodes			
Paragonimus westermani	Cough, dyspnea	Can mimic tuberculosis	Praziquantel
Fasciola hepatica	Typically asymptomatic	Biliary scarring, obstruction	Triclabendazole
Liver flukes	Acute phase nonspecific; chronic phase asymptomatic	Carcinoma of biliary tract	Praziquantel

- Volume depletion
- Electrolyte disturbances
- Nutritional deficiencies (particularly in children)
- Sepsis
- HUS

Oral Rehydration Therapy

The best studied of these nonpharmacologic treatments is oral rehydration therapy (ORT). ORT has been shown in numerous RCTs to improve outcomes in severe diarrheal illnesses, particularly cholera. Choleratoxin and related bacterial enterotoxins act by inducing hypersecretion of salts and water by intestinal crypt cells. The villi and their ability to absorb fluid are relatively preserved. Villous epithelial cells express several transport proteins that facilitate nutrient and salt absorption; one of the most highly expressed is SGLT-1, which cotransports 1 glucose molecule and 2 Na^+ ions, bringing more than 200 water molecules from the lumen into the enterocyte, leading to considerable water absorption.[12] Related cotransporters for other carbohydrates and amino acids are also active. As a result, administration of an ORT containing glucose and Na^+ in the appropriate concentrations (close to a 1:1 Molar ratio) leads to water absorption that can effectively balance out the hypersecretion, improving diarrhea and maintaining the patient's health until an appropriate immune response (or antibiotic treatment) clears the infecting organism. Standard ORT solutions also contain bicarbonate or citrate to correct acidosis and potassium to replace intestinal losses.

Progressive refinements in ORT have been made since its initial discovery. Current recommendations are found in **Table 2**. In particular, a reduction in the osmolarity has been recommended since 2004 based on several strong studies showing better control of diarrheal volume, albeit with occasional asymptomatic hyponatremia.[13,14] In addition, glucose polymers (eg, rice or wheat starch) have been shown in several large RCTs (and confirmed by a meta-analysis) to be superior to glucose in terms of duration of symptoms and need for rescue intravenous fluids.[15] However, some of these studies compared starch-based oral rehydration solution (ORS) with high-osmolarity glucose-based ORS. In addition, the differences between solutions are generally more pronounced in cholera than in other dehydrating diarrheal illnesses.

If the World Health Organization (WHO) ORS salts are not available, a simple home recipe is found in **Table 2**. The solution should taste similar to tears. Plain water or water with a bit of salt added are preferable to hyperosmolar home remedies like ginger ale or apple juice, which contain a high carbohydrate/sodium ratio, and can lead to greater intestinal fluid losses. Use of hypo-osmolar solutions can lead to asymptomatic hyponatremia, but this is preferable to potentially life-threatening dehydration.

Other Nonpharmacologic Treatments for Foodborne Illness

- Micronutrients.
  - Zinc deficiency is common in poor, developing areas with limited dietary diversity. Although young infants are relatively replete from maternal sources, older infants and children can suffer considerable gastrointestinal losses because of recurrent diarrheal episodes, leading to frank deficiency and resulting hypersusceptibility to infectious diarrhea. A recent meta-analysis of zinc supplementation trials[16] found that overall there was a small but statistically significant improvement in the duration of diarrhea with zinc administration compared with placebo. This effect was most pronounced in children older than 6 months

Table 2
Recommended oral rehydration solutions http://www.who.int/maternal_child_adolescent/ documents/fch_cah_06_1/en/

Source	Carbohydrate	Sodium Chloride	Other Salts	Indication
Recommended				
World Health Organization reduced-osmolarity ORS	Glucose 13.5 g/L (75 mM)	2.6 g/L (75 mM Na^+, 65 mM Cl^-)	KCl 1.5 g/L (20 mM K^+); trisodium citrate 2.9 g/L (10 mM citrate)	Recommended for all diarrheal illness
Acceptable range	$\geq Na^+$ concentration but <111 mM	60–90 mM Na^+; 50–80 mM Cl^-	15–25 mM K^+; 8–12 mM citrate	If World Health Organization solution not available
Starch-based ORS	50–80 g/L cooked rice powder	2.6 g/L (75 mM Na^+, 65 mM Cl^-)	KCl 1.5 g/L (20 mM K^+); trisodium citrate 2.9 g/L (10 mM citrate)	More effective than standard ORS in cholera
Home-made ORS	2 level tablespoonsful sugar (30 g)	Half a level teaspoonful salt (2.5 g)	Add 0.5 c. (125 mL) orange juice or mashed banana	Per liter of clean water
Not Recommended				
Sugared carbonated soft drink	700 mM	2 mM	Low in K^+	Osmolarity too high: can exacerbate dehydration
Apple juice	690 mM	3 mM	32 mM	Same
Gatorade	255 mM	20 mM	3 mM	Hyperosmolar
Tea	As desired	0	0	Inadequate electrolyte replacement

and in studies in Asia, where zinc-deficient diets are more common. No overall effect on mortality was identified, and zinc administration was associated with increased vomiting in children. There remains insufficient evidence to know whether zinc supplementation is beneficial in developed areas.[17]

○ Vitamin A is another micronutrient frequently low in developing areas, and deficiency is associated with xerophthalmia and blindness as well as childhood mortality. Several RCTs have examined the benefits of vitamin A supplementation to improve childhood mortality, and a meta-analysis found a significant improvement in overall mortality and specifically mortality caused by diarrhea.[18] However, use of vitamin A in the treatment of acute diarrheal episodes is not beneficial.[19]

• Feeding. Adults and older children with enteric infection often suffer from anorexia during their illness, and may experience transient weight loss, but generally recover quickly. The same is not true for young children, in whom repeated episodes of diarrheal illness, particularly persistent episodes (those lasting >14 days), can lead to permanent deficits in growth and even cognitive development.[20,21] Specific feeding approaches to prevent this situation have not yet been identified. Infants are at even greater risk, because they cannot control their own food and fluid intake. Cultural practices such as withholding breastfeeding during diarrheal illness can lead to fatal consequences, and parents should be encouraged to continue feeding infants normally as tolerated.[22]

- Infection control and public health considerations. Many foodborne infections are highly transmissible, and efforts should be made to limit spread, particularly in health care settings. The Society for Healthcare Epidemiology of America recommends that all hospitalized patients who develop diarrhea be placed on contact isolation (gown and gloves) and in a private room where possible, to reduce the spread of Clostridium difficile.[23] Often, more intensive measures such as closure of wards and banning of visitation are required during norovirus outbreaks.[3] In addition, many enteric infections must be reported to public health authorities. This strategy is instrumental for outbreak identification and also to advise people at risk of transmission (such as food service workers) when it is safe for them to resume work.
- Probiotics. There has been considerable interest in the use of nonpathogenic bacteria and yeast supplementation to prevent or treat infectious diarrhea. It is hypothesized that these organisms would colonize the intestine heavily to reduce the environmental niche for the offending pathogen, and many clinical studies have been performed. There is no solid evidence for a clear benefit of any specific probiotic preparation in the treatment of foodborne illness, although some have been proved to improve diarrheal symptoms in specific situations (such as irritable bowel syndrome[24] and antibiotic-associated diarrhea in children[25]). There is some trial evidence that addition of Lactobacillus GG to ORS can improve pediatric infectious diarrhea,[26] but not enough to warrant a universal recommendation.[22]

PHARMACOLOGIC TREATMENT OPTIONS

Pharmacologic treatments for foodborne infections include drugs used for symptomatic benefit, such as antiemetics, antispasmodics, and antimotility agents, and drugs used specifically to treat infection. Most of the latter are antimicrobials, although there are some agents that are not antibiotics per se, but either facilitate the activity of antibiotics (such as proton pump inhibitors in the treatment of Helicobacter pylori infection) or target microbial toxins (such as cholestyramine used in the treatment of Clostridium difficile infection). Antimicrobials are discussed later for each specific infectious syndrome.

Drugs used specifically to treat the symptoms of foodborne illness include:

- Antimotility agents. One of the most troubling symptoms of foodborne illness is diarrhea, particularly when prolonged. There are several available agents that act to reduce stool frequency, volume, and urgency, which can allow patients to carry out their daily activities more comfortably. These drugs are effective, particularly in relatively mild illness. For example, in combination with antibiotics, they significantly shorten the duration of illness in travelers' diarrhea.[27] However, they are not effective in high-volume secretory diarrhea (eg, cholera) or in inflammatory colitis. They are relatively contraindicated during inflammatory diarrheal illness because of a risk of potentially fatal complications such as toxic megacolon.[28] For example, rare fatal cases of Campylobacter infection were reported in association with antimotility drug use.[29] Moreover, use of antimotility drugs has been associated with worse outcomes (including HUS) in hemorrhagic colitis.[30] However, a retrospective review of patients with Clostridium difficile infection found no harmful effect of antimotility agents when coadministered with metronidazole or vancomycin.[31] The most recent Infectious Diseases Society of

America guidelines (2001) recommend avoiding these agents during bloody diarrhea or proven infection with enterohemorrhagic *E coli*.

Specific antimotility agents include:

- o Loperamide. This opioid agonist acts largely on μ-opioid receptors in the intestinal myenteric plexus, reducing intestinal motility and increasing transit time. This situation can reduce cramping and allows greater contact time with the colonic mucosa, reducing diarrheal volume.[32] It is available over the counter as a generic medication in many countries (including the United States and Canada) for treatment of adults and children older than 2 years. Side effects include constipation and bloating; in addition, coadministration with *P*-glycoprotein inhibitors (such as quinidine) can lead to accumulation in the central nervous system, with central opioid activity as a result, leading to sedation and analgesia.
- o Diphenoxylate/atropine. This combination drug, marketed for years as Lomotil, combines an opioid agonist (diphenoxylate) with the anticholinergic agent atropine. It is generally reserved for more chronic intestinal disorders rather than foodborne illness, because of its increased side effects, which include dry mouth, blurry vision, and sedation from the anticholinergic action.
- o Opiates. All opiate agonist drugs have the potential to decrease motility and reduce diarrhea as a result of their effects on intestinal neurons. Generally, their sedating qualities and potential for dependence preclude their routine use for foodborne illness in modern times, although preparations such as paregoric and tincture of opium were used through much of the twentieth century and are still available in some countries.
- Antispasmodics. These drugs are muscarinic cholinergic antagonists that act to reduce the intensity of smooth muscle contractions in the intestinal wall. These drugs can provide relief from pain caused by abdominal cramping, but are also associated with anticholinergic side effects, and the potential to induce toxic megacolon, although there are no reports of this occurring in infectious diarrhea. Currently used drugs in this class include butylscopolamine (Buscopan), hyoscyamine, dicycloverine, and the older drugs scopolamine and atropine.
- Bismuth salts. Bismuth subsalicylate is marketed worldwide as an agent to treat diarrhea, nausea, and dyspepsia. Its precise mechanism of action is unknown, but it does have antisecretory, antiinflammatory, and antibacterial properties. It is more effective than placebo in the prevention of travelers' diarrhea,[33,34] although antimicrobials are preferred for treatment based on clinical trial evidence.[35] It is a weak antacid but can reduce gastric discomfort, possibly because of the antiinflammatory activity of the salicylate moiety. Because it contains a salicylate, it should not be used in children with fever, because of risk of Reye syndrome. It also causes black discoloration of stool.
- Other antidiarrheals. Clay minerals have been used for years to treat diarrhea, and a combination of kaolin and pectin (Kaopectate) was marketed in the United States. This antidiarrheal was later (around 1990) changed to a different mineral, attapulgite. However, a review by the US Food and Drug Administration in 2003 found insufficient evidence of efficacy of attapulgite in earlier studies and withdrew approval for the drug as an antidiarrheal. The manufacturer changed the formulation in the United States to contain bismuth subsalicylate instead of attapulgite, although the latter is still available in Canada. Racecadotril is an enkephalinase inhibitor marketed in Europe but not North America; there is evidence of benefit in childhood diarrhea.[36,37]

- Antiemetics. Nausea and vomiting can be the most unpleasant symptoms of foodborne illness. They can also impair the ability to use oral rehydration, leading to hospital admissions for intravenous therapy, particularly in children. There are many different classes of antiemetics for various indications, although surprisingly few have been studied in acute gastroenteritis.
  - 5-HT$_3$ receptor antagonists. These drugs inhibit serotonin signaling in the brain chemoreceptor trigger zone, impairing the central nausea/vomiting response. They also inhibit serotonin signaling in the enteric nervous system. They were initially marketed for the prevention and treatment of chemotherapy-induced emesis, but because of their safety and efficacy, their use has expanded to other indications. The only member of this class studied in foodborne illness is ondansetron, which has been shown in several RCTs to effectively improve nausea and vomiting in children with gastroenteritis.[38] Recent meta-analyses have confirmed that this drug is safe and effective in reducing vomiting, need for intravenous hydration, and immediate hospitalization in children with acute gastroenteritis.[39,40] It can be administered orally or intravenously. Some studies have shown an increase in diarrhea, but this has been inconsistent.
  - Dopamine antagonists. Before the introduction of 5-HT$_3$ antagonists, these antagonists were the mainstay of antiemetic therapy, although they have fallen out of favor because of increased side effects, which include sedation and rare extrapyramidal neurologic symptoms (akathisia, muscle stiffness). Drugs in this class specifically used as antiemetics include prochlorperazine, domperidone, and metoclopramide. Metoclopramide also has prokinetic activity. Metoclopramide was shown to be equivalent to ondansetron in 1 RCT in children,[41] although the study was underpowered to show a significant difference. One RCT in adults found prochlorperazine to be slightly better than ondansetron in nausea scores but equivalent in terms of reducing vomiting.[42]
  - Antihistamines. Histaminergic neurons are found in the emesis pathway from the chemoreceptor trigger zone to the vomiting center in the brainstem, and numerous over-the-counter and prescription agents that block histamine 1 receptors are marketed as antiemetics. Their primary benefit is in motion sickness rather than acute gastroenteritis. Dimenhydrinate (Gravol, Dramamine) is specifically marketed for nausea, although the only RCT in acute gastroenteritis[43] found a reduction in vomiting but not need for intravenous fluids or hospitalization. These drugs are generally very sedating.
  - Ginger. Ginger root preparations have been used as a folk remedy for nausea and vomiting for years, and recent clinical trials have begun to study the activity of ginger in a rigorous fashion, but not in acute gastroenteritis. A recent meta-analysis found insufficient evidence of activity in chemotherapy-induced nausea and vomiting.[44]
  - Acupuncture/acupressure. Acupuncture by a trained practitioner or self-stimulation of the ventral surface of the wrist have been studied as treatments for anesthesia-induced and chemotherapy-induced nausea and vomiting. One small, noncontrolled study found good success in the treatment of vomiting in acute gastroenteritis in children.[45]
- Treatments for noninfectious/toxin-mediated food poisoning. The major benefit in this category is the treatment of botulism with antitoxin antibodies, which, when administered promptly, can stop symptoms from progressing but cannot reverse the effect on neurons that have already bound the toxin.[46] Equine trivalent, pentavalent, and heptavalent preparations have been used but can cause

serum sickness reactions; a human immunoglobulin Ig-based product is available for infants. Scombroid poisoning responds to antihistamine drugs, although it is self-limited regardless. There are no antitoxin agents for ciguatera and related illnesses, and supportive/symptomatic treatment is recommended. Intravenous mannitol was suggested in case reports[47] to be beneficial, but a more recent clinical trial found no efficacy, and as a result this is no longer recommended.[48]

ANTIMICROBIAL THERAPIES FOR FOODBORNE ILLNESS

Antimicrobials are of no use in toxin-mediated foodborne illness, including those caused by ingestion of bacterial, preformed toxins. In addition, there are no agents to treat viral gastroenteritis. Bacterial and protozoal agents, on the other hand, are almost always susceptible to 1 or more commercially available antibiotics. Before instituting treatment of one of these infections, is it important to consider the following:

- Does this infection need to be treated? Most causes of foodborne illness are self-limited and specific antibiotic treatment in general provides only modest benefit. Nevertheless, certain infections (Shigella, typhoid fever) have clear RCT evidence of a benefit of treatment. However, many other infections lack evidence of a benefit of antibiotic treatment, even when the isolate and drug susceptibilities are known (eg, Yersinia enterocolitica). In addition, there are some infections (nontyphoidal Salmonella) in which treatment can benefit some patients but lead to unwanted outcomes in others. There is competing evidence of both harm and benefit of antibiotics in the treatment of hemorrhagic colitis caused by enterohemorrhagic and related strains of E coli, and as a result, treatment is not generally recommended.
- Should the syndrome be treated before the cause is known? In some cases, the clinical features are enough to warrant specific antibiotic treatment even without a clear cause. The best example of this is travelers' diarrhea, in which empiric antibiotic treatment has been shown in many RCTs to shorten the severity and duration of illness (reviewed in Ref.[49]). There is also evidence that empiric treatment of severe diarrhea that persists beyond 72 hours is beneficial, although the choice of agent depends on the index of suspicion and the local susceptibility patterns (see later discussion).[50] However, treatment should generally be avoided in the syndrome of hemorrhagic colitis (frankly bloody diarrhea without fever), for reasons discussed later.
- Which antibiotic should be used? The broad variety of infectious agents that can, in many cases, produce indistinguishable clinical syndromes makes treatment challenging. Moreover, many of the drugs studied in well-designed RCTs can no longer be recommended because of increasing resistance, which can vary according to geographic area. Whenever possible, treatment should be tailored based on culture and susceptibility reports; when this is not feasible, an updated knowledge of local susceptibility patterns should guide therapy as much as possible.

A list of major bacterial and protozoal pathogens and the recommended antibiotic treatment is shown in **Tables 3** and **4**. Specific cases meriting mention are the following:

- Salmonella. Salmonella gastroenteritis is a self-limited illness, and treatment with antibiotics can prolong the duration of shedding and lead to some clinical

Table 3
Treatment of foodborne protozoal pathogens

Pathogen	Presentation of Infection	Complications if Untreated	Recommended Treatment
Giardia lamblia	Small bowel syndrome	Self-limited but often prolonged	Tinidazole, albendazole, metronidazole
Cryptosporidium	Small bowel syndrome; fulminant chronic diarrhea in AIDS	In AIDS, fatal wasting syndrome and dehydration; cholangiopathy	Nitazoxanide in immune competent; antiretroviral therapy in AIDS
Cyclospora cayetanensis	Small bowel syndrome; fatigue	Self-limited but often prolonged	TMP-SMX; ciprofloxacin if allergic
Microsporidia (Enterocytozoon bieneusi, Encephalitozoon intestinalis)	Chronic diarrhea in AIDS; rarely in transplant recipients	Wasting syndrome; cholangiopathy	Antiretrovirals or reduce immune suppression; albendazole for Encephalitozoon intestinalis
Entamoeba histolytica	Asymptomatic colonization to severe dysenteric colitis	Ameboma, liver abscess, other parenchymal abscess	Invasive disease: tinidazole or metronidazole, followed by paromomycin or iodoquinol Asymptomatic cyst passer: paromomycin or iodoquinol
Blastocystis hominis	Generally asymptomatic; some patients experience diarrhea, bloating, flatulence, and so forth	None	Treatment controversial; metronidazole, TMP-SMX, iodoquinol may be effective
Toxoplasma gondii	Acute: localized or disseminated lymphadenopathy, sometimes with fever; rarely chorioretinitis, encephalitis	Reactivation in immune compromise to encephalitis or chorioretinitis; fetal anomalies if acquired during pregnancy	Acute: treatment not clearly indicated[86] Reactivation: TMP-SMX or pyrimethamine/sulfadiazine or pyrimethamine/clindamycin
Trypanosoma cruzi	Rarely acquired through ingestion of crushed trematode bugs in food (eg, sugar cane juice)	Chronic sequelae of Chagas disease: organomegaly; chagoma in immune compromise	Acute or early chronic disease: benznidazole Late chronic disease with organomegaly: treatment benefit remains uncertain Chagoma: benznidazole

Abbreviation: TMP-SMX, trimethoprim-sulfamethoxazole.

relapses.[51] A recent meta-analysis[52] found no overall benefit of antibiotic treatment of *Salmonella* gastroenteritis in healthy adults, and confirmed increased likelihood of shedding the organism at 30 days. Most of the studies were considered to have low-quality evidence. Nevertheless, it is recommended not to use antibiotics in uncomplicated cases. Some experts do recommend treatment of severe cases (requiring hospitalization, high fever, multiple daily stools) based on efficacy in 1 RCT. In addition, treatment of children younger than 2 years and elderly patients is recommended by many experts.

One important consideration is that *Salmonella* can cause prolonged, metastatic, or lethal infection in immune-compromised hosts. These hosts include patients with AIDS, solid organ transplants, asplenia, or corticosteroid treatment. Although there are no RCT data in these cases, it is recommended that they be treated, given the relatively high risk of prolonged or recurrent bacteremia (reviewed in Ref.[53]).

- *Shigella.* Shigellosis can produce a particularly severe colitis, and is an independent risk factor for mortality in children hospitalized with diarrhea.[54] Although the illness is self-limited in most patients, antibiotics have been shown in several studies to shorten the duration of both illness and bacterial shedding, and because *Shigella* spreads readily from person to person, it is generally recommended that all cases be treated.[55] Antibiotic resistance has been increasing in different parts of the world.[56] In North America, most isolates remain susceptible to ciprofloxacin and third-generation cephalosporins.
- *Campylobacter.* Fatalities caused by *Campylobacter jejuni* gastroenteritis are rare, although bacteremias do occur, largely in immunocompromised hosts, with a mortality in those cases of 15% in 1 series.[57] A recent meta-analysis found that antibiotic treatment in uncomplicated cases does shorten the duration of illness, particularly when administered early, but the effect is modest.[58] Many patients are already better, or beyond the window of antibiotic usefulness, by the time the culture result is received. However, many experts do recommend treating severe cases and cases in immune-compromised hosts. As with most other bacterial diarrheal pathogens, *Campylobacter* is becoming increasingly resistant to first-line agents in some parts of the world, although macrolides (eg, azithromycin) remain active against most US isolates.[59]
- Enterohemorrhagic *E coli* (EHEC). The gastrointestinal symptoms of EHEC infection are self-limited, but the major complication, HUS, can be fatal or lead to permanent neurologic or renal sequelae. The predominant pathogen in this class, *E coli* O157:H7, remains antibiotic sensitive.[60] However, there is strong evidence from in vitro and animal models that antibiotics can induce increased toxin release from EHEC, leading to worse outcomes. For *E coli* O157:H7, the best evidence against the use of antibiotics was a prospective study of infected children in the United States,[61] in which antibiotic use was an independent risk factor for HUS in multivariate analysis, controlling for disease severity. However, the data were derived from only 10 HUS cases, and the antibiotics used were trimethoprim-sulfamethoxazole and β-lactam drugs. In contrast, retrospective data from the large Japanese outbreak in the late 1990s suggested that fosfomycin (the most commonly used antibiotic in that outbreak) was protective against HUS when used in the first 2 days of illness.[62] However, given the absence of RCT data and, more importantly, no good evidence of benefit, most authorities recommend against antibiotic treatment of *E coli* O157:H7 infection. In patients who do develop HUS, the C5 complement inhibitor eculizumab has been reported to be beneficial in a

Table 4
Treatment of bacterial foodborne and waterborne pathogens

Pathogen	Syndrome	Benefits of Treatment	Risks of Treatment	Recommendation	Recommended Drugs
Nontyphoidal Salmonella	Inflammatory diarrhea	Shortens duration of illness; prevents bacteremic seeding	Prolonged shedding; risk of clinical relapse	Treat only specific hosts (extremes of age, immune compromised, asplenic, and so forth)	TMP-SMX, FQ, Ceph3, amoxicillin
Typhoid fever	Enteric fever	Improves survival, eliminates shedding in most	Some patients may remain colonized and infectious	Treat	Ceph3; FQ, TMP-SMX if from area of low resistance
Shigella spp	Inflammatory diarrhea or dysentery	Reduced duration of illness, reduced shedding	Minimal	Treat	FQ, Ceph3, azithromycin; TMP-SMX if susceptible
Campylobacter spp	Inflammatory diarrhea	Reduced duration of illness if started early	Minimal	Consider treatment in severe or persistent cases	Azithromycin, FQ if from susceptible area
Enterohemorrhagic E coli	Hemorrhagic colitis	Reduces shedding; may or may not reduce risk of HUS	Increased toxin release and potential predisposition to HUS	Do not treat (from current evidence)	
Enteropathogenic E coli	Infantile diarrhea	ORS life saving; no evidence antibiotics are helpful	Unknown	Antibiotics not indicated for infantile diarrhea	
Enterotoxigenic E coli	Travelers' diarrhea	Significantly shortens duration of illness	Minimal	Empirical treatment indicated for travelers' diarrhea	Azithromycin, FQ, TMP-SMX, rifaximin

Enteroaggregative E coli	Endemic diarrhea, travelers' diarrhea, prolonged diarrhea in AIDS	Improves symptoms in AIDS; treatment of travelers' diarrhea beneficial as for ETEC	Unknown	Empirical treatment indicated for travelers' diarrhea; treat if found in persistent diarrhea	FQ, TMP-SMX, Ceph3, azithromycin
Yersinia spp	Inflammatory diarrhea or pseudoappendicitis	Reduces shedding but does not improve clinical outcomes	Unknown	No clear recommendation	Usually resistant to ampillilin and Ceph1
Listeria monocytogenes	Nonspecific gastroenteritis; bacteremia; meningitis; endocarditis	Treatment of invasive disease improves mortality	Minimal	Treat invasive disease or disease in pregnant women	Ampicillin or penicillin; TMP-SMX if allergic
Vibrio cholerae	Fulminant watery diarrhea	Self-limited without antibiotics but antibiotics shorten illness	Minimal	ORS as mainstay; antibiotics if feasible	Doxycycline, FQ, TMP-SMX
Noncholera Vibrio	Inflammatory or nonspecific diarrhea	No evidence for benefit	Minimal	Consider treating severe cases	Doxycycline, FQ
Aeromonas hydrophila	Inflammatory or nonspecific diarrhea	Most cases self-limited; case series of benefit in prolonged illness[87]	Minimal	Treat severe or prolonged cases (>7–10 d)	TMP-SMX, doxycycline, FQ

Abbreviations: Ceph1/3, first-generation/third-generation cephalosporin; FQ, fluoroquinolone; TMP-SMX, cotrimoxazole.

small case series,[63] although prospective, randomized data are lacking. Plasma exchange is frequently used, although it also lacks supporting randomized data.

- Enteroaggregative Shiga toxin–producing *E coli* O104:H4. This strain caused a large European foodborne outbreak of hemorrhagic colitis in 2011, in which the HUS rates in adults were a frightening 22%.[64] This isolate carried an extended-spectrum β-lactamase, rendering it resistant to cephalosporins, but it remained susceptible to fluoroquinolones, rifaximin, and azithromycin. There are conflicting reports as to whether antibiotics induce toxin production and release from this strain.[65,66] No randomized data are available on antibiotic use and the risk of HUS with this infection, but many patients in the outbreak received treatment with antibiotics, and no association with worse outcome was found. Treatment with ciprofloxacin was associated with reduced HUS risk in 1 case series.[67] Another case series[68] found reduced duration of shedding in patients who received azithromycin, with no apparent effect on HUS onset or outcomes, which could have implications for reducing secondary spread. There is insufficient evidence that antibiotics are either harmful or beneficial in O104:H4 infection, but the outbreak data are still being analyzed. In 1 prospective case series,[9] eculizumab was not found to be beneficial in 7 patients with severe HUS with neurologic symptoms. Plasma exchange was also not found to be beneficial in 1 case-control study.[69]

- *Giardia.* Metronidazole for 7 days has long been the recommended treatment of giardiasis, and although generally effective, it is poorly tolerated by many patients. Newer drugs active against *Giardia* have advantages of shorter treatment duration or better side-effect profile, although the studies comparing them have not been of high quality. A recent meta-analysis[70] found that tinidazole, nitazoxanide, and albendazole are likely to be as effective as metronidazole, and with generally fewer side effects. Relapses are not uncommon after metronidazole treatment, and resistance can develop. The optimal treatment in these cases remains uncertain.

- *Cryptosporidium.* This protozoan is a common cause of self-limited infections in immune-competent children and adults, although symptoms can be prolonged in some cases. In contrast, patients with advanced HIV/AIDS or other severe immune defects can develop devastating, fatal diarrheal illness. The only drug approved for this infection, nitazoxanide, provides modest symptomatic benefit in immune-competent hosts, with significantly better symptom resolution and decreased shedding at 4 days.[71] However, results in patients with HIV infection have been less encouraging, particularly in those with CD4 counts less than $50/\mu L$[72] and in children in developing areas,[73] as confirmed in 1 meta-analysis.[74] The mainstay of treatment of cryptosporidiosis in HIV/AIDS is antiretroviral therapy, which leads to lasting remission, although relapse of infection can occur if therapy is stopped.[75]

- *Entamoeba histolytica.* Metronidazole has been the mainstay of therapy for invasive amebiasis for years, although a recent meta-analysis of 8 RCTs[76] found that tinidazole is equally effective but with a shorter treatment duration and better side-effect profile. Nevertheless, metronidazole remains a first-line agent for invasive disease. It is recommended to use a luminal agent such as paromomycin to clear cysts after treatment of invasive disease, because nitroimidazoles do not reliably eradicate the cyst form. *Entamoeba histolytica* can be mistaken under microscopy for the nonpathogenic *Entamoeba dispar*, which does not require treatment.

TREATMENT RESISTANCE/COMPLICATIONS

Antibiotic resistance among enteric pathogens is continuously evolving, but large geographic differences remain. For example, fluoroquinolone resistance rates among *Campylobacter* isolates are more than 95% in Thailand,[77] but less than 20% in North America.[78] The driving forces behind evolving resistance include widespread human prescription as well as animal feed supplementation. It is important for treating practitioners to review the most recent available data on local resistance patterns when selecting empirical antibiotics to treat an enteric infection, and to follow the antibiotic sensitivity report on an isolate when available.

In general, treatment courses for foodborne infections are short and well tolerated. As with any antibiotic, allergic reactions and secondary *Clostridium difficile* infection are ever-present concerns. Among nonantibiotic agents, the greatest concern is with inappropriate use of antimotility agents during inflammatory or hemorrhagic colitis, because of a potential to increase the risk of toxic megacolon or HUS, respectively.

EVALUATION OF OUTCOME AND LONG-TERM RECOMMENDATIONS

In general, patients recover quickly from foodborne infections and permanent sequelae are relatively rare. Stool analysis for test of cure is not generally recommended for individual patients, although screening of certain individuals (such as food preparation workers) may be indicated for public health reasons.[79] Although most patients can expect to recover fully from a foodborne illness, population-based studies from large-scale outbreaks such as the *E coli* O157:H7 and *Campylobacter* outbreak in Walkerton, ON in 2000, have shown an increased risk of postinfectious irritable bowel syndrome[80,81]; moreover, the rates of chronic kidney disease and hypertension are increased in those who recover from HUS.[82] *Campylobacter* is a well-recognized trigger for Guillain-Barré syndrome.[83] Moreover, population studies suggest that an acute episode of infectious gastroenteritis is associated with about a 2-fold increased risk of developing inflammatory bowel disease.[84] Any enteric infection can precipitate reactive arthritis, which can be self-limited to a few weeks or months, or evolve into a chronic spondyloarthropathy. It is not known whether antibiotic treatment of these infections affects these long-term risks; it does not seem to improve outcomes in established reactive arthritis.[85]

SUMMARY/DISCUSSION

Foodborne illnesses come from a wide variety of infectious and noninfectious sources, and can produce several relatively distinct clinical syndromes. Recognition of these syndromes, along with a careful exposure history, can usually provide enough information to guide rational use of diagnostic testing, empiric supportive therapy, and occasionally specific antimicrobial therapy. With appropriate treatment of dehydration (ideally with ORS), the risk of mortality or long-term morbidity is generally low. Key recent advances in the management of foodborne illness include the introduction of reduced-osmolarity ORS, the benefit of zinc supplements in children in developing areas, and the usefulness of ondansetron in pediatric gastroenteritis. Antimicrobial therapy still plays a small role in enteric foodborne infections. The most worrisome foodborne illness in otherwise healthy people in developed countries is hemorrhagic colitis, with its attendant risks of HUS. Moreover, patients with immune compromise are at risk for potentially devastating consequences of enteric infection. Most of the world's children, who live in impoverished areas without appropriate sanitation, remain vulnerable to repeated bouts of foodborne illness, which are frequently fatal and in survivors produce long-term consequences that are only now beginning to be appreciated.

REFERENCES

1. Le Loir Y, Baron F, Gautier M. *Staphylococcus aureus* and food poisoning. Genet Mol Res 2003;2(1):63–76.
2. Stenfors Arnesen LP, Fagerlund A, Granum PE. From soil to gut: *Bacillus cereus* and its food poisoning toxins. FEMS Microbiol Rev 2008;32(4):579–606.
3. Division of Viral Diseases, National Center for Immunization and Respiratory Diseases, Centers for Disease Control and Prevention. Updated norovirus outbreak management and disease prevention guidelines. MMWR Recomm Rep 2011; 60(RR-3):1–18.
4. Carr ME, McKendrick GD, Spyridakis T. The clinical features of infantile gastroenteritis due to rotavirus. Scand J Infect Dis 1976;8(4):241–3.
5. Uhnoo I, Olding-Stenkvist E, Kreuger A. Clinical features of acute gastroenteritis associated with rotavirus, enteric adenoviruses, and bacteria. Arch Dis Child 1986;61(8):732–8.
6. Bresee JS, Marcus R, Venezia RA, et al. The etiology of severe acute gastroenteritis among adults visiting emergency departments in the United States. J Infect Dis 2012;205(9):1374–81.
7. Centers for Disease Control and Prevention (CDC). Recognition of illness associated with the intentional release of a biologic agent. MMWR Morb Mortal Wkly Rep 2001;50(41):893–7.
8. Wong CK, Hung P, Lee KL, et al. Features of ciguatera fish poisoning cases in Hong Kong 2004-2007. Biomed Environ Sci 2008;21(6):521–7.
9. Ullrich S, Bremer P, Neumann-Grutzeck C, et al. Symptoms and clinical course of EHEC O104 infection in hospitalized patients: a prospective single center study. PLoS One 2013;8(2):e55278.
10. Griffin PM, Ostroff SM, Tauxe RV, et al. Illnesses associated with *Escherichia coli* O157:H7 infections. A broad clinical spectrum. Ann Intern Med 1988;109(9): 705–12.
11. Thriemer K, Ley BB, Ame SS, et al. Clinical and epidemiological features of typhoid fever in Pemba, Zanzibar: assessment of the performance of the WHO case definitions. PLoS One 2012;7(12):e51823.
12. Gagnon MP, Bissonnette P, Deslandes LM, et al. Glucose accumulation can account for the initial water flux triggered by Na+/glucose cotransport. Biophys J 2004;86(1 Pt 1):125–33.
13. Multicentre evaluation of reduced-osmolarity oral rehydration salts solution. International Study Group on Reduced-osmolarity ORS solutions. Lancet 1995; 345(8945):282–5.
14. Santosham M, Fayad I, Abu Zikri M, et al. A double-blind clinical trial comparing World Health Organization oral rehydration solution with a reduced osmolarity solution containing equal amounts of sodium and glucose. J Pediatr 1996;128(1):45–51.
15. Gregorio GV, Gonzales ML, Dans LF, et al. Polymer-based oral rehydration solution for treating acute watery diarrhoea. Cochrane Database Syst Rev 2009;(2):CD006519.
16. Lazzerini M, Ronfani L. Oral zinc for treating diarrhoea in children. Cochrane Database Syst Rev 2013;(1):CD005436.
17. Salvatore S, Hauser B, Devreker T, et al. Probiotics and zinc in acute infectious gastroenteritis in children: are they effective? Nutrition 2007;23(6):498–506.

18. Mayo-Wilson E, Imdad A, Herzer K, et al. Vitamin A supplements for preventing mortality, illness, and blindness in children aged under 5: systematic review and meta-analysis. BMJ 2011;343:d5094.
19. Fischer Walker CL, Black RE. Micronutrients and diarrheal disease. Clin Infect Dis 2007;45(Suppl 1):S73–7.
20. Moore SR, Lima NL, Soares AM, et al. Prolonged episodes of acute diarrhea reduce growth and increase risk of persistent diarrhea in children. Gastroenterology 2010;139(4):1156–64.
21. Oria RB, Patrick PD, Zhang H, et al. APOE4 protects the cognitive development in children with heavy diarrhea burdens in Northeast Brazil. Pediatr Res 2005; 57(2):310–6.
22. Guarino A, Albano F, Ashkenazi S, et al. European Society for Paediatric Gastroenterology, Hepatology, and Nutrition/European Society for Paediatric Infectious Diseases evidence-based guidelines for the management of acute gastroenteritis in children in Europe. J Pediatr Gastroenterol Nutr 2008;46(Suppl 2):S81–122.
23. Cohen SH, Gerding DN, Johnson S, et al. Clinical practice guidelines for *Clostridium difficile* infection in adults: 2010 update by the Society for Healthcare Epidemiology of America (SHEA) and the Infectious Diseases Society of America (IDSA). Infect Control Hosp Epidemiol 2010;31(5):431–55.
24. Whelan K. Probiotics and prebiotics in the management of irritable bowel syndrome: a review of recent clinical trials and systematic reviews. Curr Opin Clin Nutr Metab Care 2011;14(6):581–7.
25. Johnston BC, Goldenberg JZ, Vandvik PO, et al. Probiotics for the prevention of pediatric antibiotic-associated diarrhea. Cochrane Database Syst Rev 2011;(11):CD004827.
26. Szajewska H, Mrukowicz JZ. Probiotics in the treatment and prevention of acute infectious diarrhea in infants and children: a systematic review of published randomized, double-blind, placebo-controlled trials. J Pediatr Gastroenterol Nutr 2001;33(Suppl 2):S17–25.
27. Riddle MS, Arnold S, Tribble DR. Effect of adjunctive loperamide in combination with antibiotics on treatment outcomes in traveler's diarrhea: a systematic review and meta-analysis. Clin Infect Dis 2008;47(8):1007–14.
28. Butler T. Loperamide for the treatment of traveler's diarrhea: broad or narrow usefulness? Clin Infect Dis 2008;47(8):1015–6.
29. Smith GS, Blaser MJ. Fatalities associated with *Campylobacter jejuni* infections. JAMA 1985;253(19):2873–5.
30. Bell BP, Griffin PM, Lozano P, et al. Predictors of hemolytic uremic syndrome in children during a large outbreak of *Escherichia coli* O157:H7 infections. Pediatrics 1997;100(1):E12.
31. Koo HL, Koo DC, Musher DM, et al. Antimotility agents for the treatment of *Clostridium difficile* diarrhea and colitis. Clin Infect Dis 2009;48(5):598–605.
32. Baker DE. Loperamide: a pharmacological review. Rev Gastroenterol Disord 2007;7(Suppl 3):S11–8.
33. Steffen R. Worldwide efficacy of bismuth subsalicylate in the treatment of travelers' diarrhea. Rev Infect Dis 1990;12(Suppl 1):S80–6.
34. DuPont HL, Ericsson CD, Farthing MJ, et al. Expert review of the evidence base for prevention of travelers' diarrhea. J Travel Med 2009;16(3):149–60.
35. Shlim DR. Update in traveler's diarrhea. Infect Dis Clin North Am 2005;19(1): 137–49.
36. Lehert P, Cheron G, Calatayud GA, et al. Racecadotril for childhood gastroenteritis: an individual patient data meta-analysis. Dig Liver Dis 2011;43(9):707–13.

37. Szajewska H, Ruszczynski M, Chmielewska A, et al. Systematic review: racecadotril in the treatment of acute diarrhoea in children. Aliment Pharmacol Ther 2007;26(6):807–13.
38. Freedman SB, Adler M, Seshadri R, et al. Oral ondansetron for gastroenteritis in a pediatric emergency department. N Engl J Med 2006;354(16):1698–705.
39. Carter B, Fedorowicz Z. Antiemetic treatment for acute gastroenteritis in children: an updated Cochrane systematic review with meta-analysis and mixed treatment comparison in a Bayesian framework. BMJ Open 2012;2(4). http://dx.doi.org/10.1136/bmjopen, 2011-000622.
40. Fedorowicz Z, Jagannath VA, Carter B. Antiemetics for reducing vomiting related to acute gastroenteritis in children and adolescents. Cochrane Database Syst Rev 2011;(9):CD005506.
41. Al-Ansari K, Alomary S, Abdulateef H, et al. Metoclopramide versus ondansetron for the treatment of vomiting in children with acute gastroenteritis. J Pediatr Gastroenterol Nutr 2011;53(2):156–60.
42. Patka J, Wu DT, Abraham P, et al. Randomized controlled trial of ondansetron vs. prochlorperazine in adults in the emergency department. West J Emerg Med 2011;12(1):1–5.
43. Uhlig U, Pfeil N, Gelbrich G, et al. Dimenhydrinate in children with infectious gastroenteritis: a prospective, RCT. Pediatrics 2009;124(4):e622–32.
44. Lee J, Oh H. Ginger as an antiemetic modality for chemotherapy-induced nausea and vomiting: a systematic review and meta-analysis. Oncol Nurs Forum 2013;40(2):163–70.
45. Anders EF, Findeisen A, Lode HN, et al. Acupuncture for treatment of acute vomiting in children with gastroenteritis and pneumonia. Klin Padiatr 2012; 224(2):72–5.
46. Tacket CO, Shandera WX, Mann JM, et al. Equine antitoxin use and other factors that predict outcome in type A foodborne botulism. Am J Med 1984;76(5): 794–8.
47. Palafox NA, Jain LG, Pinano AZ, et al. Successful treatment of ciguatera fish poisoning with intravenous mannitol. JAMA 1988;259(18):2740–2.
48. Schnorf H, Taurarii M, Cundy T. Ciguatera fish poisoning: a double-blind randomized trial of mannitol therapy. Neurology 2002;58(6):873–80.
49. Kollaritsch H, Paulke-Korinek M, Wiedermann U. Traveler's diarrhea. Infect Dis Clin North Am 2012;26(3):691–706.
50. Dryden MS, Gabb RJ, Wright SK. Empirical treatment of severe acute community-acquired gastroenteritis with ciprofloxacin. Clin Infect Dis 1996; 22(6):1019–25.
51. Neill MA, Opal SM, Heelan J, et al. Failure of ciprofloxacin to eradicate convalescent fecal excretion after acute salmonellosis: experience during an outbreak in health care workers. Ann Intern Med 1991;114(3):195–9.
52. Onwuezobe IA, Oshun PO, Odigwe CC. Antimicrobials for treating symptomatic non-typhoidal Salmonella infection. Cochrane Database Syst Rev 2012;(11):CD001167.
53. Gordon MA. Salmonella infections in immunocompromised adults. J Infect 2008; 56(6):413–22.
54. Uysal G, Sokmen A, Vidinlisan S. Clinical risk factors for fatal diarrhea in hospitalized children. Indian J Pediatr 2000;67(5):329–33.
55. Metzler AE, Burri HR. The etiology of "malignant catarrhal fever" originating in sheep: serological findings in cattle and sheep with ruminant gamma herpesviruses. Tierarztl Prax 1991;19(2):135–40.

56. Rahman M, Shoma S, Rashid H, et al. Increasing spectrum in antimicrobial resistance of *Shigella* isolates in Bangladesh: resistance to azithromycin and ceftriaxone and decreased susceptibility to ciprofloxacin. J Health Popul Nutr 2007;25(2):158–67.

57. Fernandez-Cruz A, Munoz P, Mohedano R, et al. *Campylobacter* bacteremia: clinical characteristics, incidence, and outcome over 23 years. Medicine (Baltimore) 2010;89(5):319–30.

58. Ternhag A, Asikainen T, Giesecke J, et al. A meta-analysis on the effects of antibiotic treatment on duration of symptoms caused by infection with *Campylobacter* species. Clin Infect Dis 2007;44(5):696–700.

59. Wang X, Zhao S, Harbottle H, et al. Antimicrobial resistance and molecular subtyping of *Campylobacter jejuni* and *Campylobacter coli* from retail meats. J Food Prot 2011;74(4):616–21.

60. Beier RC, Poole TL, Brichta-Harhay DM, et al. Disinfectant and antibiotic susceptibility profiles of *Escherichia coli* O157:H7 strains from cattle carcasses, feces, and hides and ground beef from the United States. J Food Prot 2013; 76(1):6–17.

61. Wong CS, Jelacic S, Habeeb RL, et al. The risk of the hemolytic-uremic syndrome after antibiotic treatment of *Escherichia coli* O157:H7 infections. N Engl J Med 2000;342(26):1930–6.

62. Ikeda K, Ida O, Kimoto K, et al. Effect of early fosfomycin treatment on prevention of hemolytic uremic syndrome accompanying *Escherichia coli* O157:H7 infection. Clin Nephrol 1999;52(6):357–62.

63. Lapeyraque AL, Malina M, Fremeaux-Bacchi V, et al. Eculizumab in severe Shiga-toxin-associated HUS. N Engl J Med 2011;364(26):2561–3.

64. Frank C, Werber D, Cramer JP, et al. Epidemic profile of Shiga-toxin-producing *Escherichia coli* O104:H4 outbreak in Germany. N Engl J Med 2011;365(19):1771–80.

65. Corogeanu D, Willmes R, Wolke M, et al. Therapeutic concentrations of antibiotics inhibit Shiga toxin release from enterohemorrhagic *E. coli* O104:H4 from the 2011 German outbreak. BMC Microbiol 2012;12:160.

66. Bielaszewska M, Idelevich EA, Zhang W, et al. Effects of antibiotics on Shiga toxin 2 production and bacteriophage induction by epidemic *Escherichia coli* O104:H4 strain. Antimicrob Agents Chemother 2012;56(6):3277–82.

67. Geerdes-Fenge HF, Lobermann M, Nurnberg M, et al. Ciprofloxacin reduces the risk of hemolytic uremic syndrome in patients with *Escherichia coli* O104:H4-associated diarrhea. Infection 2013;41(3):669.

68. Nitschke M, Sayk F, Hartel C, et al. Association between azithromycin therapy and duration of bacterial shedding among patients with Shiga toxin-producing enteroaggregative *Escherichia coli* O104:H4. JAMA 2012;307(10):1046–52.

69. Menne J, Nitschke M, Stingele R, et al. Validation of treatment strategies for enterohaemorrhagic *Escherichia coli* O104:H4 induced haemolytic uraemic syndrome: case-control study. BMJ 2012;345:e4565.

70. Granados CE, Reveiz L, Uribe LG, et al. Drugs for treating giardiasis. Cochrane Database Syst Rev 2012;(12):CD007787.

71. Rossignol JF, Kabil SM, el-Gohary Y, et al. Effect of nitazoxanide in diarrhea and enteritis caused by *Cryptosporidium* species. Clin Gastroenterol Hepatol 2006; 4(3):320–4.

72. Rossignol JF, Hidalgo H, Feregrino M, et al. A double-'blind' placebo-controlled study of nitazoxanide in the treatment of cryptosporidial diarrhoea in AIDS patients in Mexico. Trans R Soc Trop Med Hyg 1998;92(6):663–6.

73. Amadi B, Mwiya M, Sianongo S, et al. High dose prolonged treatment with nitazoxanide is not effective for cryptosporidiosis in HIV positive Zambian children: a randomised controlled trial. BMC Infect Dis 2009;9:195.

74. Abubakar I, Aliyu SH, Arumugam C, et al. Prevention and treatment of cryptosporidiosis in immunocompromised patients. Cochrane Database Syst Rev 2007;(1):CD004932.

75. Carr A, Marriott D, Field A, et al. Treatment of HIV-1-associated microsporidiosis and cryptosporidiosis with combination antiretroviral therapy. Lancet 1998; 351(9098):256–61.

76. Gonzales ML, Dans LF, Martinez EG. Antiamoebic drugs for treating amoebic colitis. Cochrane Database Syst Rev 2009;(2):CD006085.

77. Boonmar S, Morita Y, Fujita M, et al. Serotypes, antimicrobial susceptibility, and gyr A gene mutation of *Campylobacter jejuni* isolates from humans and chickens in Thailand. Microbiol Immunol 2007;51(5):531–7.

78. Thakur S, Zhao S, McDermott PF, et al. Antimicrobial resistance, virulence, and genotypic profile comparison of *Campylobacter jejuni* and *Campylobacter coli* isolated from humans and retail meats. Foodborne Pathog Dis 2010;7(7): 835–44.

79. Guerrant RL, Van Gilder T, Steiner TS, et al. Practice guidelines for the management of infectious diarrhea. Clin Infect Dis 2001;32(3):331–51.

80. Thabane M, Simunovic M, Akhtar-Danesh N, et al. An outbreak of acute bacterial gastroenteritis is associated with an increased incidence of irritable bowel syndrome in children. Am J Gastroenterol 2010;105(4):933–9.

81. Zanini B, Ricci C, Bandera F, et al. Incidence of post-infectious irritable bowel syndrome and functional intestinal disorders following a water-borne viral gastroenteritis outbreak. Am J Gastroenterol 2012;107(6):891–9.

82. Clark WF, Sontrop JM, Macnab JJ, et al. Long term risk for hypertension, renal impairment, and cardiovascular disease after gastroenteritis from drinking water contaminated with *Escherichia coli* O157:H7: a prospective cohort study. BMJ 2010;341:c6020.

83. Kalra V, Chaudhry R, Dua T, et al. Association of *Campylobacter jejuni* infection with childhood Guillain-Barre syndrome: a case-control study. J Child Neurol 2009;24(6):664–8.

84. Garcia Rodriguez LA, Ruigomez A, Panes J. Acute gastroenteritis is followed by an increased risk of inflammatory bowel disease. Gastroenterology 2006;130(6): 1588–94.

85. Fryden A, Bengtsson A, Foberg U, et al. Early antibiotic treatment of reactive arthritis associated with enteric infections: clinical and serological study. BMJ 1990;301(6764):1299–302.

86. Gilbert RE, See SE, Jones LV, et al. Antibiotics versus control for toxoplasma retinochoroiditis. Cochrane Database Syst Rev 2002;(1):CD002218.

87. Vila J, Ruiz J, Gallardo F, et al. *Aeromonas* spp. and traveler's diarrhea: clinical features and antimicrobial resistance. Emerg Infect Dis 2003;9(5):552–5.

Treatment of Shiga Toxin–Producing *Escherichia coli* Infections

T. Keefe Davis, MD[a], Ryan McKee, MD[b],
David Schnadower, MD, MPH[b], Phillip I. Tarr, MD[c],*

KEYWORDS

* Shiga-toxin * *Escherichia coli* O157:H7 * Hemolytic uremic syndrome * Antibiotics
* Microbiologic diagnosis

KEY POINTS

* *Escherichia coli* O157:H7 remains the chief precipitant of the hemolytic uremic syndrome worldwide, among all of the Shiga toxin–producing organisms that have been implicated in human disease.
* Optimal diagnosis of this pathogen in 2013 remains dependent on plating of all specimens on receipt on sorbitol MacConkey agar; reliance on a toxin assay to screen specimens to evaluate for pathogens to the exclusion of agar plating is inappropriate.
* Clinical profiling of patients who might be infected with *E coli* O157:H7 and other Shiga toxin–producing *E coli*, and empirical, vigorous, and closely monitored intravenous volume expansion with isotonic crystalloid is associated with better outcomes, probably because of the nephroprotective effect of volume expansion.
* Antibiotics are contraindicated in patients acutely infected with Shiga toxin–producing *E coli*.

INTRODUCTION

Shiga toxin (Stx)-producing *Escherichia coli* (STEC) causes a spectrum of disease, ranging from asymptomatic carriage (rare)[1–3] to diarrhea, bloody diarrhea, and the hemolytic uremic syndrome (HUS).[4] HUS, which is a microangiopathic hemolytic

Disclosures: Dr Tarr has received an honorarium for a lecture at Cepheid corporate headquarters. Part of his laboratory effort is supported by a grant to another investigator at Washington University from Alexion Corporation (makers of eculizumab).
[a] Division of Nephrology, Department of Pediatrics, Washington University School of Medicine, 660 South Euclid, St Louis, MO 63110, USA; [b] Division of Emergency Medicine, Department of Pediatrics, Washington University School of Medicine, 660 South Euclid, St Louis, MO 63110, USA; [c] Division of Gastroenterology, Hepatology, and Nutrition, Department of Pediatrics, Washington University School of Medicine, 660 South Euclid, St Louis, MO 63110, USA
* Corresponding author. Division of Gastroenterology, Hepatology, and Nutrition, Department of Pediatrics, Washington University School of Medicine, Campus Box 8208, 660 South Euclid, St Louis, MO 63110.
E-mail address: tarr@wustl.edu

Infect Dis Clin N Am 27 (2013) 577–597
http://dx.doi.org/10.1016/j.idc.2013.05.010
0891-5520/13/$ – see front matter © 2013 Elsevier Inc. All rights reserved.

id.theclinics.com

anemia with thrombocytopenia and renal failure, is predominantly caused by a single serotype of E coli, namely, O157:H7. For this reason alone, E coli O157:H7 causes one of the most highly feared gut infections in North America. These infections are medical emergencies.

In this article, the treatment of STEC infections is reviewed, but there are no specific treatments for these illnesses. Nonetheless, certain management practices optimize the likelihood of good outcomes. Overall, the successful management of STEC infections is based on recognition that a patient might have an STEC infection. The timeliness of STEC identification cannot be overemphasized, because it avoids therapies prompted by inappropriate additional testing, and directs the clinician to focus on appropriate management strategies. The opportunities during STEC infections to avert the worst outcomes are brief, and this article emphasizes practical matters relevant to making a diagnosis, anticipating the trajectory of illness, and optimizing care.

BACKGROUND
Nomenclature

Confusing nomenclature plagues STEC. **Table 1** defines the often interchangeable terms that are used when describing these organisms. E coli that contain genes encoding Stx are described as Stx-producing E coli (STEC), and the subset of STEC that have shown their virulence in humans as enterohemorrhagic E coli (EHEC).

Pathogenesis

The cardinal virulence property of EHEC is their ability to produce Stxs.[4] These organisms do not invade the bloodstream. Rather, the vascular perturbations that occur during EHEC infections are almost certainly a consequence of toxemia from Stx absorbed from the gut. Toxemia occurs early in illness, is short-lived,[5] and is likely cleared by the time patients present. Well before overt renal injury in children who develop HUS, and even in children whose course resolves without severe microangiopathy, there is evidence of thrombin generation, increased plasminogen activator inhibitor type 1 activity, intravascular fibrin accretion, and shearing of von Willebrand factor multimers.[6,7] At this point in illness, there is a paucity of biologically active Stx, or Stx antigen, in stool, despite an abundance of E coli O157:H7. A trial of monoclonal antibody against Stx is under way in Argentina[8] in an attempt to avert HUS in infected children, but it is possible that the interval in which an antitoxin therapy might be effective has already passed by the time of presentation.

E COLI O157:H7 VERSUS NON-O157:H7 EHEC: DIAGNOSIS AND COMPARATIVE OUTCOMES

E coli O157:H7 is the EHEC that has, decade after decade and on multiple continents, been the predominant cause of HUS.[9–19] This single serotype, representing a highly circumscribed clade of organisms,[20] causes epidemic and sporadic illness, although sporadic infections are more common. Most clinical data pertain to E coli O157:H7, and therefore this article is heavily weighted toward infections caused by this serotype. However, there are practical considerations to differentiating O157:H7 from non-O157:H7 EHEC. E coli O157:H7 is best diagnosed by plating all fresh stools submitted for microbiological culture on sorbitol MacConkey agar, with or without cefixime-tellurite.[21] Unlike most commensal E coli and almost all non-O157:H7 EHEC, E coli O157:H7 fails to ferment sorbitol on these agar plates after overnight incubation. These pathogens are usually easy to detect if stool is plated appropriately on

Table 1
Nomenclature used to describe Stxs and the *E coli* that produce them

Term	Definition	Synonyms	Comments
Stx-producing *E coli* (STEC)	*E coli* that contain genes encoding 1 or more Stxs[75,76]	Verocytotoxin-producing, verotoxin-producing, Shiga-like toxin (archaic)–producing *E coli*	
Stx (as elaborated by Shigella)[77]	The principal extracellular toxin of *Shigella dysenteriae* serotype 1. Variants of Stx are found in *E coli*		
Stxs 1 and 2[77]	Variants of Stx produced by *E coli*. Stx1 and its variants are closely related to Stx of *Shigella dysenteriae* serotype 1. Stx2 is less orthologous to Stx than is Stx1	Verocytotoxin, verotoxin, Shiga-like toxin (archaic)	Stx1 and its variants are closely related to Stx of *Shigella dysenteriae* serotype 1. Stx2 is less orthologous to Stx than is Stx1
Enterohemorrhagic *E coli* (EHEC)[78]	The subset of STEC that cause human disease		Virulence is customarily established by causation of an outbreak, or repeated bona fide (recovered from stool, in the absence of other pathogens or a serologic response to *E coli* O157:H7) associations with human diseases. Generally infers that an organism contains the locus of enterocyte effacement.[79]

receipt (**Fig. 1**). Hence, all diagnostic priorities, as discussed later, should be directed toward confirming or refuting the presence of *E coli* O157:H7 in a stool culture.

Failure to make, or delay in making, a microbiological diagnosis of *E coli* O157:H7 infection is usually related to not obtaining a culture at initial presentation, slow transport to a laboratory, or failure to seek *E coli* O157:H7 on all incoming specimens. It is a dangerous misconception to rely on toxin assay screening to detect *E coli* O157:H7, because for unclear reasons, sorbitol MacConkey agar screening is more sensitive than toxin enzyme immunoassays (EIAs)[1,14,22–26] for detecting this pathogen. Also, using the toxin EIA as a screen for O157:H7 as well as non-O157:H7 EHEC, with culture pursuit only of specimens in which the assay is positive, delays informing the physician if a patient is infected with a highly actionable EHEC (ie, *E coli* O157:H7), or one of the many non-O157:H7 EHEC that in any individual case are less likely to cause HUS. We believe that using toxin assays as a screen to the exclusion of sorbitol MacConkey agar plating is a threat to public health and to efficient and effective clinical medicine. For these reasons, we concur with the recommendation of the US Centers for Disease Control and Prevention that all stools be simultaneously plated for *E coli* O157:H7 on selective agar and tested for non-O157:H7 EHEC[27] with an appropriate toxin detection system.

Serology and immunomagnetic bead separation are alternative ways to diagnose *E coli* O157:H7 infections when stool cultures are negative.[19] These tests are not available rapidly, and often require facilitation by local health departments but can provide clarity in situations in which microbiology is not definitive. We also encourage attempts to take possession of the original agar plates if they are not in your institution, and repeat the cultures using sorbitol MacConkey agar and toxin EIAs on broth outgrowths.

Although some non-O157:H7 EHEC can cause severe disease, the context of their prevalence in various case series shows the primacy of *E coli* O157:H7. In many regions of the world, when a causative enteric pathogen is discovered, 95% or more of all patients with diarrhea-related HUS have microbiological evidence of infection with *E coli* O157:H7.[9–19] Several studies are particularly instructive: Banatvala and colleagues[13] reported that among 83 patients in a nationwide study of HUS, 70 patients had stool cultures with bacterial growth, with stools obtained a median of 8 days after

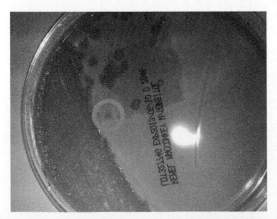

Fig. 1. Colorless colony of *E coli* O157:H7 (*green circle*) on a sorbitol MacConkey agar plate. Specimen was plated on receipt in laboratory, and incubated overnight. A rapid agglutination test determined that this colony contained the O157 LPS antigen.

illness onset. Thirty STEC were recovered from these stools, and 25 were *E coli* O157. This finding is similar to early data showing that stools of two-thirds of patients with HUS are negative for *E coli* O157:H7 if cultured on admission to hospital with HUS.[10] Four of the 5 patients from whom non-O157:H7 were recovered also had serologic testing during convalescence, and 3 of these 4 had evidence of a recent exposure to O157 lipopolysaccharide (LPS). Moreover, two-thirds of the cases from whom no STEC were recovered were seropositive for O157. In a recent 11-center study, Hickey and colleagues[17] showed that of 50 children with HUS, 27 were positive for *E coli* O157:H7, and 1 was positive for *E coli* O121:H19; microbiological data were negative or incomplete on the remainder. It is likely that all or almost all of the negative cases were infected with *E coli* O157:H7.[10] A recent focused and intensive analysis of FoodNet sets reiterated these data.[19] Taken together, and in combination with additional reports,[9–12,14–16,18] these data suggest that if *E coli* O157:H7 is not recovered from a patient with HUS, the most likely explanation is that timely and appropriate microbiological assessment of the stool for this pathogen was not performed.

Non-O157:H7 EHEC clearly do cause severe human disease, as shown by the tragic *E coli* O104:H4 outbreak in Germany in 2011.[28,29] However, this event was a combination of the expansion of the population of a single pathogen in conditions conducive to growth (sprouting facilities), and contamination of a product (sprouts) that are not typically subjected to bactericidal processes before consumption. In contrast, when thorough testing is implemented in prospective studies, the frequency with which non-O157:H7 EHEC are identified is inversely proportional to the acuity of the illness in the patients whose stools are being tested. For example, as noted earlier, *E coli* O157:H7 remains the near exclusive cause of HUS.[9–19] Also, in 3 different studies of cohorts exclusively[1,30] or largely[31] identified in pediatric emergency departments, non-O157:H7 accounted for about one-third of all diagnosed EHEC infections. However, when extended to the state level,[18,32] the proportion of non-O157:H7 EHEC exceeds that of *E coli* O157:H7 (although O157:H7 remains the most common of all serotypes). The Connecticut study[18] is a case in point. Of the 229 patients infected with non-O157:H7 EHEC, only 1 developed HUS. In contrast, 45 of the 434 patients infected with *E coli* O157 developed HUS. Hence, the toxin EIA, when added to sorbitol MacConkey agar screening, is likely to detect cases that are at less risk of developing HUS.

Spectrum of Illness

E coli O157:H7 infections pass through recognizable phases (**Table 2**). After a several-day incubation period, patients usually present with nonbloody diarrhea. In only rare cases is the first loose stool bloody. In about 80% of culture-positive cases, the diarrhea turns bloody after about 2 days of nonbloody diarrhea.

Critical Points in Illness and Symptom Definition

It is important to determine the day of onset of illness, because clinical decisions are often intimately related to time points in illness evaluation (see **Table 4** in Ref.[33]), and clinical and pathophysiology data are related to this metric.[6,7,17,34–38] We have used the calendar day on which the first loose stool occurred as the first day of diarrhea, because it is difficult to know if antecedent signs and symptoms, such as abdominal pain, vomiting, or transient fever, really reflect the earliest signs of the infection. Bloody diarrhea is defined by visible, and not occult, blood in stool. HUS occurs when laboratory tests reach a simultaneous set of abnormal values (platelet count <150,000/mm^3, hematocrit level <30%, and creatinine level > upper limit of normal for age). Critical defining points in EHEC illnesses are provided in **Table 3**.

Table 2
Phases of *E coli* O157:H7 infections. Day-by-day laboratory courses are portrayed in other publications

Phase	1	2	3	4	5
Description	Incubation Period	Nonbloody diarrhea[a]	Bloody diarrhea	HUS[b,c]	Oligoanuric HUS
Onset and intervals	About 3 d before first loose stool →	Day 1[d] of illness, lasts for 2–3 d →	Day 3 of illness, lasts 3–5 d →	Days 5–13 of illness. Patients are generally hospitalized for 1–2 wk from this point forward, if there is no need for dialysis,[35] although interinstitutional practices might vary →	Onset generally by day 10 of illness. Patients requiring dialysis are generally hospitalized for 2–3 wk from this point forward,[35] although interinstitutional practices might vary
Comments	Based on outbreak analyses[41,80]	Based on personal experience and early series.[81] Almost all infected patients have diarrhea	Based on personal experience and early case series. Bloody diarrhea occurs in approximately 80% of culture-proven cases[41,81,82]	Based on recent case series of HUS[6,17,34,35,38] 15%–20% of culture-proven cases of *E coli* O157:H7 develop HUS	Based on a case series.[17] Overall, about two-thirds of EHEC-related HUS in children is oligoanuric, and requires dialysis

[a] Minimally symptomatic cases of *E coli* O157:H7 infection can occur, but are unusual.[84]

[b] HUS is defined stringently as hemolytic anemia (hematocrit level <30% with smear evidence of hemolysis), thrombocytopenia (platelet count <150,000/mm³), and renal insufficiency (serum creatinine level higher than the upper limit of normal for age).

[c] Occasionally, HUS caused by *E coli* O157:H7 occurs without antecedent diarrhea,[12,85] but is unusual.

[d] Day 1 of illness is the first day of diarrhea. See **Table 3** for definition of clinical terms.

Data from Tarr PI, Bass DM, Hecht GA. Bacterial, viral, and toxic causes of diarrhea, gastroenteritis, and anorectal infections. In: Yamada T, editor. Textbook of gastroenterology. (NJ): Blackwell; 2009. p. 1157; and Ahn CK, Holt NJ, Tarr PI. Shiga-toxin producing *Escherichia coli* and the hemolytic uremic syndrome: what have we learned in the past 25 years? Adv Exp Med Biol 2009;634:1–17.

Table 3
Definitions of clinical events during EHEC infection

Terms	Definitions	Comments
Diarrhea	Loose stool, independent of number of bowel movements per day	Many diarrhea studies use a gradient of loose stools such as are shown on the Bristol stool chart,[86] but it is critical to date the first day of diarrhea for case management, and we prefer the first day of the first loose stool, even if it is the only loose stool that day. We also prefer not to dwell on semiquantitative fluidity specifications
First day of illness	First day of diarrhea	This definition is important, because it is important to anticipate the likely evolution of this disease, and particularly of the onset of anuria if HUS ensues, and the best data relate to the first day of diarrhea.[17,35] There are often symptoms before the first loose stool, but such symptoms are vague (nausea), or nonspecific (vomiting), and are difficult to factor into attempts to measure subsequent points of illness
Bloody diarrhea	Visible blood in the stool	Stool that has occult blood is not bloody diarrhea
Fever	Temperature determined by any modality in a health care setting that is $\geq$38.0°C	About half of all families report that children infected with EHEC have had a fever before evaluation, but such fevers are almost never documented in health care settings[38]
HUS	HUS is defined stringently as hemolytic anemia (hematocrit level <30% with smear evidence of hemolysis), thrombocytopenia (platelet count <150,000/mm³), and renal insufficiency (serum creatinine level higher than the upper limit of normal for age)[7,13,14,17,32,35–37,87,88,89–97]	This is a urinalysis-independent definition. Using urinalysis as a criterion for HUS is inappropriate because of the risk of fecal contamination, leading to spurious proteinuria, hemoglobinuria, and pyuria
First day of HUS	First day on which the above criteria are all met	Thrombocytopenia generally occurs first, followed by anemia, followed by renal insufficiency[6,83]
Oligoanuric HUS	HUS in which the patient has urine output <0.5 mL/kg/h for at least 24 consecutive hours[17,34,35]	Oligoanuric HUS is categorically worse than nonoligoanuric HUS

MANAGEMENT OF EHEC INFECTIONS

The initial assessment of patients infected with EHEC is important, because tests and interventions that are chosen at this point in illness might well ordain the outcome. In the next sections, an overview is provided of the various scenarios of such first encounters, and subsequent management considerations.

Clinical Presentation

Patients infected with EHEC can present to care at any point in illness, and even in the resolution phase of HUS. However, independent of the timing of presentation, it is critical to gather certain baseline data and remain focused in the evaluation. In the history, we determine the first day of diarrhea, if the diarrhea is painful (it almost always is), identify concurrently ill contacts, and try to learn where tests (blood and stool) might have been performed before evaluation. We do not try to determine the source (epidemiologic attribution is better left to the local disease investigation authorities) or family history (beyond ill contacts who might need to be encouraged to seek medical attention). In the physical examination, we focus on the vital signs and abdominal examination and do not encourage digital rectal examination.

Table 4 portrays the history and studies that should be obtained on presentation, and evaluations that we discourage because, if positive or negative, they do not help manage infected patients. Also, by pursuing extraneous laboratory testing, the provider runs the risk of receiving data that are irrelevant at best, and harmful at worst, because misleading results could lead to inappropriate actions. Examples of test-driven misadventures that we encounter several times each year include obtaining a urinalysis that is contaminated with stool, or that has mild abnormalities, or seeking presence of *Clostridium difficile* (a result that is often returned before the results of the stool culture are known and that is difficult to interpret in children), with both such results prompting the use of antibiotics.

Table 4
Evaluations that are recommended at presentation, and evaluations that are not appropriate, or rarely helpful

Laboratory Tests at Presentation	Laboratory Tests Discouraged at Presentation	Imaging Studies that Might be Helpful, if Intussusception is Suspected	Imaging Studies that are Rarely Necessary or Helpful
Stool culture[a]	Urinalysis	Ultrasonography	Computed tomography scans
Complete blood count	Parasite testing	Plain abdominal radiographs	Contrast studies
Electrolytes, blood urea nitrogen, creatinine	Viral studies Lactate dehydrogenase Coagulation studies Complement studies von Willebrand factor analysis		

[a] Stool culture is defined as an appropriate test for bacterial enteric pathogens, including *E coli* O157:H7 (ie, sorbitol MacConkey agar plating) as well as a test to detect non-O157:H7 EHEC, per Centers of Disease Control recommendations. The toxin test should not be used as a screen, with the plating performed only on positives.[27]

Initial Management

Regardless of when in the course of an EHEC infection a patient enters your care, it is important to support that patient's intravascular perfusion. This support means intravenous volume expansion, in an attempt to provide nephroprotection. Patients can appear deceptively well hydrated and have on standard tests no evidence of microangiopathy, yet be undergoing a massive prothrombotic process manifest as increased circulating D-dimers, plasminogen activator inhibitor type 1 (PAI-1) activity, PAI-1/tissue plasminogen activator antigen complexes,[6] and sheared von Willebrand factor multimers.[7]

Nephroprotection is not conferred by oral rehydration; it must be administered by intravenous infusion of isotonic crystalloid. The details of fluid therapy are provided in a recent review by Holtz and colleagues,[33] modified slightly in our review of phase 3 of EHEC infection (see later discussion).

Antibiotics should not be given to patients who are, or who might be, infected with E coli O157:H7, while they are still at risk of developing HUS. In multiple case-cohort studies, antibiotics have shown either no beneficial effect on the course of this infection or a greater risk of developing HUS (**Table 5**).

PHASE-SPECIFIC CONSIDERATIONS
Phase 1: the Patient is in the Incubation Period

Profile of patients
People at risk of being infected with E coli O157:H7, but yet to have diarrhea. Occasionally, in outbreaks and in households in which a patient is diagnosed as being infected with E coli O157:H7, the question arises as to the risk of becoming symptomatic, and to the advisability of prescribing antibiotics to avert a symptomatic case.

Diagnostic considerations
We generally do not perform stool cultures before diarrhea.

Interventions
In view of considerable data showing the adverse effects of antibiotics in terms of increasing the risk of HUS (discussed later), and in the absence of any data showing benefit in this situation, we discourage such interventions. Some data from infected adults suggest that presymptomatic antibiotic use in E coli O157:H7 infections is associated with a worse outcome.[39,40]

Comment
It is reassuring that the attack rate among people exposed to contaminated food products is low: only about 1 in 300 Washingtonians who consumed contaminated hamburger in the massive 1993 outbreak attributable to poorly cooked product at a fast food restaurant chain developed symptomatic infection.[41] However, one should keep in mind that hamburger and other foods may not be homogenously contaminated and proper cooking and preparation of food is important.

Phase 2: the Patient has Nonbloody Diarrhea

Patients who present in phase 2 fit 1 of 2 profiles:

Profile A
Symptomatic contacts of patients with known or possible E coli O157:H7 infection.

Table 5
Summary of antibiotic experience in multiple case control studies of children

Study	Year Performed, Setting	Ages of Patients	Predominant Antibiotics Given	HUS Rate in Group Receiving Antibiotics	HUS Rate in Group not Receiving Antibiotics
Carter et al,[39] 1987	1985 Outbreak analysis, Canada	16–67 y	Amoxicillin, tetracycline	Does not specify*	Does not specify*
Pavia et al,[99] 1990	1988 Outbreak, case control study, Utah	6–39 y	Predominantly trimethoprim-sulfamethoxazole	5/8 (63%)	0/7 (0%)
Proulx et al,[98] 1992	1989–1990 Randomized controlled trial, Canada, antibiotics administered late in illness	5 y ± 4 y (average)	Trimethoprim-sulfamethoxazole (1)	2/22 (8%)	4/25 (16%)
Bell et al,[82] 1997	1993 Outbreak, retrospective cohort, Washington State	<16 y	Trimethoprim-sulfamethoxazole (62%), ampicillin or amoxicillin (26%), cephalosporins (12%), metronidazole (8%)	8/50 (16%)	28/218 (13%)

Study	Years, study type	Age	Antibiotic		
Wong et al,[38] 2000	1997–1999 Multistrain, prospective cohort study, 4 states	<10 y	Trimethoprim-sulfamethoxazole (2/5), β-lactams (3/5)	5/9 (56%)	5/62 (8%)
Dundas et al,[40] 2001	1996 Outbreak, retrospective cohort study, Scotland	18 m to 94 y Mean = 63 y	Ciprofloxacin	8/14 (57%) treated with antibiotics in the 4 wk before illness onset 7/15 (47%) treated with antibiotics within 4 d after illness onset	26/104 (25%)
Wong et al,[34] 2012	1997–2006 Multistrain, prospective cohort study, 5 states	<10 y	Trimethoprim-sulfamethoxazole (9/25), β-lactams (9/25), metronidazole (3/25), azithromycin (4/25)	9/25 (36%)	27/234 (12%)
Smith et al,[100] 2012	1996–2002 Multistrain, age-matched, case-case comparison	<20 y	β-lactams (22% case 4% controls), sulfonamides (14% case 24% control), metronidazole (6% case 2% control)	27/63 (43%)	38/125 (30%)

* Rate of HUS not provided, but risk ratios were, and were 8.5 (95% CI 2.7–27.5), in favor of antibiotics associated with HUS development.

Diagnostic considerations

We recommend that such patients be evaluated in the same manner as those who present in phase 3 (see later discussion).

Interventions

If and when the culture is positive, the interventions described in phase 3 should be started (if patient has not been receiving this treatment) or continued (if intravenous hydration was started on initial evaluation).

Comments

The earlier intravenous volume expansion is commenced, the better the outcome.[17,35] It is not appropriate to await bloody diarrhea or results of a stool culture if a contact of a patient infected with E coli O157:H7 has acute diarrhea, because a valuable opportunity to provide volume expansion is lost.

Profile B

Patients with nonbloody diarrhea who present without knowledge of other patients being infected. There is usually considerable abdominal pain.

Diagnostic considerations

It is difficult to recommend a uniform diagnostic and therapeutic approach to patients with nonbloody diarrhea, if there is no reason to suspect an EHEC infection. Indications for stool culture to detect patients who are infected with bacterial enteric pathogens are difficult to formulate, but provider judgment is reasonably predictive in a pediatric emergency department setting.[33] The site of presentation is also a potential factor to consider: in the past decade, we have noticed that at least in childhood, infected patients almost always present to emergency facilities, so short of a blanket stool culture policy in these settings for all patients with diarrhea, it is difficult to rapidly identify such at-risk individuals.

Interventions

We have observed that severe pain is the retrospective justification of admission in these cases, and we would not hesitate to use intravenous isotonic crystalloid in such patients to provide volume expansion, before the infecting organism has been identified. There is literature in support of the use of isotonic intravenous fluids in hospitalized children with gastroenteritis.[42,43]

If the laboratory reports presumptive E coli O157:H7, intravenous volume expansion should be commenced as recommended later (phase 3), if it is not already under way.

Comments

The severity of illness in children infected with E coli O157:H7 whose diarrhea is not bloody is often underestimated, and these patients' stools might not undergo microbiological analysis. The subset who develop HUS might be at added risk of worse outcome because without bloody diarrhea or a positive stool culture, the provider is not aware that intravenous volume expansion is warranted.[35]

Phase 3: the Patient has Bloody Diarrhea

Profile

Patients with painful diarrhea that becomes bloody after 1 to 3 days of nonbloody diarrhea. Such patients usually present to emergency facilities. They are usually afebrile at first medical evaluation, their pain is worse immediately before, during, or after defecation, and abdominal tenderness is usually noted on examination.

Comments

About 80% of patients infected with culture-proven *E coli* O157:H7 have bloody diarrhea.[6,34,38] For patients infected with non-O157:H7 EHEC, this percentage is lower.[14,32] We have written extensively about presentations of patients with acute bloody diarrhea, and summarized our approach in a recent publication.[33] Because of space considerations, we refer readers to this review of the topic. Our recommendations remain unchanged, except that we now also encourage blood counts every 12 hours for the first several days of hospitalization, until there is evidence of therapeutic hemodilution (0.5 g/dL/12 h is our goal), or the platelet count is increasing (see **Table 4** in Ref.[33]). The justification for aggressive use of intravenous fluids is based on emerging data that if HUS ensues, early-in-illness volume expansion is nephroprotective,[17,35] and absolute or relative hemoconcentration in early HUS is associated with worse outcomes.[44–46]

Phase 4: the Patient has HUS

Profile

The patient on presentation has met the case definition of HUS. This definition consists of thrombocytopenia (platelet count <150,000/mm³), anemia (hematocrit level <30%), and renal insufficiency (creatinine level > upper limit of normal for age). At this point, *E coli* O157:H7 might or might not have been isolated, and the patient is still urinating. The trend in the creatinine is not yet known.

Diagnostic considerations

If the culture is pending at another facility, a repeat culture is probably advisable. If a culture has not been obtained, it is important to obtain one, because this pathogen is often cleared by this point in illness.[10] We encourage a rectal swab culture on admission, rather than waiting for a specimen to be produced. If the patient is prediagnosed, there is no major imperative to make a microbiological diagnosis. However, it is helpful to obtain 1 or more subsequent cultures during the hospitalization, so as to remove contact precautions if they are negative and facilitate return to settings in which transmission might occur, such as day care. We do not recommend seeking rare causes of thrombotic microangiopathy in children or adults if the story is classic (bloody diarrhea), or the stool yields an EHEC.

Intervention

If patients are still urinating, we continue intravenous volume expansion, although in these situations, the risk of fluid overload is greater than earlier in illness (ie, before azotemia develops). Assiduous monitoring is critical. Except in rare situations (ie, symptomatic cardiopulmonary overload), we do not use diuretics in this phase.

Comments

Oligoanuric HUS is worse than nonoligoanuric HUS.[44,47–60] This situation provides the rationale for intravenous volume expansion, even if the creatinine level is already increased (if the patient is still urinating and does not have cardiopulmonary overload), but volume expansion in this setting must be accompanied by careful clinical monitoring. If oligoanuria does not ensue by day 10 of illness (not day 10 of HUS), patients are highly likely to continue to urinate during their episode of HUS.[17]

Phase 5: Profile: a Patient has Oligoanuric HUS

Diagnostic considerations

As described in phase 4.

Interventions

If HUS is oligoanuric, dialysis is the mainstay of therapy. There is no role for anti-complement treatment (see later discussion) or therapeutic plasma exchange, because such interventions are not justified by current data. For plasma therapies, the microangiopathy-driven shearing of von Willebrand factor during HUS suggests that there might be some risk to giving plasma that would contain larger forms of this molecule, which are presumably more thrombogenic than native multimers in infected patients.[7,61] EHEC-related HUS is not caused by the same processes as thrombotic thrombocytopenic purpura, for which plasma exchange is warranted.

Comment

The detailed description of the management of EHEC-related HUS is beyond the scope of this article. However, various non-EHEC infections that can complicate EHEC-related HUS are described in the next section.

INFECTIOUS COMPLICATIONS DURING HUS, INDEPENDENT OF EHEC
Use of Antibiotics in Patients Who Already Have HUS

We are often asked if antibiotics are contraindicated after HUS develops. If oligoanuric HUS is already established, there is no contraindication to using antibiotics, if the indications for the antibiotics are appropriate. However, if anuria has not yet ensued, it is theoretically possible that a second wave of toxemia from viable EHEC in the gut could add injury to the vasculature. As always, the use of antibiotics in severely ill patients should be balanced against their general risk, irrespective of the HUS. In the 2011 E coli O104:H4 outbreak, 1 analysis suggested an association between using antibiotics during HUS and a milder course of HUS.[62] This is an observation worthy of validation in randomized controlled studies.

Infections Related to Peritoneal Dialysis

Patients undergoing peritoneal dialysis for HUS are at risk for infectious complications. In 2 retrospective, single-center studies in which peritoneal dialysis was used almost exclusively, the rates of peritonitis were 20% and 24%.[63,64] The use of intravenous prophylactic antibiotics at time of surgical placement or revision is standard,[65] but prophylactic intraperitoneal antibiotics are not recommended. Additional measures for preventing dialysis-associated peritonitis include minimizing manipulation of the catheter and anchoring the catheter using adhesive tape and nonocclusive dressing rather than placing a surgical stitch at the exit site. All exit site dressing changes should be performed in a sterile fashion by specially trained personnel. Hydrogen peroxide and povidone iodine solutions should not be used; chlorhexidine or normal saline are appropriate, and the application of topical antibiotics to the catheter exit site can be considered.[65]

Risk factors for HUS-related peritonitis are fluid leak and catheter manipulation, specifically surgical revisions.[63,64] Leakage from the incision site is minimized by initiating dialysis with low volumes. Avoidance of catheter manipulation can be accomplished by delaying use (rarely possible in acute renal failure) and prescribing continuous dialysis, thereby avoiding multiple connections and disconnections.

Peritonitis is more common in children than adults,[65] and the incidence of peritonitis during dialysis for HUS is higher than for chronic peritoneal dialysis.[66] The diagnosis of peritonitis is made by fever and a turbid effluent, and, variably, abdominal pain, chills, rigors, anorexia, vomiting, or abdominal distension. Delayed diagnosis of peritonitis can present as septic shock. Because HUS has clinical features similar to dialysis-associated peritonitis, a high index of suspicion for infection must be maintained.

Clear fluid does not exclude the diagnosis of peritonitis, and if the diagnosis is considered, peritoneal fluid should be sent for cell count, differential count, Gram stain, and culture.

Ideally, peritoneal fluid/dialysate that has dwelled in the abdominal cavity for at least 1 hour should be sent for analysis if infection is suspected. If the white blood cell count in the uncentrifuged fluid is greater than 100/mm³, and more than 50% of the cells are neutrophils, a diagnosis of peritonitis should be considered, and empirical antibiotics should be started.[65] If the 1-hour dwell time cannot be accomplished, then the presence of 50% neutrophils or greater, even if the total cell count is less than 100/mm³, suggests peritonitis. A Gram stain may guide empirical therapy if positive, but its sensitivity is low.[65] One might think that HUS peritonitis is caused by enteric organisms, but most peritoneal infections are from streptococci and staphylococci, again highlighting the importance of sterile technique in catheter care. If multiple organisms are identified in culture, a perforated viscus should be considered.

Treatment of Dialysis-Associated Peritonitis

Intraperitoneal instillation of antibiotics is the preferred route of administration for dialysis-associated peritonitis. Most antibiotics are absorbed from the peritoneum and achieve therapeutic levels that can be used to confirm adequate dosing. Current guidelines recommend empirical monotherapy with intraperitoneal cefepime. Intraperitoneal vancomycin should be added if the patient is colonized with methicillin-resistant *Staphylococcus aureus* (MRSA), or if center-specific resistance rates to MRSA are greater than 10%.[65]

Clostridium difficile Infections

Clostridium difficile infections are occasionally diagnosed before or during HUS,[67] or on presentation. Many children carry *C difficile* without symptoms,[1] so we do not respond to a positive result early in illness before we know the results of a stool culture, or during HUS unless we are convinced that colonic symptoms are truly caused by *C difficile* colitis (this would be unusual).

The Empirical Use of Eculizumab

During the 2011 *E coli* O104:H4 outbreak, many clinicians used eculizumab to treat HUS, based on a letter to the *New England Journal of Medicine* attributing sudden recoveries to this monoclonal antibody to C5 in 3 children with HUS.[68] However, these 3 patients were already showing improvement in their serum lactate dehydrogenase concentrations or platelet count. Therefore, we do not believe that the data provided in this letter showed sufficient evidence of efficacy to recommend its use, especially because patients with HUS often make sudden and spontaneous improvement 1 to 2 weeks after HUS is established. Moreover, 3 analyses of the use of eculizumab in the O104:H4 outbreak concluded that there was no benefit in the infected adults.[62,69,70] In the unlikely event that eculizumab use can be justified, appropriate antimeningococcal precautions should be instituted.

Postinfectious Decolonization

An analysis from the 2011 *E coli* O111:H4 outbreak suggested that azithromycin hastens decolonization after HUS.[71] We do not think that late-in-illness decolonization has much merit, because there are few data that postsymptomatic excretion is an important source of human infection. Decolonization brings no medical benefit to the host at this point in illness,[72] and there might be some risk, because of the association between use of azithromycin and sudden death.[73,74] The observation that azithromycin might reduce complications during HUS[62] should not be extrapolated to individuals presenting early in illness, because azithromycin does not unequivocally prevent the development of HUS,[34] although the number of cases treated in illness phase 2 or 3 with azithromycin who have been reported so far is small.

SUMMARY

EHEC infections remain challenging to clinicians. Good management begins at the many different points of presentation, and is critically dependent on accurate and rapid microbiology. There are no specific treatments for such illnesses, but admission to hospital, intravenous volume expansion, and avoidance of antibiotics are associated with averting HUS, and, in particular, oligoanuric HUS.

ACKNOWLEDGMENTS

The authors wish to thank Ms Ariana Jasarevic for expert assistance with article preparation.

REFERENCES

1. Denno DM, Shaikh N, Stapp JR, et al. Diarrhea etiology in a pediatric emergency department: a case control study. Clin Infect Dis 2012;55(7):897–904.
2. Watanabe H, Terajima J, Izumiya H, et al. Molecular analysis of enterohemorrhagic Escherichia coli isolates in Japan and its application to epidemiological investigation. Pediatr Int 1999;41(2):202–8.
3. Stephan R, Untermann F. Virulence factors and phenotypical traits of verotoxin-producing Escherichia coli strains isolated from asymptomatic human carriers. J Clin Microbiol 1999;37(5):1570–2.
4. Tarr PI, Gordon CA, Chandler WL. Shiga-toxin-producing Escherichia coli and haemolytic uraemic syndrome. Lancet 2005;365(9464):1073–86.
5. Lopez EL, Contrini MM, Glatstein E, et al. An epidemiologic surveillance of Shiga-like toxin-producing Escherichia coli infection in Argentinean children: risk factors and serum Shiga-like toxin 2 values. Pediatr Infect Dis J 2012;31(1):20–4.
6. Chandler WL, Jelacic S, Boster DR, et al. Prothrombotic coagulation abnormalities preceding the hemolytic-uremic syndrome. N Engl J Med 2002;346(1): 23–32.
7. Tsai HM, Chandler WL, Sarode R, et al. Von Willebrand factor and von Willebrand factor-cleaving metalloprotease activity in Escherichia coli O157:H7-associated hemolytic uremic syndrome. Pediatr Res 2001;49(5):653–9.
8. Bitzan M, Mellmann A, Karch H, et al. Shigatec: A phase II study evaluating shigamabs in STEC-infected children. Zoonoses and Public Health 2012; 59(Suppl 1):2–18.
9. Neill MA, Tarr PI, Clausen CR, et al. Escherichia coli O157:H7 as the predominant pathogen associated with the hemolytic uremic syndrome: a prospective study in the Pacific Northwest. Pediatrics 1987;80(1):37–40.
10. Tarr PI, Neill MA, Clausen CR, et al. Escherichia coli O157:H7 and the hemolytic uremic syndrome: importance of early cultures in establishing the etiology. J Infect Dis 1990;162(2):553–6.
11. Rowe PC, Orrbine E, Lior H, et al. Risk of hemolytic uremic syndrome after sporadic Escherichia coli O157:H7 infection: results of a Canadian collaborative study. Investigators of the Canadian Pediatric Kidney Disease Research Center. J Pediatr 1998;132(5):777–82.

12. Miceli S, Jure MA, de Saab OA, et al. A clinical and bacteriological study of children suffering from haemolytic uraemic syndrome in Tucuman, Argentina. Jpn J Infect Dis 1999;52(2):33–7.

13. Banatvala N, Griffin PM, Greene KD, et al. The United States National Prospective Hemolytic Uremic Syndrome Study: microbiologic, serologic, clinical, and epidemiologic findings. J Infect Dis 2001;183(7):1063–70.

14. Klein EJ, Stapp JR, Clausen CR, et al. Shiga toxin-producing *Escherichia coli* in children with diarrhea: a prospective point-of-care study. J Pediatr 2002;141(2):172–7.

15. Rivas M, Miliwebsky E, Chinen I, et al. Characterization and epidemiologic subtyping of Shiga toxin-producing *Escherichia coli* strains isolated from hemolytic uremic syndrome and diarrhea cases in Argentina. Foodborne Pathog Dis 2006;3(1):88–96.

16. Pollock KG, Young D, Beattie TJ, et al. Clinical surveillance of thrombotic microangiopathies in Scotland, 2003-2005. Epidemiol Infect 2008;136(1):115–21.

17. Hickey CA, Beattie TJ, Cowieson J, et al. Early volume expansion during diarrhea and relative nephroprotection during subsequent hemolytic uremic syndrome. Arch Pediatr Adolesc Med 2011;165(10):884–9.

18. Hadler JL, Clogher P, Hurd S, et al. Ten-year trends and risk factors for non-O157 Shiga toxin-producing *Escherichia coli* found through Shiga toxin testing, Connecticut, 2000-2009. Clin Infect Dis 2011;53(3):269–76.

19. Mody RK, Luna-Gierke RE, Jones TF, et al. Infections in pediatric postdiarrheal hemolytic uremic syndrome: factors associated with identifying Shiga toxin-producing *Escherichia coli*. Arch Pediatr Adolesc Med 2012;166(10):902–9.

20. Leopold SR, Magrini V, Holt NJ, et al. A precise reconstruction of the emergence and constrained radiations of *Escherichia coli* O157 portrayed by backbone concatenomic analysis. Proc Natl Acad Sci U S A 2009;106(21):8713–8.

21. Chapman PA, Siddons CA. A comparison of immunomagnetic separation and direct culture for the isolation of verocytotoxin-producing *Escherichia coli* O157 from cases of bloody diarrhoea, non-bloody diarrhoea and asymptomatic contacts. J Med Microbiol 1996;44(4):267–71.

22. Fey PD, Wickert RS, Rupp ME, et al. Prevalence of non-O157:H7 Shiga toxin-producing *Escherichia coli* in diarrheal stool samples from Nebraska. Emerg Infect Dis 2000;6(5):530–3.

23. Carroll KC, Adamson K, Korgenski K, et al. Comparison of a commercial reversed passive latex agglutination assay to an enzyme immunoassay for the detection of Shiga toxin-producing *Escherichia coli*. Eur J Clin Microbiol Infect Dis 2003;22(11):689–92.

24. Manning SD, Madera RT, Schneider W, et al. Surveillance for Shiga toxin-producing *Escherichia coli*, Michigan, 2001-2005. Emerg Infect Dis 2007;13(2):318–21.

25. Teel LD, Daly JA, Jerris RC, et al. Rapid detection of Shiga toxin-producing *Escherichia coli* by optical immunoassay. J Clin Microbiol 2007;45(10):3377–80.

26. Park CH, Kim HJ, Hixon DL, et al. Evaluation of the duopath verotoxin test for detection of Shiga toxins in cultures of human stools. J Clin Microbiol 2003;41(6):2650–3.

27. Gould LH, Bopp C, Strockbine N, et al. Recommendations for diagnosis of Shiga toxin–producing *Escherichia coli* infections by clinical laboratories. MMWR Recomm Rep 2009;58(RR-12):1–14.

28. Bielaszewska M, Mellmann A, Zhang W, et al. Characterisation of the *Escherichia coli* strain associated with an outbreak of haemolytic uraemic syndrome in Germany, 2011: a microbiological study. Lancet Infect Dis 2011;11(9): 671–6.

29. Buchholz U, Bernard H, Werber D, et al. German outbreak of *Escherichia coli* o104:H4 associated with sprouts. N Engl J Med 2011;365(19):1763–70.

30. Klein EJ, Boster DR, Stapp JR, et al. Diarrhea etiology in a children's hospital emergency department: a prospective cohort study. Clin Infect Dis 2006; 43(7):807–13.

31. Bokete TN, O'Callahan CM, Clausen CR, et al. Shiga-like toxin-producing *Escherichia coli* in Seattle children: a prospective study. Gastroenterology 1993; 105(6):1724–31.

32. Jelacic JK, Damrow T, Chen GS, et al. Shiga toxin-producing *Escherichia coli* in Montana: bacterial genotypes and clinical profiles. J Infect Dis 2003;188(5): 719–29.

33. Holtz LR, Neill MA, Tarr PI. Acute bloody diarrhea: a medical emergency for patients of all ages. Gastroenterology 2009;136(6):1887–98.

34. Wong CS, Mooney JC, Brandt JR, et al. Risk factors for the hemolytic uremic syndrome in children infected with *Escherichia coli* O157:H7: a multivariable analysis. Clin Infect Dis 2012;55(1):33–41.

35. Ake JA, Jelacic S, Ciol MA, et al. Relative nephroprotection during *Escherichia coli* O157:H7 infections: association with intravenous volume expansion. Pediatrics 2005;115(6):e673–80.

36. Smith JM, Jones F, Ciol MA, et al. Platelet-activating factor and *Escherichia coli* O157:H7 infections. Pediatr Nephrol 2002;17(12):1047–52.

37. Cornick NA, Jelacic S, Ciol MA, et al. *Escherichia coli* O157:H7 infections: discordance between filterable fecal Shiga toxin and disease outcome. J Infect Dis 2002;186(1):57–63.

38. Wong CS, Jelacic S, Habeeb RL, et al. The risk of the hemolytic-uremic syndrome after antibiotic treatment of *Escherichia coli* O157:H7 infections. N Engl J Med 2000;342(26):1930–6.

39. Carter AO, Borczyk AA, Carlson JA, et al. A severe outbreak of *Escherichia coli* O157:H7–associated hemorrhagic colitis in a nursing home. N Engl J Med 1987; 317(24):1496–500.

40. Dundas S, Todd WT, Stewart AI, et al. The Central Scotland *Escherichia coli* O157:H7 outbreak: risk factors for the hemolytic uremic syndrome and death among hospitalized patients. Clin Infect Dis 2001;33(7):923–31.

41. Bell BP, Goldoft M, Griffin PM, et al. A multistate outbreak of *Escherichia coli* O157:H7-associated bloody diarrhea and hemolytic uremic syndrome from hamburgers. The Washington experience. JAMA 1994;272(17):1349–53.

42. Moritz ML, Ayus JC. Improving intravenous fluid therapy in children with gastroenteritis. Pediatr Nephrol 2010;25(8):1383–4.

43. Hanna M, Saberi MS. Incidence of hyponatremia in children with gastroenteritis treated with hypotonic intravenous fluids. Pediatr Nephrol 2010;25(8):1471–5.

44. Balestracci A, Martin SM, Toledo I, et al. Dehydration at admission increased the need for dialysis in hemolytic uremic syndrome children. Pediatr Nephrol 2012; 27(8):1407–10.

45. Coad NA, Marshall T, Rowe B, et al. Changes in the postenteropathic form of the hemolytic uremic syndrome in children. Clin Nephrol 1991;35(1):10–6.

46. Oakes RS, Siegler RL, McReynolds MA, et al. Predictors of fatality in postdiarrheal hemolytic uremic syndrome. Pediatrics 2006;117(5):1656–62.

47. Gianantonio CA, Vitacco M, Mendilaharzu F, et al. The hemolytic-uremic syndrome. Nephron 1973;11(2):174–92.
48. Oakes RS, Kirkham JK, Nelson RD, et al. Duration of oliguria and anuria as predictors of chronic renal-related sequelae in post-diarrheal hemolytic uremic syndrome. Pediatr Nephrol 2008;23(8):1303–8.
49. Loirat C. Post-diarrhea hemolytic-uremic syndrome: clinical aspects. Arch Pediatr 2001;8(Suppl 4):776s–84s [in French].
50. Siegler RL, Pavia AT, Christofferson RD, et al. A 20-year population-based study of postdiarrheal hemolytic uremic syndrome in Utah. Pediatrics 1994;94(1):35–40.
51. Siegler RL, Milligan MK, Burningham TH, et al. Long-term outcome and prognostic indicators in the hemolytic-uremic syndrome. J Pediatr 1991;118(2): 195–200.
52. Garg AX, Suri RS, Barrowman N, et al. Long-term renal prognosis of diarrhea-associated hemolytic uremic syndrome: a systematic review, meta-analysis, and meta-regression. JAMA 2003;290(10):1360–70.
53. Tonshoff B, Sammet A, Sanden I, et al. Outcome and prognostic determinants in the hemolytic uremic syndrome of children. Nephron 1994;68(1):63–70.
54. Huseman D, Gellermann J, Vollmer I, et al. Long-term prognosis of hemolytic uremic syndrome and effective renal plasma flow. Pediatr Nephrol 1999;13(8): 672–7.
55. Mizusawa Y, Pitcher LA, Burke JR, et al. Survey of haemolytic-uraemic syndrome in Queensland 1979-1995. Med J Aust 1996;165(4):188–91.
56. Spizzirri FD, Rahman RC, Bibiloni N, et al. Childhood hemolytic uremic syndrome in Argentina: long-term follow-up and prognostic features. Pediatr Nephrol 1997;11(2):156–60.
57. Gianantonio CA, Vitacco M, Mendilaharzu F, et al. The hemolytic-uremic syndrome. Renal status of 76 patients at long-term follow-up. J Pediatr 1968; 72(6):757–65.
58. Dolislager D, Tune B. The hemolytic-uremic syndrome: spectrum of severity and significance of prodrome. Am J Dis Child 1978;132(1):55–8.
59. de Jong MC, Monnens LA. Recurrent haemolytic uraemic syndrome. Padiatr Padol 1976;11(3):521–7.
60. Mencia Bartolome S, Martinez de Azagra A, de Vicente Aymat A, et al. Uremic hemolytic syndrome. Analysis of 43 cases. An Esp Pediatr 1999;50(5):467–70 [in Spanish].
61. Tarr PI. Shiga toxin-associated hemolytic uremic syndrome and thrombotic thrombocytopenic purpura: distinct mechanisms of pathogenesis. Kidney Int Suppl 2009;112:S29–32.
62. Menne J, Nitschke M, Stingele R, et al. Validation of treatment strategies for enterohaemorrhagic Escherichia coli O104:H4 induced haemolytic uraemic syndrome: case-control study. BMJ 2012;345:e4565.
63. Grisaru S, Morgunov MA, Samuel SM, et al. Acute renal replacement therapy in children with diarrhea-associated hemolytic uremic syndrome: a single center 16 years of experience. Int J Nephrol 2011;2011:930539.
64. Adragna M, Balestracci A, Garcia Chervo L, et al. Acute dialysis-associated peritonitis in children with D+ hemolytic uremic syndrome. Pediatr Nephrol 2012;27(4):637–42.
65. Warady BA, Bakkaloglu S, Newland J, et al. Consensus guidelines for the prevention and treatment of catheter-related infections and peritonitis in pediatric patients receiving peritoneal dialysis: 2012 update. Perit Dial Int 2012; 32(Suppl 2):S32–86.

66. Chadha V, Schaefer FS, Warady BA. Dialysis-associated peritonitis in children. Pediatr Nephrol 2010;25(3):425–40.
67. Burgner DP, Rfidah H, Beattie TJ, et al. *Clostridium difficile* after haemolytic uraemic syndrome. Arch Dis Child 1993;69(2):239–40.
68. Lapeyraque AL, Malina M, Fremeaux-Bacchi V, et al. Eculizumab in severe Shiga-toxin-associated HUS. N Engl J Med 2011;364(26):2561–3.
69. Kielstein JT, Beutel G, Fleig S, et al. Best supportive care and therapeutic plasma exchange with or without eculizumab in Shiga-toxin-producing *E. coli* O104:H4 induced haemolytic-uraemic syndrome: an analysis of the German STEC-HUS registry. Nephrol Dial Transplant 2012;27(10):3807–15.
70. Samuelsson O, Follin P, Rundgren M, et al. HUS-epidemin sommaren 2011 var allvarlig. Tyska och svenska erfarenheter av EHEC-utbrottet [The HUS epidemic in the summer of 2011 was severe. German and Swedish experiences of the EHEC outbreak]. Läkartidningen 2012;109(25):1230–4 [in Swedish].
71. Nitschke M, Sayk F, Hartel C, et al. Association between azithromycin therapy and duration of bacterial shedding among patients with Shiga toxin-producing enteroaggregative *Escherichia coli* O104:H4. JAMA 2012;307(10): 1046–52.
72. Seifert ME, Tarr PI. Therapy: azithromycin and decolonization after HUS. Nat Rev Nephrol 2012;8(6):317–8.
73. Ray WA, Murray KT, Hall K, et al. Azithromycin and the risk of cardiovascular death. N Engl J Med 2012;366(20):1881–90.
74. Seifert ME, Tarr PI. Azithromycin decolonization of STEC–a new risk emerges. Nat Rev Nephrol 2012;8(7):429.
75. Konowalchuk J, Speirs JI, Stavric S. Vero response to a cytotoxin of *Escherichia coli*. Infect Immun 1977;18(3):775–9.
76. Calderwood S, Acheson DW, Keusch G, et al. Proposed new nomenclature for Shiga-like toxin (verotoxin) family. ASM News 1996;62:118–9.
77. Calderwood SB, Auclair F, Donohue-Rolfe A, et al. Nucleotide sequence of the Shiga-like toxin genes of *Escherichia coli*. Proc Natl Acad Sci U S A 1987; 84(13):4364–8.
78. Levine MM. *Escherichia coli* that cause diarrhea: enterotoxigenic, enteropathogenic, enteroinvasive, enterohemorrhagic, and enteroadherent. J Infect Dis 1987;155(3):377–89.
79. Jarvis KG, Giron JA, Jerse AE, et al. Enteropathogenic *Escherichia coli* contains a putative type III secretion system necessary for the export of proteins involved in attaching and effacing lesion formation. Proc Natl Acad Sci U S A 1995; 92(17):7996–8000.
80. Tango T. Maximum likelihood estimation of date of infection in an outbreak of diarrhea due to contaminated foods assuming lognormal distribution for the incubation period. Nihon Koshu Eisei Zasshi 1998;45(2):129–41 [in Japanese].
81. Ostroff SM, Kobayashi JM, Lewis JH. Infections with *Escherichia coli* O157:H7 in Washington state. The first year of statewide disease surveillance. JAMA 1989; 262(3):355–9.
82. Bell BP, Griffin PM, Lozano P, et al. Predictors of hemolytic uremic syndrome in children during a large outbreak of *Escherichia coli* O157:H7 infections. Pediatrics 1997;100(1):E12.
83. Ahn CK, Holt NJ, Tarr PI. Shiga-toxin producing *Escherichia coli* and the hemolytic uremic syndrome: what have we learned in the past 25 years? Adv Exp Med Biol 2009;634:1–17.

84. Rodrigue DC, Mast EE, Greene KD, et al. A university outbreak of *Escherichia coli* O157:H7 infections associated with roast beef and an unusually benign clinical course. J Infect Dis 1995;172(4):1122–5.

85. Brandt JR, Fouser LS, Watkins SL, et al. *Escherichia coli* O157:H7-associated hemolytic-uremic syndrome after ingestion of contaminated hamburgers. J Pediatr 1994;125(4):519–26.

86. Lewis SJ, Heaton KW. Stool form scale as a useful guide to intestinal transit time. Scand J Gastroenterol 1997;32(9):920–4.

87. Jelacic S, Wobbe CL, Boster DR, et al. ABO and P1 blood group antigen expression and stx genotype and outcome of childhood *Escherichia coli* O157:H7 infections. J Infect Dis 2002;185(2):214–9.

88. Thayu M, Chandler WL, Jelacic S, et al. Cardiac ischemia during hemolytic uremic syndrome. Pediatr Nephrol 2003;18(3):286–9.

89. Zimmerhackl LB, Rosales A, Hofer J, et al. Enterohemorrhagic *Escherichia coli* O26:H11-associated hemolytic uremic syndrome: bacteriology and clinical presentation. Semin Thromb Hemost 2010;36(6):586–93.

90. Gerber A, Karch H, Allerberger F, et al. Clinical course and the role of Shiga toxin-producing *Escherichia coli* infection in the hemolytic-uremic syndrome in pediatric patients, 1997-2000, in Germany and Austria: a prospective study. J Infect Dis 2002;186(4):493–500.

91. Bielaszewska M, Middendorf B, Kock R, et al. Shiga toxin-negative attaching and effacing *Escherichia coli*: distinct clinical associations with bacterial phylogeny and virulence traits and inferred in-host pathogen evolution. Clin Infect Dis 2008;47(2):208–17.

92. Bielaszewska M, Kock R, Friedrich AW, et al. Shiga toxin-mediated hemolytic uremic syndrome: time to change the diagnostic paradigm? PLoS One 2007; 2(10):e1024.

93. Friedrich AW, Zhang W, Bielaszewska M, et al. Prevalence, virulence profiles, and clinical significance of Shiga toxin-negative variants of enterohemorrhagic *Escherichia coli* O157 infection in humans. Clin Infect Dis 2007;45(1):39–45.

94. Bielaszewska M, Friedrich AW, Aldick T, et al. Shiga toxin activatable by intestinal mucus in *Escherichia coli* isolated from humans: predictor for a severe clinical outcome. Clin Infect Dis 2006;43(9):1160–7.

95. Sonntag AK, Prager R, Bielaszewska M, et al. Phenotypic and genotypic analyses of enterohemorrhagic *Escherichia coli* o145 strains from patients in Germany. J Clin Microbiol 2004;42(3):954–62.

96. Ikeda K, Ida O, Kimoto K, et al. Effect of early fosfomycin treatment on prevention of hemolytic uremic syndrome accompanying *Escherichia coli* O157:H7 infection. Clin Nephrol 1999;52(6):357–62.

97. Loos S, Ahlenstiel T, Kranz B, et al. An outbreak of Shiga toxin-producing *Escherichia coli* o104:H4 hemolytic uremic syndrome in Germany: presentation and short-term outcome in children. Clin Infect Dis 2012;55(6):753–9.

98. Proulx F, Turgeon JP, Delage G, et al. Randomized, controlled trial of antibiotic therapy for *Escherichia coli* O157:H7 enteritis. J Pediatr 1992;121(2):299–303.

99. Pavia AT, Nichols CR, Green DP, et al. Hemolytic-uremic syndrome during an outbreak of *Escherichia coli* O157:H7 infections in institutions for mentally retarded persons: clinical and epidemiologic observations. J Pediatr 1990;116(4):544–51.

100. Smith KE, Wilker PR, Reiter PL, et al. Antibiotic treatment of *Escherichia coli* O157 infection and the risk of hemolytic uremic syndrome, Minnesota. Pediatr Infect Dis J 2012;31(1):37–41.

Long-Term Consequences of Foodborne Infections

Michael B. Batz, MSc[a],*, Evan Henke, PhD[b],
Barbara Kowalcyk, PhD[c,d]

KEYWORDS

- Chronic bowel disorders • Autoimmune disorders • Neurologic dysfunction
- Renal failure

KEY POINTS

- Foodborne infections with *Campylobacter*, *Escherichia coli* O157:H7, *Listeria monocytogenes*, *Salmonella*, *Shigella*, *Toxoplasma gondii*, and other pathogens can result in long-term sequelae to numerous organ systems.
- Prominent sequelae of foodborne infection include irritable bowel syndrome, inflammatory bowel diseases, reactive arthritis, hemolytic-uremic syndrome, chronic kidney disease, Guillain-Barré Syndrome, neurologic disorders from acquired and congenital listeriosis and toxoplasmosis, and cognitive and developmental deficits due to severe acute illness or diarrheal malnutrition.
- Evidence-based patient management and estimates of burden of disease used in public health and food policy should incorporate established and quantified long-term outcomes.
- For many chronic sequelae, disease mechanisms and the etiologic role of specific pathogens need further elucidation, as do the relative risks of sequelae following infection.
- Well-designed, large-scale, long-running prospective studies that account for the complicated interactions of host, environment, and microorganism are critical to improving our understanding of the long-term consequences of foodborne infection.

INTRODUCTION

Foodborne pathogens are a significant cause of infectious disease, resulting in an estimated 48 million illnesses, 128,000 hospitalizations, and 3000 deaths annually in

Funding Sources: None.
Conflicts of Interest: None.
[a] Emerging Pathogens Institute, University of Florida, PO Box 100009, Gainesville, FL 32610, USA; [b] 3M Food Safety Department, 3M Corporation, 3M Center Building 275-05-W-05, St. Paul, MN 55144, USA; [c] Department of Food, Bioprocessing and Nutrition Sciences, North Carolina State University, 100 Schaub Hall, Campus Box 7624, Raleigh, NC 27695, USA; [d] Centre for Foodborne Illness Research & Prevention, North Carolina State University, 1017 Main Campus Drive, Suite 1500, Raleigh, NC 27606, USA
* Corresponding author.
E-mail address: mbatz@ufl.edu

Infect Dis Clin N Am 27 (2013) 599–616
http://dx.doi.org/10.1016/j.idc.2013.05.003
0891-5520/13/$ – see front matter © 2013 Elsevier Inc. All rights reserved.

id.theclinics.com

the United States.[1,2] In addition to these acute illnesses, however, many foodborne bacteria, viruses, and parasites can result in long-term sequelae to gastrointestinal, immune, nervous, respiratory, cardiovascular, endocrine, and hepatic systems. However, because these manifestations may not arise for weeks, months, or even years after infection, they are difficult to characterize and therefore too often neglected by clinicians and public health officials alike.

Considering the long-term consequences of foodborne infections is important for patient management and setting priorities for public health. The aforementioned incidence estimates from the Centers for Disease Control and Prevention (CDC) are invaluable for the latter, but provide only a limited picture, as they include only acute illnesses and do not include any accounting of latent, chronic, or congenital sequelae. Integrated approaches to estimating the burden of foodborne disease, on the other hand, such as those that estimate annual disability-adjusted life years (DALYs), quality-adjusted life years (QALYs), or economic costs, are better able to capture the full scope of symptoms, severities, and outcomes of foodborne disease.[3–7] These studies develop disease outcome trees that resemble the decision trees used in medical decision making; they characterize the likelihoods of major outcomes based on available evidence. When long-term sequelae are included in burden of disease studies, the impacts are significant. Over half of the estimated costs in the United States associated with *Campylobacter*, for example, are due to subsequent Guillain-Barré syndrome (GBS).[5] In Dutch estimates more inclusive of sequelae, chronic morbidity is responsible for 42% of the total disease burden of 14 major foodborne pathogens.[7]

Burden-of-disease studies and clinical guidelines both rely on evidence of the etiologic role of specific agents in specific long-term sequelae. These data, drawn from epidemiologic studies and clinical practice, range from convincing to anecdotal. For many long-term conditions, the disease mechanism and the relative risk associated with specific microbial causes require further elucidation. There are several challenges to establishing causality for postinfectious chronic conditions, including, but not limited to: (1) latency between infection and sequelae; (2) complicated disease mechanisms with environmental, host genetic, and microbial genetic factors; (3) the role of coinfection and acquired host characteristics; (4) technical barriers to detecting or isolating certain pathogens; (5) the lack of systematic data collection on long-term follow-up care; and (6) the lack of necessary prospective epidemiologic studies.[8–11]

This brief overview of long-term consequences of acute foodborne illness centers on the most prominent sequelae: irritable bowel syndrome (IBS), inflammatory bowel diseases (IBDs), reactive arthritis, GBS, neurologic disorders from acquired and congenital listeriosis and toxoplasmosis, hemolytic-uremic syndrome (HUS), and attendant systemic sequelae, as well as a few others. Pathogens include *Campylobacter*, *Escherichia coli* O157:H7, *Listeria monocytogenes*, *Salmonella*, *Shigella*, *Toxoplasma gondii*, and *Yersinia enterocolitica*, among others. **Table 1** presents the most prominent sequelae associated with major foodborne pathogens while **Table 2** lists sequelae for less common infections and intoxications. This review is neither comprehensive nor systematic, and reflects a body of scientific literature that often lacks consensus. The authors use best judgment, and characterize the strength of etiologic evidence where possible. References are limited and tend toward reviews, as length restrictions prevent a fuller account of relevant primary sources.

CHRONIC BOWEL AND GASTROINTESTINAL DYSFUNCTION

The symptoms of acute gastrointestinal illness are generally self-limiting, although persistent infection is common with foodborne parasites such as *Cryptosporidium*,

Cyclospora, and *Giardia* if left untreated.[12] Chronic, severe diarrhea lasting months or years has also been documented with *Salmonella, Campylobacter, Klebsiella, Enterobacter, Aeromonas*, and others.[8] *Clostridium difficile* can cause a chronic, relapsing colitis following antibiotic therapy; foodborne transmission of *C difficile* is hypothesized but unproven.[13] Persistent diarrhea is a particular concern for immunocompromised patients. Transplant recipients and patients with AIDS, leukemia, and other hematologic malignancies have higher risk for prolonged cryptosporidiosis, among other pathogens.[14] Foodborne pathogens have also been associated with functional gastrointestinal disorders (FGID) and IBD.

Irritable Bowel Syndrome

FGID are a range of chronic gastrointestinal syndromes of unknown etiology, including functional dyspepsia, functional constipation, and noncardiac chest pain.[15] The most common FGID is IBS, a broad-spectrum disorder characterized by abdominal discomfort and altered bowel habits that affects between 10% and 20% of Western populations.[16,17] Up to 33% of reported cases have a prior acute enteric infection, with *Salmonella, Campylobacter, Shigella*, and *E coli* O157:H7 the most commonly linked pathogens.[16–22] Other pathogens linked to postinfectious IBS (PI-IBS) include *Giardia, Trichinella*, and *Norovirus*, although these associations are not as well established.[16–18,21,22] The incidence of PI-IBS varies by pathogen, but reviews of prospective cohort studies and studies of sporadic cases place the relative risk following gastroenteritis centered around 15% with a range of 4% to 36%.[16,18,19,21,22] Risk of PI-IBS is higher in the first year, but can remain elevated for longer time periods. Up to 7 years following the 2000 Walkerton, Ontario, outbreak of *E coli* O157:H7 and *Campylobacter*, patients displayed a nearly 5-fold higher risk of IBS than controls (10.5%–2.5%, odds ratio 4.6, 95% confidence interval [CI] 1.63–13.33).[20]

Diagnosis of IBS is difficult, and misclassification bias often confounds attempts to characterize its associations and pathogenesis. It is hypothesized that exposure to an infectious agent alters the gut flora, increases intestinal permeability, and triggers an inappropriate immune response, modulated by environmental, genetic, microbiome, and psychosocial factors.[16,22] Identified risk factors include family history, age, gender, severity of infection, prior antibiotic use, smoking, education level, psychosocial factors (eg, stress, neuroses, and hypochondrias) and health care–seeking behaviors. Three candidate gene variants (TLR9, IL6, CDH1) that encode epithelial barrier function and innate immune response have been associated with increased risk of IBS following foodborne illness even after controlling for other clinical risk factors.[23] Conversely, a Dutch study identified an association between chronic intestinal disease and a single nucleotide polymorphism in the *IFNG* gene suggesting that preexisting IBS may instead predispose to gastroenteritis.[24] Foodborne pathogens such as *Salmonella, Campylobacter, Shigella*, and *E coli* O157:H7 have also been associated with postinfectious dyspepsia, although the literature is thinner.

Inflammatory Bowel Disease

Crohn disease (CD) and ulcerative colitis (UC) constitute the 2 major forms of IBD.[25–27] Although CD and UC are distinct diseases, they have overlapping diagnostic criteria and are both characterized by chronic, intermittent periods of abdominal pain, diarrhea, fever, and weight loss. Genetic risk factors are evident and environmental factors are suspected.[26,28] Several retrospective studies using national patient databases have found increased risk of IBD following infection with *Campylobacter, Salmonella, Yersinia, Shigella*, and certain pathogenic *E coli*, but results are inconsistent.[29,30]

Table 1
Reported long-term consequences for major foodborne pathogens in the United States[a]

Pathogen	Long-Term Consequences[b]
Campylobacter	Severe complications (sepsis, meningitis, carditis, endocarditis, hepatitis, cholecystitis, pancreatitis, abortion, and neonatal sepsis)[57,97,98]. Chronic diarrhea[8,12]. Guillain-Barré syndrome (inflammatory demyelinating polyradiculoneuropathy, muscle weakness, ascending paralysis, respiratory failure, permanent paraplegia, and walking difficulties)[42–45]; irritable bowel syndrome, dyspepsia[16–22]; inflammatory bowel disease[29–31]; reactive arthritis[33–41]; glomerulonephritis and other renal diseases[34,87]
Cryptosporidium	Chronic diarrhea[8,12]; reactive arthritis[36]; cognitive, developmental, and fitness deficits in small children[8,53]
Escherichia coli O157:H7[c]	Hemolytic-uremic syndrome, chronic kidney disease, and renal failure[79–84]; systemic sequelae (hypertension, cardiovascular disease, stroke, endothelial injury, pancreatitis, diabetes, splenic abscesses, gall stones, gastrointestinal disruption)[78,88,89,91–93]; CNS dysfunction following D+HUS (coma, seizures, hemiplegia, cortical blindness, and psychomotor retardation)[94]; irritable bowel syndrome, dyspepsia[16,18,20,22]; reactive arthritis[36,37,39,40]
Giardia lamblia	Chronic diarrhea[8,12]; irritable bowel syndrome[16,18]; inflammatory bowel disease[30]; reactive arthritis[36]; Severe malabsorption leading to cognitive, developmental, and fitness deficits in small children[8,53,97]; disaccharide intolerance (most frequently lactose)[97]
Listeria monocytogenes	Severe complications (encephalitis, meningitis, seizures, bacteremia, sepsis, endocarditis, pulmonary infection, septic arthritis)[57,58,97,98]; chronic neurologic manifestations (cranial nerve palsies, epilepsy, impaired executive and cognitive function, memory loss, aphasia, vision and hearing loss, attention deficits, depression)[60–63]; congenital acute conditions (miscarriage, preterm birth, meningitis, sepsis, respiratory distress, pneumonia)[60,63]; congenital neurologic sequelae (cerebral palsy, epilepsy, hearing loss, cognitive deficits, chronic lung disease)[60,63,64]
Norovirus	Irritable bowel syndrome[18,21]
Salmonella enterica (nontyphoidal)	Severe complications (bacteremia, sepsis, meningitis, septic arthritis, spondylitis, cholangitis, pneumonia, septic metastases, arterial infection, aortitis, aortic aneurysm, endocarditis, osteomyelitis and bone sequelae, splenic abscesses, pancreatitis)[29,57,97–99]; chronic diarrhea[8,12,57]; irritable bowel syndrome, dyspepsia[16–19,21,22]; inflammatory bowel disease[29–31]; reactive arthritis[33,36,38–41]; hemolytic uremic syndrome[85]

Shigella	Severe complications (intestinal perforation, toxic megacolon, bacteremia, sepsis)[57,97,98]; Hemolytic-uremic syndrome, chronic kidney disease, and renal failure[79-84]; systemic sequelae following D+HUS (hypertension, cardiovascular disease, endothelial injury, pancreatitis, diabetes, splenic abscesses, gallstones, gastrointestinal disruption)[78,88,89,91-93]; CNS dysfunction following D+HUS (coma, seizures, hemiplegia, cortical blindness, and psychomotor retardation)[94]; irritable bowel syndrome, dyspepsia[16-19,21,22]; inflammatory bowel disease[30]; reactive arthritis[33,36,38-41]
Toxoplasma gondii	Severe complications (meningitis, encephalitis, myocarditis)[56,65,66]; ocular manifestations due to acquired or congenital infection (chorioretinitis, vitritis, retinal vasculitis, optical nerve involvement)[65,66,70,71]; congenital toxoplasmosis (miscarriage, preterm birth, low birth weight, hydrocephalus, intercranial calcifications, chorioretinitis and other aforementioned ocular symptoms, hearing impairment, cognitive deficits, learning disabilities, epilepsy, palsies, growth retardation, developmental delays)[65-69]; psychiatric sequelae (schizophrenia, depression)[56,72-76]; behavior and physiology (morphologic and personality changes associated with increased testosterone or estrogen, reduced concentration, psychomotor deficits including slow reaction time)[73,74]; Alzheimer disease[75]
Vibrio vulnificus	Sepsis, secondary lesions with necrotizing fasciitis or vasculitis necessitating debridement or amputation, altered mental status, hypotension, pneumonia, endometritis[57,97,98]
Yersinia enterocolitica	Severe complications (appendicitis-like mesenteric lymphadenitis leading to unnecessary laparotomy, intestinal perforation, intussusception, toxic megacolon, mesenteric vein thrombosis, osteomyelitis, sinusitis, pneumonia, empyema, bacteremia, sepsis, endocarditis, meningitis, abscesses in kidney, lung, liver, or spleen)[57,97,98]; chronic diarrhea (enterocolitis)[98]; autoimmune thyroid disease (Graves disease: fatigue, irregular heartbeat, weight loss, goiters, proptosis)[34,46-49]; reactive arthritis[33,34,36,38,40,41]

Abbreviations: CNS, central nervous system; D+HUS, diarrhea-associated hemolytic-uremic syndrome.

[a] This table is not comprehensive, nor the result of systematic review. It reflects the authors' judgment on reported outcomes based on available literature, and reflects variable strength in etiologic evidence: for some, etiology is established while for others it is merely suspected. References include both those supporting and those disputing etiology.

[b] Long-term consequences include chronic sequelae, congenital effects, and severe acute conditions with long-term impacts on health.

[c] In addition, some non-O157 Shiga toxin–producing *E coli* cause HUS and O157-like sequelae.

Table 2
Reported long-term consequences of foodborne infections and intoxications uncommon in the United States[a]

Bacteria and Viruses	Outcomes[b]
Aeromonas	Chronic diarrhea[8,12]
Brucella	Endocarditis, epididymo-orchitis, arthralgias including reactive arthritis, myalgias, spondylitis, neurobrucellosis (meningitis, encephalitis, stroke, motor deficits, cranial nerve deficits, seizures, psychological disturbances), spontaneous abortion, enlarged spleen, enlarged liver[41,54]
Clostridium difficile[c]	Chronic colitis[12,100], reactive arthritis[33,36], inflammatory bowel disease[30], hemolytic-uremic syndrome[86]
Enterobacter	Chronic diarrhea[8]
Helicobacter pylori[c]	Chronic gastritis, gastric cancer[8,10,34]
Hepatitis A virus	Liver disease; chronic or relapsing infection may trigger an active, deteriorating hepatitis[8,101]
Klebsiella spp[c]	Chronic diarrhea[8], ankylosing spondylitis (chronic, inflammatory arthritis of the spine and sacroiliac joints; fusion of the spine)[8,102]
Salmonella Typhi and Salmonella Paratyphi	Chronic carriage may lead to gallbladder carcinoma[34]

Parasites	Outcomes[b]
Ascaris	Malnutrition, and resulting sequelae[55]
Cyclospora cayetanensis	Chronic diarrhea[12]
Diphyllobothrium latum	Megaloblastic anemia, vitamin B12 deficiency, subacute combined degeneration (degeneration of lateral and dorsal columns of spinal cord with peripheral nerve involvement, resulting in paresthesia, ataxia, memory loss, dementia, hallucinations, and personality change)[55,56]
Echinococcus	E granulosus: cystic echinococcosis (cysts in liver, lung, bone, brain, spleen, kidneys, or heart, with resulting organ diseases and symptoms)[55,56]; E multilocularis: alveolar echinococcosis (larval cystic infestation of liver, hematogenous metastases to lung and brain)[55,56]

Entamoeba histolytica	Amebiasis: colitis, chronic diarrhea[55]
Fasciola	Chronic bile duct inflammation[55]
Opisthorchis and *Chlonorchis sinensis*	Hepatobiliary disease, bile duct cancer, pancreatitis, cholangiocarcinoma (*C sinensis* only)[55,98]
Paragonimus	Chronic cough, hemoptysis[55]
Spirometra	Chronic sparganosis (CNS manifestations: chronic degeneration of cortex and white matter, ventricular dilation, vasculitis, hemorrhage, calcification; resulting in confusion, focal deficits, or grand-mal seizures)[55,56]
Taenia solium	Cysticercosis (myocardiopathy, vision loss, cystic nodules in skeletal muscle with intense inflammation and pain)[55,56]; neurocysticercosis (seizures, intracranial hypertension, hemiparesis, dysphasia, blindness, ependymitis, cognitive dysfunction, movement disorders, psychosocial sequelae)[55,56]
Toxocara	Visceral larval migrans (focal retinal inflammation, chronic neurologic symptoms such as absence attacks, convulsions, focal deficits, and paraplegia)[55,56]
Trichinella	Severe complications (cardiomyopathy, neurologic sequelae including seizures, polyneuritis, meningitis, and psychotic symptoms, respiratory distress, cyanosis, coma)[56,57,98], irritable bowel syndrome[18,21,22]
Natural Toxins	**Outcomes[b]**
Ciguatoxin	Chronic ciguatera: neurologic disorders lasting weeks, months, or years, including paresthesia of the extremities, temperature perception reversal, severe localized itching, dental pain, and arthralgias[103]
Mycotoxins	Primarily aflatoxins and fumonisins: chronic exposure may lead to cancers of the liver, kidney, and esophagus, CNS malfunctions, and growth impairment[104]

[a] This table is not comprehensive, nor the result of systematic review. It reflects the authors' judgment on reported outcomes based on available literature, and reflects variable strength in etiologic evidence: for some, etiology is established while for others it is merely suspected. References include both those supporting and those disputing etiology.

[b] Long-term consequences include chronic sequelae, congenital effects, and severe acute conditions with long-term impacts to health.

[c] Enteric pathogen, though generally not considered foodborne.

Conversely, one recent retrospective cohort study found patterns that suggested that estimates of increased risk of IBD following infection were primarily due to detection bias.[31] The pathogenesis of IBD is unclear, but evidence suggests that it results from an inappropriate host response to intestinal microbes. Whether this response is activated by an intrinsic defect or is due to a change in the epithelial mucosal barrier (possibly caused by acute infection) is unknown, and remains a point of active research.[25,26,28,30]

IBDs are associated with a long list of extraintestinal manifestations, including arthropathies, ocular inflammation, skin diseases, osteoporosis, kidney stones, thromboembolism, and hepatobiliary diseases.[32] The pathogeneses of most are unclear, and the role of infection is unknown. IBDs have also been associated with increased risk of colorectal cancer, small-bowel cancer, and bile-duct cancer.[27,32] In addition, many treatments for IBDs are associated with important side effects.

AUTOIMMUNE DISORDERS

Infection with foodborne pathogens can trigger autoimmune responses weeks after acute illness, which include reactive arthritis, GBS, and possibly autoimmune thyroid disease.

Reactive Arthritis

Reactive arthritis is generally characterized by a pattern of sterile arthritis of the lower limbs, often involving other inflammatory ailments such as tendonitis, skin lesions, and inflammatory back pain.[33] When these symptoms present together with conjunctivitis or uveitis and urethritis/cervicitis, it is sometimes referred to as Reiter syndrome. Patients with reactive arthritis are typically young adults of either sex, with a mean age of 30 to 40 years. Symptoms generally begin within a month of infection (which can be asymptomatic) and resolve within a year, although some patients may have symptoms after 5 years.[34,35] Susceptibility and severity of symptoms are associated with both the immunogenetic marker HLA-B27 and the severity of antecedent infection.[33,36,37]

Campylobacter, *Salmonella*, *Shigella*, and *Yersinia*, along with *Chlamydia*, are the classic etiologic triggers for reactive arthritis, although recent studies also suggest a role for *E coli* O157:H7.[33,36] The risk of developing reactive arthritis following infection varies widely in the literature, depending on study type, case definition, and location.[36] Rates outside of Scandinavia are often summarized in the 1% to 7% range, although there are differences by pathogen.[34,37,38] Two United States population studies of culture-confirmed enteric infections have estimated the risk of reactive arthritis following culture-confirmed infections. The risk of reactive arthritis in these studies varies by study and by pathogen, giving the following ranges: *Campylobacter* (3%–13%), *E coli* O157:H7 (0%–9%), *Salmonella* (2%–15%), *Shigella* (1%–10%), and *Yersinia* (0%–14%).[39,40] Some other enteric pathogens are thought to trigger reactive arthritis, though with a more diverse pattern of symptoms with fewer extraarticular features, including *C difficile*, *Brucella*, *Giardia*, *Cryptosporidium*, *Staphylococcus*, and *Vibrio parahaemolyticus*.[33,36,41]

Guillain-Barré Syndrome

GBS is a spectrum of acute peripheral neuropathies, with the leading type in North America being an acute inflammatory demyelinating polyradiculoneuropathy characterized by a 4-week onset of progressive muscle weakness, sensory loss, and ascending paralysis.[42,43] One-fourth of cases may require mechanical ventilation,[43] and mortality is 4% to 15% in the first year.[44] A majority of cases recover, but about a quarter of patients suffer persistent disability that is slow to resolve, and 10% to 20% of patients never regain the capability to walk unaided.[43]

Overall incidence of GBS in the United States is estimated between 1 and 2 cases per 100,000,[34,42] resulting in about $1.7 billion in annual medical costs, productivity losses, and premature mortality.[45] About 20% to 40% of these cases are estimated to be caused by a preceding infection with *Campylobacter jejuni*[42,44]; the risk of GBS following campylobacteriosis has been estimated at 30 to 100 per 100,000.[44] Onset of GBS usually occurs within 6 weeks of enteric infection, and *C jejuni*–associated GBS is generally more severe and has a poorer prognosis.[42] Although the pathogenesis of GBS is not fully understood, the cause is thought to be an autoimmune response whereby antibodies to foreign antigens (such as *C jejuni*) are cross-reactive with nerve-tissue molecules.[42,43]

Autoimmune Thyroid Disease

Also known as Graves disease, autoimmune thyroid disease (AITD) is the leading cause of hyperthyroidism, a condition that occurs when autoantibodies bind to and chronically stimulate the thyrotropin receptor.[46,47] It causes a wide range of symptoms, including fatigue, irregular heartbeat, weight loss, diffuse goiters, proptosis, and pretibial myxedema.[34,46] *Y enterocolitica* has long been suspected of having an etiologic role in AITD, an association supported by some cross-sectional and laboratory studies.[34,47] However, more recent case-control and prospective cohort studies have concluded that yersiniosis does not cause AITD; the documented association may be instead caused by a shared genetic susceptibility to both illnesses, or risk conferred by shared environmental exposures.[48,49]

NEUROLOGIC DYSFUNCTION

Indirect neurologic sequelae can result from several foodborne infections. Invasive infections from foodborne pathogens such as *Salmonella*, *Campylobacter*, *Shigella*, and *L monocytogenes* can cause severe sepsis and acute respiratory distress syndrome, resulting, in turn, in cognitive impairment, overall functional impairment, and increased risk of mortality from unrelated causes.[50–52] Some studies suggest that malnourishment caused by early childhood diarrheas, particularly infections with *Cryptosporidium*, *Giardia*, and rotavirus in the first 2 years of life, have lasting impacts on cognitive development, fitness, growth, and immunologic status.[8,53]

Certain pathogens invade the central nervous system (CNS) directly, resulting in serious acute illness as well as long-term sequelae. These pathogens include *Brucella* and several parasites that are rare in the United States but important globally, such as *Taenia solium*, *Trichinella*, *Echinococcus*, *Diphyllobothrium*, *Paragonimus*, *Spirometra*, and *Toxocara*.[54–57] In the United States, however, the 2 most prominent pathogens with neurologic sequelae are the bacteria *L monocytogenes* and the protozoan *T gondii*.

Listeriosis

Listeriosis remains an uncommon but serious infection, causing about 1600 foodborne cases and 250 deaths annually.[1] It predominantly affects the elderly, the immunocompromised, pregnant women, and neonates. In adults, *L monocytogenes* often invades the brainstem, meninges, and other parts of the CNS, resulting in meningitis, encephalitis, and sepsis, among other conditions.[58] One-fourth of these patients suffer seizures. An estimated 7% of patients relapse after hospital discharge, and 14% to 32% suffer a range of significant neurologic and psychological sequelae such as cranial nerve palsies, paresis, epilepsy, impaired executive and cognitive function, memory loss, aphasia, vision and hearing loss, attention deficits, decreased motivation, and depression.[59–62]

Listeriosis in pregnant women generally presents with mild flu-like symptoms, but can result in early-onset neonatal infection via transplacental transmission. About 20% to 25% of perinatal cases result in miscarriage or stillbirth, and the majority of remaining pregnancies are delivered preterm with septic conditions leading to respiratory distress, pneumonia, meningitis, and/or hydrocephalus.[60,63] About half of surviving cases of sepsis and meningitis incur neurodevelopmental sequelae including cerebral palsy, mild to severe cognitive deficits, and hearing loss. There are some indications that perinatal listeriosis also increases risk of chronic lung disease (bronchopulmonary dysplasia), likely as a result of maternal chorioamnionitis.[64]

Toxoplasmosis

T gondii is a parasitic protozoan that is estimated to infect about 10% to 20% of the United States population.[65] About half of these infections are assumed to be foodborne, making it the second leading cause of foodborne deaths.[1] As with *Listeria*, infection can be congenital or acquired.

Congenital toxoplasmosis occurs via placental transmission, resulting in miscarriage, premature birth, and an array of ocular and neurologic symptoms.[56,66–68] About 70% to 90% of infected newborns are asymptomatic at birth,[67] but a review of 12 studies found that in the first year, 13% developed chorioretinitis, 11% intercranial calcification, 2% hydrocephalus, and 3% CNS abnormalities.[69] Sequelae such as visual impairment, hearing problems, mental and cognitive abnormalities, learning disabilities, epilepsy, palsies, growth retardation, and developmental delays may not become apparent for years. Risk factors for severe outcomes include strain virulence, inoculum size, the stage of pregnancy at time of infection, and the host's age, genetic background, and immunologic status.[66–68]

Most acquired toxoplasmosis is asymptomatic in immunocompetent persons, although about 10% present with a mild self-limiting illness and less than 1% are estimated to develop ocular toxoplasmosis characterized by chorioretinitis, vitritis, retinal vasculitis, optic nerve involvement, and other manifestations.[70,71] Reactivation of latent infection in immunocompromised patients, such as AIDS patients or organ transplant recipients, causes an array of life-threatening complications and high mortality.[56,65,66]

Latent *T gondii* infection in the brain may have more subtle impacts to human personality and behavior.[72–75] A recent meta-analysis of 23 of more than 40 studies revealed an odds ratio of 2.73 (CI 2.1–3.6) for *T gondii* seroprevalence and schizophrenia.[76] *Toxoplasma* has also been associated with depression, suicide, personality shifts, changes to physical appearance associated with testosterone and estrogen levels, slow reaction time, reduced concentration, cognition deficits, and, in some very preliminary work, Alzheimer disease.[75] Animal studies support the hypothesis that the parasite may be manipulating human host behavior in an effort to complete its life cycle.[72,73]

RENAL FAILURE AND ASSOCIATED SEQUELAE

Infection with some foodborne pathogens, most notably *E coli* O157:H7 and other Shiga toxin–producing *E coli* (STEC), can cause HUS, which can develop into chronic kidney disease and end-stage renal disease. In addition, Shiga toxins are known to produce thrombocytopenia, hemolytic anemia, endothelial damage, microthrombi formation, and ischemic necrosis, which can result in long-term deficits to many organs including the gastrointestinal tract, brain, liver, heart, adrenals, spleen, and pancreas.[77,78]

Hemolytic-Uremic Syndrome

HUS is a spectrum disorder characterized by a triad of acute hemolytic anemia, thrombocytopenia, and nephropathy.[79] Postdiarrheal HUS (D+HUS) is associated with STECs and, to a lesser extent, *Shigella dysenteriae*; Shiga toxins bind to tubular epithelium and glomerular endothelial cells rich in globotriaosylceramide (Gb3) membrane receptors and trigger apoptosis, necrosis, and thrombotic microangiopathy, thus contributing to acute kidney failure.[80,81] It has been estimated that about 15% of children diagnosed with STECs develop HUS,[82] although the overall rate found in a 2009 review of 3464 STEC O157 infections (of all ages) found a 6.3% likelihood.[83] D+HUS has been associated with infections with *Salmonella* and non–foodborne *Streptococcus pneumoniae* and *C difficile*.[84–86] *Campylobacter* has been associated with glomerulonephritis and other renal diseases.[87]

Long-Term Systemic Sequelae Secondary to Renal Failure

D+HUS is associated with several long-term systemic sequelae, most notably chronic kidney disease, end-stage renal disease, and chronic hypertension. A 2003 meta-analysis of 3467 HUS patients who were younger than 18 years at presentation from 1950 to 2001 found that 5% to 11% suffer impaired kidney function (a glomerular filtration rate [GFR] of <80 mL/min), 8% to 12% suffered hypertension, and 10% to 20% suffered proteinuria a median of 4.4 years after an acute episode of D+HUS.[79] A follow-up (median 6.5 years) of 72 pediatric cases in Utah found at least 1 systemic abnormality in 51% of cases; 5.6% with hypertension, 31% with proteinuria, and 31% with GFR lower than 90 mL/min.[88] A follow-up (mean 13 years) of 118 pediatric cases in Argentina found 17.7% of cases had proteinuria without hypertension, 16.1% had a reduced GFR, and 3.4% had end-stage renal failure.[89] Young age, elevated white blood cell count on admission, prolonged oligioanuria, persistent proteinuria, and persistent microalbuminuria are thought to be predictors of poor long-term outcome.[90]

In 2010, the Walkerton Health Study detected a statistically significant association between gastroenteritis after drinking water contaminated with *E coli* O157:H7 and self-reported cardiovascular disease among 1977 Canadian adults a median of 7.9 years after infection. Although this finding has not been replicated in other cohorts to date, it is possible that endothelial damage caused by microthrombotic and inflammatory incidents contributes to an increased risk for cardiovascular events in the long term.[91]

Pancreatitis and diabetes mellitus (DM) have been reported during acute episodes of D+HUS. A 2005 meta-analysis of 1189 pediatric HUS cases from 5 countries found a pooled incidence of DM of 3.2%, with point estimates from 21 studies ranging from 0% to 15%.[92] In a retrospective study of 29 Canadian children, 21% were found to have elevated pancreatic enzymes with supportive evidence of pancreatitis during and after an acute episode of HUS. When present, pancreatitis during the acute phase of HUS is typically mild, but may occasionally involve extensive pancreatic necrosis.[78]

Several gastrointestinal sequelae are also associated with D+HUS. Twenty-one percent of 29 survivors of an outbreak of D+HUS reported rectal prolapse, colonic perforation, intussusception, gastric stricture, or cholelithiasis 2 to 3 years after the acute phase of HUS.[78,93] Gastrointestinal complications may require surgical intervention that can further affect the patient's long-term prognosis.

D+HUS is occasionally accompanied by CNS dysfunction, including coma. Seizures, hemiplegia, cortical blindness, and psychomotor retardation have been noted in 2% to 3% of D+HUS survivors. It is possible that hypernatremia, hypertension, uremia, and endothelial injury contribute to the development of CNS dysfunction during the acute phase of D+HUS, and severe acute neurologic involvement is a portent for long-term CNS dysfunction.[94]

ADDITIONAL SEQUELAE

Although most of this article focuses on the most prominent long-term health outcomes of the most prevalent foodborne infections, there are several less well recognized sequelae that have been reported. Some are well documented while others are not. However, the list presented in **Table 2** serves to present a more complete picture of the long-term consequences of acute foodborne infection and intoxication.

An additional emerging area of interest in characterizing the sequelae of foodborne infection is the relationship between gastrointestinal and psychological health. Although research is nascent, it is hypothesized that the 2-way gut-brain axis plays an important role in some diseases: psychological distress has been associated with certain gastrointestinal diseases, and enteric infection has been associated with psychological disorders. For example, as previously described, psychosocial factors are associated with diagnosis and severity of FGID.[95] On the other hand, group A streptococcal infections have been hypothesized as causing PANDAS (Pediatric Autoimmune Neuropsychiatric Disorders Associated with Streptococcal infections), a syndrome primarily characterized by a rapid and recurrent onset of a variable combination of obsessive-compulsive and tic disorders.[96] There are also numerous anecdotal stories of personality changes, psychiatric problems, and behavioral disorders following other cases of severe foodborne illness. Clearly this is a research area with far more questions than answers, but which may eventually prove important for both characterizing long-term outcomes associated with foodborne infection and developing effective treatments for these sequelae.

SUMMARY

The long-term consequences of foodborne infection can be more significant than those of acute illness. Malnutrition caused by profuse diarrhea in young children may cause long-term deficits in cognition and development, and in adults acute diarrhea may become chronic. IBS, IBDs, reactive arthritis, and GBS have been associated with foodborne pathogens. Pregnant women who become infected with L monocytogenes or T gondii may miscarry or give birth to preterm infants with permanent neurologic and ocular disorders. Invasive and enterotoxic pathogens can cause life-threatening conditions in the acute phase such as sepsis, meningitis, and respiratory distress that can lead to lifelong deficits in cognition, immunity, cardiovascular health, renal function, and other functions. In particular, D+HUS caused by STEC infection has been associated with a wide range of sequelae including hypertension, pancreatitis, diabetes, seizures, partial paralysis, blindness, and psychomotor retardation.

For many of these long-term conditions, disease mechanisms and the etiologic role of specific pathogens needs further illumination. Well-designed, large-scale prospective studies that account for the complicated interactions of host, environment, and microorganism are critical to improving our understanding. Only with increased funding of research geared toward elucidating the long-term health outcomes of foodborne infection will we be able to develop effective evidence-based clinical treatments or fully characterize the public health burden of foodborne disease.

ACKNOWLEDGMENTS

The authors thank Sandra A. Hoffmann and J. Glenn Morris Jr for collaboration on disease burden estimates that informed this work. The authors are doubly thankful to Dr Morris for also providing comments on a draft of this article. Thanks also to Robert Herrick, Alida Sorrenson, and Elizabeth Allen for sharing their posters on systematic reviews they conducted on sequelae associated with *Salmonella*, *Listeria monocytogenes*, and *Campylobacter*.

REFERENCES

1. Scallan E, Hoekstra RM, Angulo FJ, et al. Foodborne illness acquired in the United States—major pathogens. Emerg Infect Dis 2011;17:7–15.
2. Scallan E, Griffin PM, Angulo FJ, et al. Foodborne illness acquired in the United States—unspecified agents. Emerg Infect Dis 2011;17:16–22.
3. Mangen MJ, Batz MB, Käsbohrer A, et al. Integrated approaches for the public health prioritization of foodborne and zoonotic pathogens. Risk Anal 2010;30(5): 782–97.
4. Batz MB, Hoffmann S, Morris JG. Ranking the disease burden of 14 pathogens in food sources in the United States using attribution data from outbreak investigations and expert elicitation. J Food Prot 2012;75(7):1278–91.
5. Hoffmann S, Batz MB, Morris JG. Annual cost of illness and quality-adjusted life year losses in the United States due to 14 foodborne pathogens. J Food Prot 2012;75:1292–302.
6. Scharff RL. Economic burden from health losses due to foodborne illness in the United States. J Food Prot 2012;75:123–31.
7. Havelaar AH, Haagsma JA, Mangen MJ, et al. Disease burden of foodborne pathogens in the Netherlands, 2009. Int J Food Microbiol 2012;156(3):231–8.
8. Lindsay JA. Chronic sequelae of foodborne disease. Emerg Infect Dis 1997;3: 443–52.
9. Carbone KM. Infectious causes of chronic disease: from hypothesis to proof. In: Fratamico PM, Smith JL, Brogden KA, editors. Sequelae and long-term consequences of infectious diseases. Washington, DC: ASM Press; 2009. p. 1–8.
10. Institute of Medicine. The infectious etiology of chronic diseases: defining the relationship, enhancing the research, and mitigating the effects: workshop summary. Washington, DC: National Academies Press; 2004.
11. Roberts T, Kowalcyk B, Buck P, et al. The long-term health outcomes of selected foodborne pathogens. Grove City (PA): Center for Foodborne Illness Research and Prevention; 2009.
12. Lee SD, Surawicz CM. Infectious causes of chronic diarrhea. Gastroenterol Clin North Am 2001;30(3):679–92.
13. Rodriguez-Palacios A, Borgmann S, Kline TR, et al. *Clostridium difficile* in foods and animals: history and measures to reduce exposure. Anim Health Res Rev 2013;14(1):11–9.
14. Lund BM, O'Brien SJ. The occurrence and prevention of foodborne disease in vulnerable people. Foodborne Pathog Dis 2011;8(9):961–73.
15. Drossman DA. The functional gastrointestinal disorders and the Rome III process. Gastroenterology 2006;130:1377–90.

16. Smith JL, Bayles D. Postinfectious irritable bowel syndrome: a long-term consequence of bacterial gastroenteritis. J Food Prot 2007;70:1762–9.
17. Haagsma JA, Siersema PD, De Wit NJ, et al. Disease burden of post-infectious irritable bowel syndrome in The Netherlands. Epidemiol Infect 2010;138: 1650–6.
18. Schwille-Kiuntke J, Frick JS, Zanger P, et al. Post-infectious irritable bowel syndrome—a review of the literature. Z Gastroenterol 2011;49:997–1003.
19. Halvorson HA, Schlett CD, Riddle MS. Postinfectious irritable bowel syndrome—a meta-analysis. Am J Gastroenterol 2006;101:1894–9 [quiz: 1942].
20. Thabane M, Simunovic M, Akhtar-Danesh N, et al. An outbreak of acute bacterial gastroenteritis is associated with an increased incidence of irritable bowel syndrome in children. Am J Gastroenterol 2010;105:933–9.
21. Thabane M, Kottachchi DT, Marshall JK. Systematic review and meta-analysis: the incidence and prognosis of post-infectious irritable bowel syndrome. Aliment Pharmacol Ther 2007;26(4):535–44.
22. Thabane M, Marshall JK. Post-infectious irritable bowel syndrome. World J Gastroenterol 2009;15(29):3591–6.
23. Villani AC, Lemire M, Thabane M, et al. Genetic risk factors for post-infectious irritable bowel syndrome following a waterborne outbreak of gastroenteritis. Gastroenterology 2010;138:1502–13.
24. Doorduyn Y, Van Pelt W, Siezen CL, et al. Novel insight in the association between salmonellosis or campylobacteriosis and chronic illness, and the role of host genetics in susceptibility to these diseases. Epidemiol Infect 2008; 136:1225–34.
25. Podolsky DK. Inflammatory bowel disease. N Engl J Med 2002;347:417–29.
26. Baumgart DC, Carding SR. Inflammatory bowel disease: cause and immunobiology. Lancet 2007;369:1627–40.
27. Baumgart DC, Sandborn WJ. Inflammatory bowel disease: clinical aspects and established and evolving therapies. Lancet 2007;369(9573):1641–57.
28. Xavier RJ, Podolsky DK. Unravelling the pathogenesis of inflammatory bowel disease. Nature 2007;448:427–34.
29. Ternhag A, Törner A, Svensson A, et al. Short- and long-term effects of bacterial gastrointestinal infections. Emerg Infect Dis 2008;14(1):143–8.
30. Verdu EF, Riddle MS. Chronic gastrointestinal consequences of acute infectious diarrhea: evolving concepts in epidemiology and pathogenesis. Am J Gastroenterol 2012;107(7):981–9.
31. Jess T, Simonsen J, Nielsen NM, et al. Enteric Salmonella or Campylobacter infections and the risk of inflammatory bowel disease. Gut 2011;60:318–24.
32. Danese S, Semeraro S, Papa A, et al. Extraintestinal manifestations in inflammatory bowel disease. World J Gastroenterol 2005;11(46):7227–36.
33. Hannu T. Reactive arthritis. Best Pract Res Clin Rheumatol 2011;25(3):347–57.
34. Rees JR. Enteric pathogens. In: Fratamico PM, Smith JL, Brogden KA, editors. Sequelae and long-term consequences of infectious diseases. Washington, DC: ASM Press; 2009. p. 53–68.
35. Bremell T, Bjelle A, Svedhem A. Rheumatic symptoms following an outbreak of Campylobacter enteritis: a five year follow up. Ann Rheum Dis 1991;50: 934–8.
36. Townes JM. Reactive arthritis after enteric infections in the United States: the problem of definition. Clin Infect Dis 2010;50(2):247–54.
37. Garg AX, Pope JE, Thiessen-Philbrook H, et al. Arthritis risk after acute bacterial gastroenteritis. Rheumatology (Oxford) 2008;47:200–4.

38. Sieper J, Rudwaleit M, Khan MA, et al. Concepts and epidemiology of spondyloarthritis. Best Pract Res Clin Rheumatol 2006;20:401–17.
39. Rees JR, Pannier MA, McNees A, et al. Persistent diarrhea, arthritis, and other complications of enteric infections: a pilot survey based on California FoodNet surveillance, 1998-1999. Clin Infect Dis 2004;38(Suppl 3):S311–7.
40. Townes JM, Deodhar AA, Laine ES, et al. Reactive arthritis following culture-confirmed infections with bacterial enteric pathogens in Minnesota and Oregon: a population-based study. Ann Rheum Dis 2008;67(12):1689–96.
41. Girschick HJ, Guilherme L, Inman RD, et al. Bacterial triggers and autoimmune rheumatic diseases. Clin Exp Rheumatol 2008;26(1 Suppl 48):S12–7.
42. Hughes RA, Cornblath DR. Guillain-Barré syndrome. Lancet 2005;366:1653–66.
43. Lehmann HC, Hughes RA, Kieseier BC, et al. Recent developments and future directions in Guillain-Barré syndrome. J Peripher Nerv Syst 2012;17(Suppl 3): 57–70.
44. Poropatich KO, Walker CL, Black RE. Quantifying the association between Campylobacter infection and Guillain-Barré syndrome: a systematic review. J Health Popul Nutr 2010;28:545–52.
45. Frenzen PD. Economic cost of Guillain-Barré syndrome in the United States. Neurology 2008;71:21–7.
46. Weetman AP. Graves' disease. N Engl J Med 2000;343:1236–48.
47. Prummel MF, Strieder T, Wiersinga WM. The environment and autoimmune thyroid diseases. Eur J Endocrinol 2004;150:605–18.
48. Hansen PS, Wenzel BE, Brix TH, et al. Yersinia enterocolitica infection does not confer an increased risk of thyroid antibodies: evidence from a Danish twin study. Clin Exp Immunol 2006;146:32–8.
49. Effraimidis G, Tijssen JG, Strieder TG, et al. No causal relationship between Yersinia enterocolitica infection and autoimmune thyroid disease: evidence from a prospective study. Clin Exp Immunol 2011;165:38–43.
50. Benjamim CF, Hogaboam CM, Kunkel SL. The chronic consequences of severe sepsis. J Leukoc Biol 2004;75:408–12.
51. Yende S, Angus DC. Long-term outcomes from sepsis. Curr Infect Dis Rep 2007;9:382–6.
52. Iwashyna TJ, Ely EW, Smith DM, et al. Long-term cognitive impairment and functional disability among survivors of severe sepsis. JAMA 2010;304(16):1787–94.
53. Guerrant RL, Kosek M, Moore S, et al. Magnitude and impact of diarrheal diseases. Arch Med Res 2002;33:351–5.
54. Dean AS, Crump L, Greter H, et al. Clinical manifestations of human brucellosis: a systematic review and meta-analysis. PLoS Negl Trop Dis 2012; 6(12):e1929.
55. Ortega YR. Foodborne parasites. New York: Springer; 2006.
56. Fratamico PM, Smith JL, Brogden KA. Sequelae and long-term consequences of infectious diseases. Washington, DC: ASM Press; 2009.
57. Riemann HP, Cliver DO, editors. Foodborne infections and intoxications. 3rd edition. Amsterdam (NL): Academic Press; 2006.
58. Schlech WF 3rd. Foodborne listeriosis. Clin Infect Dis 2000;31:770–5.
59. Mylonakis E, Hohmann EL, Calderwood SB. Central nervous system infection with Listeria monocytogenes: 33 years' experience at a general hospital and review of 776 episodes from the literature. Medicine (Baltimore) 1998;77:313–36.
60. Aouaj Y, Spanjaard L, Van Leeuwen N, et al. Listeria monocytogenes meningitis: serotype distribution and patient characteristics in The Netherlands, 1976-95. Epidemiol Infect 2002;128:405–9.

61. Brouwer MC, Van de Beek D, Heckenberg SG, et al. Community-acquired *Listeria monocytogenes* meningitis in adults. Clin Infect Dis 2006;43:1233–8.
62. Schmidt H, Heimann B, Djukic M, et al. Neuropsychological sequelae of bacterial and viral meningitis. Brain 2006;129:333–45.
63. Mylonakis E, Paliou M, Hohmann EL, et al. Listeriosis during pregnancy: a case series and review of 222 cases. Medicine (Baltimore) 2002;81:260–9.
64. Hsieh WS, Tsai LY, Jeng SF, et al. Neonatal listeriosis in Taiwan, 1990-2007. Int J Infect Dis 2009;13:193–5.
65. Jones JL, Dubey JP. Foodborne toxoplasmosis. Clin Infect Dis 2012;55:845–51.
66. Montoya JG, Liesenfeld O. Toxoplasmosis. Lancet 2004;363:1965–76.
67. Rorman E, Zamir CS, Rilkis I, et al. Congenital toxoplasmosis—prenatal aspects of *Toxoplasma gondii* infection. Reprod Toxicol 2006;21:458–72.
68. Kaye A. Toxoplasmosis: diagnosis, treatment, and prevention in congenitally exposed infants. J Pediatr Health Care 2011;25:355–64.
69. Havelaar AH, Kemmeren JM, Kortbeek LM. Disease burden of congenital toxoplasmosis. Clin Infect Dis 2007;44(11):1467–74.
70. Butler NJ, Furtado JM, Winthrop KL, et al. Ocular toxoplasmosis II: clinical features, pathology and management. Clin Experiment Ophthalmol 2013;41: 95–108.
71. Burnett AJ, Shortt SG, Isaac-Renton J, et al. Multiple cases of acquired toxoplasmosis retinitis presenting in an outbreak. Ophthalmology 1998;105: 1032–7.
72. Yolken RH, Dickerson FB, Fuller Torrey E. *Toxoplasma* and schizophrenia. Parasite Immunol 2009;31:706–15.
73. Flegr J. Influence of latent *Toxoplasma* infection on human personality, physiology and morphology: pros and cons of the *Toxoplasma*-human model in studying the manipulation hypothesis. J Exp Biol 2013;216:127–33.
74. Flegr J. Effects of toxoplasma on human behavior. Schizophr Bull 2007;33:757–60.
75. Hurley RA, Taber KH. Latent *Toxoplasma gondii*: emerging evidence for influences on neuropsychiatric disorders. J Neuropsychiatry Clin Neurosci 2012; 24:376–83.
76. Torrey EF, Bartko JJ, Lun ZR, et al. Antibodies to *Toxoplasma gondii* in patients with schizophrenia: a meta-analysis. Schizophr Bull 2007;33:729–36.
77. Koster F, Levin J, Walker L, et al. Hemolytic-uremic syndrome after shigellosis. Relation to endotoxemia and circulating immune complexes. N Engl J Med 1978;298:927–33.
78. Grodinsky S, Telmesani A, Robson WL, et al. Gastrointestinal manifestations of hemolytic uremic syndrome: recognition of pancreatitis. J Pediatr Gastroenterol Nutr 1990;11:518–24.
79. Garg AX, Suri RS, Barrowman N, et al. Long-term renal prognosis of diarrhea-associated hemolytic uremic syndrome: a systematic review, meta-analysis, and meta-regression. JAMA 2003;290:1360–70.
80. Mayer CL, Leibowitz CS, Kurosawa S, et al. Shiga toxins and the pathophysiology of hemolytic uremic syndrome in humans and animals. Toxins (Basel) 2012;4:1261–87.
81. Karpman D, Håkansson A, Perez MT, et al. Apoptosis of renal cortical cells in the hemolytic-uremic syndrome: in vivo and in vitro studies. Infect Immun 1998;66: 636–44.
82. Wong CS, Mooney JC, Brandt JR, et al. Risk factors for the hemolytic uremic syndrome in children infected with *Escherichia coli* O157:H7: a multivariable analysis. Clin Infect Dis 2012;55:33–41.

83. Gould LH, Demma L, Jones TF, et al. Hemolytic uremic syndrome and death in persons with *Escherichia coli* O157:H7 infection, foodborne diseases active surveillance network sites, 2000-2006. Clin Infect Dis 2009;49:1480–5.
84. Siegler R, Oakes R. Hemolytic uremic syndrome; pathogenesis, treatment, and outcome. Curr Opin Pediatr 2005;17:200–4.
85. Srivastava RN, Moudgil A, Bagga A, et al. Hemolytic uremic syndrome in children in northern India. Pediatr Nephrol 1991;5:284–8.
86. Alvarado AS, Brodsky SV, Nadasdy T, et al. Hemolytic uremic syndrome associated with Clostridium difficile infection. Clin Nephrol, in press.
87. Lim A, Lydia A, Rim H, et al. Focal segmental glomerulosclerosis and Guillain-Barré syndrome associated with Campylobacter enteritis. Intern Med J 2007; 37(10):724–8.
88. Siegler RL, Pavia AT, Christofferson RD, et al. A 20-year population-based study of postdiarrheal hemolytic uremic syndrome in Utah. Pediatrics 1994; 94:35–40.
89. Spizzirri FD, Rahman RC, Bibiloni N, et al. Childhood hemolytic uremic syndrome in Argentina: long-term follow-up and prognostic features. Pediatr Nephrol 1997;11:156–60.
90. Lou-Meda R, Oakes RS, Gilstrap JN, et al. Prognostic significance of microalbuminuria in postdiarrheal hemolytic uremic syndrome. Pediatr Nephrol 2007;22: 117–20.
91. Clark WF, Sontrop JM, Macnab JJ, et al. Long term risk for hypertension, renal impairment, and cardiovascular disease after gastroenteritis from drinking water contaminated with *Escherichia coli* O157:H7: a prospective cohort study. BMJ 2010;341:c6020.
92. Suri RS, Clark WF, Barrowman N, et al. Diabetes during diarrhea-associated hemolytic uremic syndrome: a systematic review and meta-analysis. Diabetes Care 2005;28:2556–62.
93. Brandt JR, Joseph MW, Fouser LS, et al. Cholelithiasis following *Escherichia coli* O157: H7-associated hemolytic uremic syndrome. Pediatr Nephrol 1998;12: 222–5.
94. Schlieper A, Orrbine E, Wells GA, et al. Neuropsychological sequelae of haemolytic uraemic syndrome. Investigators of the HUS Cognitive Study. Arch Dis Child 1999;80:214–20.
95. Collins SM, Surette M, Bercik P. The interplay between the intestinal microbiota and the brain. Nat Rev Microbiol 2012;10:735–42.
96. Mell LK, Davis RL, Owens D. Association between streptococcal infection and obsessive-compulsive disorder, Tourette's syndrome, and tic disorder. Pediatrics 2005;116:56–60.
97. U.S. Food and Drug Administration. Bad Bug Book: foodborne pathogenic microorganisms and natural toxins handbook [Internet]. 2nd edition. Washington, DC: 2012. Available at: http://www.fda.gov/food/foodsafety/foodborneillness/ foodborneillnessfoodbornepathogensnaturaltoxins/badbugbook/default.htm. Accessed February 12, 2013.
98. Doyle MP, Beuchat LR, Montville TJ, editors. Food microbiology: fundamentals and frontiers. Washington, DC: ASM Press; 1997.
99. Hohmann EL. Nontyphoidal salmonellosis. Clin Infect Dis 2001;32(2):263–9.
100. Rodríguez LA, Ruigómez A. Increased risk of irritable bowel syndrome after bacterial gastroenteritis: cohort study. BMJ 1999;318(7183):565–6.
101. Tabak F, Ozdemir F, Tabak O, et al. Autoimmune hepatitis induced by the prolonged hepatitis A virus infection. Ann Hepatol 2008;7:177–9.

102. Rashid T, Ebringer A. Ankylosing spondylitis is linked to *Klebsiella*—the evidence. Clin Rheumatol 2007;26(6):858–64.
103. Dickey RW, Plakas SM. Ciguatera: a public health perspective. Toxicon 2010;56: 123–36.
104. Reddy KR, Salleh B, Saad B, et al. An overview of mycotoxin contamination in foods and its implications for human health. Toxin Rev 2010;29:3–26.

Iatrogenic High-Risk Populations and Foodborne Disease

David Acheson, MD, FRCP

KEYWORDS

- Foodborne illness • Immunocompromised • Food safety • Vulnerable populations
- Patient susceptibility

KEY POINTS

- Various immune conditions can make individuals either more susceptible to foodborne illness, can result in increased severity of the illness, or both.
- Approximately 20% of the population has suppressed immune function, because of age, reproductive status, pharmacologic therapy, or disease.
- Vulnerable populations should be made aware of the risks and provided with education on how to avoid foodborne illness.
- High risk patients need to understand the need to take food safety seriously and have a low threshold for seeking medical attention when foodborne illness strikes.

INTRODUCTION

Some of the key emerging trends in relation to foodborne illness have been described in other articles elsewhere in this issue. In a healthy adult, the symptoms often resolve spontaneously without the need for significant medical intervention and without long-term consequence or exposure to a foodborne pathogen does not even result in symptoms. However, certain subsets of the population are at a greater risk of acquiring foodborne infections and have a greater propensity to develop serious complications.

Both as a patient and a physician, answering the question "Am I at higher risk of foodborne illness?" can be challenging. Although we may be able to identify who is at risk, quantifying the risk may not be straightforward. There are varying degrees of vulnerability to the same pathogen amongst those deemed at higher risk of a foodborne illness, and there may be greater vulnerability to a given pathogen in 1 vulnerable population than in another vulnerable population. The degree to which an individual is considered vulnerable and the pathogens from which that person has increased risk vary depending on a wide range of factors. Some of these factors relate to the properties of the pathogen in question, others relate to the immune status of the individual concerned, and yet others are determined by how food is stored and prepared.

The Acheson Group, 1 Old Frankfort Way, Frankfort, IL 60423, USA
E-mail address: david@achesongroup.com

Infect Dis Clin N Am 27 (2013) 617–629
http://dx.doi.org/10.1016/j.idc.2013.05.008
0891-5520/13/$ – see front matter © 2013 Elsevier Inc. All rights reserved.

id.theclinics.com

Regarding managing risk in vulnerable populations, one key need is to communicate the most appropriate risk-based information to the patient. Such information may provide the patient with specific advice regarding certain types of food to avoid, or offer recommendations on food preparation and storage that reduce the likelihood of the food containing harmful pathogens.

PHYSIOLOGIC DEFENSES

Susceptibility to foodborne infection is dependent on numerous factors that largely relate to the status of an individual's defense systems in regard to both preventing and mitigating foodborne illness. The human host has several barriers that offer protection from infection with orally acquired agents. These barriers include the physical barriers and components of the gastrointestinal tract that either block or destroy foodborne agents.

The Intestinal Mucosal Barrier

The intestinal mucosal barrier has an enormous surface area, approximately 400 m², and comprises a variety of cellular and noncellular elements.[1] Structurally, the barrier is formed by an epithelial cell lining with a complex array of agents on its luminal surface, and by organized lymphoid tissues designed to assist in the protective function against harmful foreign antigens. Although the epithelial barrier consists of only a single layer of columnar cells, it serves the balanced function of providing a physical deterrent as well as providing the portal for uptake of important nutrients. Epithelial cells in the intestine have microvilli on their apical surfaces, with a filamentous brush border glycocalyx at the tips.[1] This cellular anatomy helps to prevent penetration by foreign antigens, and these cells simultaneously express major histocompatibility complex class II receptors to facilitate antigen presentation to immune cells as needed. Moreover, cells of this villous epithelium produce a variety of functional molecules, such as defensins,[2] trefoil factors, and mucins, which help to further protect the human host.[3] Mucins are the principal components of mucus, which lines the surface epithelium throughout the intestinal tract.[4] Microbes of all types (ie, bacteria, viruses, and protozoa) become trapped in the mucus layer and are expelled from the intestine by peristalsis.

Interspersed with the villous epithelial monolayer is the follicle-associated epithelia (FAE), which overlies a vast network of organized mucosa-associated lymphoid tissue, including M cells.[5] This specialized epithelia is distributed throughout the intestinal tract as part of the gut-associated lymphoid tissue (GALT) and is found in a more organized fashion in areas reflecting a high presence of foreign materials and microorganisms, such as the Peyer patches in the distal small intestine, the palatine tonsils, and the pharyngeal mucosa of the Waldeyer ring and the appendix. The GALT also contains important regulatory cells of the mucosal immune system, such as lymphocytes and phagocytes. Lymphocytes organize and mount rapid, selective, and potent immune responses against harmful foreign pathogens, and phagocytes play a role in the sampling, presentation, and destruction of pathogens.

The GALT comprises 4 distinct lymphoid compartments: Peyer patches and other lymphoid follicles associated with the FAE; lamina propria (LP); intraepithelial lymphocytes (IELs); and mesenteric lymph nodes (MLNs).[6] Lymphoid follicles are characterized by aggregates of immature B cells and CD4 (+) helper T cells sitting within specific pockets of the M cell[5] and resemble lymph nodes without the afferent lymphatics. Thus, these lymphoid aggregates come into contact solely with antigens from the gut lumen and serve as inductive sites for intestinal immune responses.[7] Another unique feature of these lymphoid tissues is the propensity for IgA production.

Populations of IELs, predominantly cytotoxic T cells, inhabit the interdigitating spaces between epithelial cells above the basement membrane. Natural killer–like lymphocytes have also been detected in these spaces.[8] The role of IELs in immune defense remains to be fully elucidated. However, because of their location and the observation that most cells are cytotoxic, IELs are believed to play an important role in innate defense and tumor surveillance in the gut. The MLNs and the vascular endothelium also serve important functions in the GALT. After ingestion of foreign antigen, dendritic cells and macrophages often migrate to MLN and present antigen to MLN T cells. These interactions aid MLN B-cell differentiation into primarily IgA-producing plasma cells and induce a systemic response to the foreign antigen. The plasma cells are released into the bloodstream to then home back through the gut vascular endothelium to populate the LP, where they are needed to release IgA into the gut lumen. Furthermore, killing and removal of pathogens also occur in the MLN. Pathogens able to bypass immune defenses and reach these targets have an optimal chance to spread systemically through the bloodstream or lymphatic system.

Breakdown of Mucosal Barrier Function

The mucosal barrier helps maintain symbiosis between microbes residing in the gut and the host animal. The integrity of this barrier is regulated by a complex network of physical, physiologic, and immune factors, which includes dietary influences, the host environment (which can be modified by age, external factors such as antibiotics, and immune competency), and the indigenous microbial flora (IMF) of the gut.[9] Modification or breakdown of these factors leads to ineffective clearance or degradation of harmful ingested antigens or disruption of regulatory cell function, resulting in mucosal damage, increased gut permeability, and overgrowth of harmful pathogens, which may result in disease.

Diet not only introduces carcinogens or toxins that may be directly toxic to the gut mucosa but also provides nutrients that modify the physiologic environment and allow growth of certain bacteria in the gut. For example, infant diets comprising solely breast milk are rich in acetic/propionic acids, which induce an acidic environment, whereas diets comprising infant formula have increased isobutyric, isovaleric, and isocaproic acids, favoring higher pH. Lower pH seems to inhibit growth of certain *Escherichia coli* and *Vibrio cholera* strains, and this has been postulated as a reason for the decreased incidence of intestinal symptoms or diseases in breastfed compared with formula-fed infants. Also, starvation leads to a gut environment with unconjugated bile acids and decreased short-chain fatty acid concentrations, which tend to inhibit anaerobic bacterial growth and favor growth of pathogenic coliform bacteria, such as *E coli*.[10]

Age or stage of gut development may dictate which pathogens colonize the gut mucosa and contribute to disease. Infants tend to have a higher prevalence of gastrointestinal disease than adults, especially from enteric viruses. Developmental immaturity of the infant gut plays a factor. Newborns typically lack IgA and IgM in exocrine secretions until a few months of age, and secretory IgA is found in low levels in the saliva and gut after birth.[11] These low antibody levels may provide an inefficient barrier to microbes. Moreover, porous villous membranes, low basal acid output, and immature proteolyic activity in the gut are additional factors that lead to altered clearance of potentially harmful microbes.[11] Infants are further colonized by a unique repertoire of bacteria compared with adults, and this difference has been suggested to make the infant more susceptible to botulism following ingestion of *Clostridium botulinum* spores.[9,12] Up to 90% of infants are colonized with *Clostridium difficile*, but rarely develop disease from this organism.[9]

Antibiotics are beneficial in treating illness caused by certain enteric pathogens. However, they may also contribute to disease by eliminating from the IMF certain microbes that inhibit or suppress the growth of other pathogenic microbes in the gut. Moreover, prolonged use of antibiotics may favor colonization by antibiotic-resistant strains of bacteria, which can pose serious consequences if these strains become pathogenic. A prime example of the suppressive phenomenon of antibiotics is infection with *C difficile*, leading to pseudomembranous colitis.

Disease states or pathogens are kept in check by competent cells or pathways of the immune system. Immune competency can be altered by drugs (eg, steroids), age (ie, infants and elderly individuals), acquired disease states (eg, infections, malignancies), stressors (eg, trauma, surgery), and germline immunodeficiency. The result is naive, delayed or defective IgA, phagocytic, or T-cell effector immune responses leading to ineffective neutralization of pathogens and increased susceptibility to disease. IgA represents a first line of defense by blocking the association of certain nonindigenous microbes, namely *Salmonella, Vibrio cholera*, and enteric viruses, with the gut epithelium,[13] and therefore reducing penetration of these pathogens into the LP. Phagocytes and T cells offer a second line of defense against cellular invasive organisms and help eliminate pathogens from cellular tissues. Also, interactions between these cells and epithelial cells help elaborate cytokines or other factors that support the symbiotic relationship with the IMF. Thus, immune deficiency leads not only to acute microbial disease but also favors chronic persistence of these pathogens in diseased tissues because of ineffective measures to clear offending pathogens, contributing to malignancies, inflammatory disorders, or other systemic illness.[7]

Translocation of Pathogens

Breakdown of the mucosal barrier network also facilitates the invasion or entry through host cells by pathogenic organisms, some of which would not otherwise normally cause disease. Factors that favor translocation include bacterial overgrowth, immune deficiencies, and mucosal injury, with loss of barrier integrity. Evidence of increased translocation of pathogens has been observed in a variety of disease states[14] and has been shown to be associated with cases of postoperative sepsis[15] and with spontaneous bacterial peritonitis in cirrhotic rats.[16] The ability of a pathogen to translocate efficiently through cells, coupled with mechanisms to avoid immune detection or destruction, seems to provide a survival advantage for a pathogen and may account for the systemic spread of certain organisms.

WHO IS VULNERABLE?

The simple answer to the question of who constitutes the population vulnerable to foodborne illness is the young, the elderly and the immunocompromised. However, there are significant nuances with this broad categorization. Not all these populations are equally susceptible to the same range of specific agents. Susceptibility to a pathogen may mean higher likelihood of getting sick if exposed, it may mean the individual has a more prolonged or severe illness compared with a nonsusceptible person, or it may mean both. Specific definitions of young and elderly may be different for different pathogens.

The populations most at risk for foodborne illness and subsequent death are collectively characterized by suppressed immune function, whether because of age (the very young or the very old), reproductive status (pregnancy), pharmacologic therapy (chemotherapy or organ transplantation), or disease (human immunodeficiency virus [HIV] infection).[17] Together, these groups represent approximately 20% of the American population.[17,18] Although each of these high-risk groups is immune suppressed or compromised, they differ in the length of time that immune function is affected and in the source of the physiologic insult on the immune system.[19] **Box 1** summarizes the main groups. There are 2 principal types of immune deficiency: congenital and acquired. Congenital immune deficiencies are caused by disorders in which a portion of the immune system is either not present or not functioning properly. The risk of foodborne illness in these primary immunodeficiencies is related to which aspect(s) of the immune system are not functioning properly. For example, patients with common variable immunodeficiency are at higher risk of severe infection with enteric viruses and *Giardia*; patients with chronic granulomatous disease are at higher risk of infection with nontyphoidal salmonellosis. Acquired immune deficiencies occur as a result of 1 or more secondary event(s), which may be natural, age related or caused by some medical treatments or medical condition (see **Box 1**). In the next sections, specific common vulnerable populations at risk are discussed.

AGE-RELATED IMMUNE DEFICIENCY
Elderly

The population in the United States and in many other countries throughout the world is aging. Life expectancy has increased during the past century, from 47 years for

---

Box 1
Examples of conditions that may result in increased susceptibility to foodborne infections

- Acquired or secondary
  - Age
    - Young
    - Elderly
  - Temporary
    - Pregnancy
  - Chronic disease
    - End-stage renal disease
    - Cirrhosis
    - Diabetes mellitus
    - Inflammatory bowel disease
    - HIV/AIDS
  - Malignancy
    - Solid tumors
    - Hematologic malignancy
  - Iatrogenic (medication induced)
    - Reduced gastric acidity
    - Immunosuppressive medications
    - Anti–tumor necrosis factor

Americans born in 1900 to 77 years for those born in 2001.[20] Not only are people in the United States living longer, but the proportion of the population that is aged 65 years and older is also growing, a trend that will continue to increase as baby boomers (ie, born between 1946 and 1964) reach age 65 years. Since 1900, the population of the United States has tripled; however, the number of older adults has increased 11-fold, from 3.1 million in 1900 to 35 million in 2000. By 2030, when all of the baby boomers have reached age 65 years, the number of older Americans is expected to reach 71 million, or roughly 20% of the population.[21]

Infectious diseases are a major problem in the elderly, as a result of senescence of both humoral and cellular immunity, age-related changes in the gastrointestinal tract, malnutrition, lack of exercise, comorbidities, use of acid-suppressing or immunosuppressive medications, entry into nursing homes, and excessive use of antibiotics.[22–24] Specific pathogens to which the elderly are more vulnerable are listeriosis, *Salmonella* and *Campylobacter* bacteremia, death from infection with *E coli* O157:H7, and norovirus (reviewed in Ref.[36]). With poorer health status, higher rates of chronic disease, greater exposure to risk-increasing medications, exposure to centralized food preparation, and higher potential for fecal soiling of the environment, elderly people living in long-term care facilities are likely at even higher risk than community-based elderly individuals. Most epidemiologic studies concerning a specific agent in the elderly are focused on nursing homes, because the impact can be more easily observed with a confined group of individuals. Case fatality rates for specific enteric pathogens are frequently markedly greater in this group than the general population.[18] Although many cases of gastrointestinal distress may be short-lived, secondary long-term complications may arise that are life-threatening and require hospitalization. Gordon and colleagues[25] reported a mortality of 1.3% among a retirement community during a foodborne outbreak of the Snow Mountain agent, a norovirus. The investigators noted that several of the residents sustained serious injuries from falling because of near-syncopal episodes caused by dehydration from the gastroenteritis.

Hepatitis A virus usually causes a mild and often asymptomatic infection in children. However, in adults the virus typically produces clinical illness, which can lead to death.[26] Waterborne outbreaks are often characterized by high attack rates, with all or most of the infected individuals showing clinical illness.[27] In an 8-year review of hepatitis A cases from England, Wales, and Ireland, the case fatality rate of hepatitis A for patients younger than 55 years was 0.02% to 0.03%, 0.9% at 55 to 64 years of age, and 1.5% for older patients. The median age of those dying from hepatitis A is higher than 60 years in the United Kingdom.[28]

Children

Children deserve added attention, because the risks of some foodborne illnesses, such as salmonellosis, are relatively higher for children than for any other demographic group. Children are at higher risks because of a less-developed, more permeable gut tissue, less gastrointestinal reserve capacity, lower body weight (ie, it takes a smaller quantity of pathogens to make them sick), potential for rapid dehydration, and limited recognition of thirst.[29,30]

AIDS

Enteric pathogens are among the many agents that take advantage of an impaired or destroyed immune system to develop persistent and generalized infections in the immunocompromised host. Such infections are difficult to treat, tend to be long-term, add to the burden of the debilitation in the patient, and can result in a significantly higher mortality than in immunocompetent persons.[31] Many studies have shown that the rates of diarrheal disease in developing countries among individuals infected with the HIV virus are higher than the rates in developed countries, probably reflecting more frequent exposure to enteric pathogens by contaminated food and water. Adenoviruses and rotaviruses are the most common enteric viruses isolated in the stools of HIV-infected persons. A comprehensive study of Australian men showed that 54% of diarrheal illnesses in patients with AIDS were caused by viruses and that 37% of the viral diarrheas were adenovirus related.[31]

In addition, enteric bacterial infections are more severe in patients with AIDS. For example, patients with *Salmonella, Shigella*, and *Campylobacter* infection often develop bacteremia.[32,33] *Cryptosporidium* is also a serious problem among patients with AIDS. A severe and protracted diarrhea results, with fluid losses of several liters per day in some cases. Symptoms may persist for months, resulting in severe weight loss and mortality. Mortality of 50% has been reported for this organism.[34] Although patients with AIDS may not have more severe illness with *Giardia*, they do show impaired immune response to the parasite.

TRANSPLANT RECIPIENTS AND PATIENTS WHO HAVE CANCER

Patients who have cancer undergo intensive chemotherapy with cytotoxic and immunosuppressive drugs and often radiation treatment in an attempt to destroy neoplastic growth. These measures also attack the immune system, leaving the patient with little defense against opportunistic pathogens.[18] Patients who have undergone either bone marrow or solid organ transplantation are also at increased risk, because of use of immunosuppressive agents with varying effects against T cells, B cells, or both, in order to maintain the transplanted organ(s). Examples of agents affecting primarily T cells include OKT-3 (anti-CD3) and calcineurin inhibitors (eg, tacrolimus or cyclosporine). Rituximab (monoclonal anti-CD20) affects primarily B cells. Sirolimus, mycophenolic acid, azathiaprine, and corticosteroids have effects on both B cells and T cells.

Low-microbial diets are recommended for hematopoietic stem cell transplant recipients before engraftment of the donor marrow. If autologous, the suggested duration is 3 months. If allogeneic, a low-microbial diet is suggested until all immunosuppressive drugs are discontinued.[35] Solid organ transplant recipients remain at relatively higher lifelong risk, because of need for chronic immunosuppression.

Foodborne illnesses to which people with hematologic malignancy or transplants are more vulnerable include *Listeria, Toxoplasma, Salmonella* bacteremia, *Cryptosporidium, Giardia*, norovirus, and hepatitis E (reviewed in Ref.[36]).

Both patients with cancer and transplant recipients are believed to be at the highest risk for listeriosis, even amongst other populations termed vulnerable.[37] Data from France estimated the risk of listeriosis in transplant recipients and patients with hematologic malignancy as being more than 2500 times and 1000 time higher, respectively, than the risk of an individual younger than 65 years with no underlying medical conditions. (In comparison, alcoholics were estimated to be approximately 20 times more vulnerable, and dialysis recipients about 500 times more vulnerable than the average population.)

Bone marrow transplant recipients are believed to be particularly vulnerable to enteric viral infections, such as norovirus, or adenovirus (which can be transmitted by water). The case fatality rates for adenoviruses in bone marrow transplant recipients has been reported to range from 53% to 69%, depending on subgenus.[38] Children with bone marrow and solid organ transplants seem to be at the highest risk,[39] and diagnosis and management are not straightforward.[40] Both bone marrow and solid organ recipients are at risk for more severe and prolonged infections with norovirus, as are those with HIV and certain primary immunodeficiencies (reviewed in Ref.[41]). Again, diagnosis and treatment may not be straightforward. Dramatic weight loss and diarrhea can persist for months, with an extended period of viral shedding and more rapid evolution of the virus, presumably caused by limited immune pressure. In transplant recipients, decreasing immunosuppressive therapy must be considered, and passive administration of postpyloric immunoglobulin has been tried, with reports of anecdotal success.

PREGNANCY-RELATED IMMUNE SUPPRESSION

During pregnancy, alteration of cellular immune function leads to increased susceptibility to intracellular infections, most notably toxoplasmosis and listeriosis.[42] It is difficult to obtain an accurate assessment of the number of pregnancies in which either toxoplasmosis or listeriosis result in morbidity or mortality. However, studies in France estimate that close to 25% of listeriosis cases are maternal-fetal infections.[43] Listeriosis during pregnancy remains a significant problem in the United States. FoodNet Data from 2004 to 2009 describe epidemiology and overall and specific incidence rates and compares pregnancy-associated and non–pregnancy-associated cases. These data show that 12 of 762 cases were pregnancy related (17%), with increases in both pregnant Hispanic (5.09–12.37 cases per 100,000 for periods of 2004–2006 and 2007–2009, respectively) and non-Hispanic women (1.74–2.80 cases per 100,000 over the study period).[44]

Women may also be at an increased risk during pregnancy from enteric viruses and may act as a source of infection for neonates. At least 30 outbreaks of hepatitis E have been documented in 17 countries caused by contaminated water,[45] and foodborne outbreaks have been suspected. Although outbreaks of hepatitis E have not been reported in the United States, cases do occur among tourists returning from developing countries. Waterborne outbreaks have at times involved thousands of individuals. Overall, the case fatality ratios have ranged from 1% to 2% during outbreaks, which is significantly higher than that for the hepatitis A virus. However, for pregnant women, the ratio is generally between 10% and 20% and can be as high as 40%.[45,46]

Infection during pregnancy may also result in the transmission of infection from mother to child in utero, during birth, or shortly thereafter, with a potentially serious outcome.[18] This situation is especially true with *Listeria monocytogenes*. Neonates are uniquely susceptible to enterovirus infections, and this group of viruses can cause severe disease and death when infection occurs within the first l0 to 14 days of life. Enteroviruses are often acquired from the fecal-oral route, and one of the most significant viruses in this group with regard to children is coxsackie B. Acquisition of coxsackie B infections early in life is the most significant risk factor leading to fatal disease. The most fatal cases caused by this virus are probably transmitted transplacentally at term.[47]

FACTORS CONTRIBUTING TO FOODBORNE INFECTION

Although it may not be possible to protect all immunocompromised individuals from all foodborne infections, there are several steps that can be undertaken to minimize the potential risk. At the outset, it is important to recognize that certain groups are at greater risk than others.

According to the Council for Agricultural Science and Technology, most foodborne illnesses can be attributed to improper food-handling behaviors.[48] Leading causal behaviors are failure to (1) hold and cool foods appropriately, (2) practice proper personal hygiene, (3) prevent cross-contamination, (4) cook to proper internal temperatures, and (5) procure food from safe sources.

BASIC FOOD-HANDLING PRACTICES

Irrespective of the type of immune deficiency a person may have, and even if their immune systems are normal, there are 4 basic rules that should be followed to prevent foodborne illness: appropriate cleaning, proper separation of foods, adequate cooking, and maintaining foods at safe temperatures. A summary of the critical issues for each can be found in the subsequent sections.

Clean: Wash Hands and Surfaces Often

Wash hands and surfaces often with hot, soapy water (for at least 20 seconds) before and after handling food and after using the bathroom, changing diapers, and handling pets. Always wash hands, cutting boards, countertops, dishes, utensils, and spills in the refrigerator with hot, soapy water after they come in contact with raw foods and ready-to-eat foods (eg, hot dogs, luncheon meats, cold cuts, fermented and dry sausage, and other deli-style meat and poultry products). Wash hands after use of the bathroom or after handling animals or animal waste. Thorough washing helps eliminate any bacteria that might get on hands or other surfaces from food before it is reheated. Consider using paper towels to clean up kitchen surfaces. If you use cloth towels, wash them often in the hot cycle of your washing machine.

Separate: Do Not Cross-Contaminate

Cross-contamination is how bacteria can be spread. Ready-to-eat foods and raw meat, poultry, and seafood can contain dangerous bacteria. As a result, keep these foods and their juices separate from vegetables, fruits, breads, and other foods that are already prepared for eating. For example, separate raw meat, poultry, seafood and eggs from other foods in your grocery shopping cart, grocery bags, and in your refrigerator. Use 1 cutting board for fresh produce and a separate 1 for raw meat, poultry, and seafood. Never place cooked food on a plate that previously held raw meat, poultry, seafood, or eggs.

Cook: Cook to Proper Temperatures

Food is safely cooked when it reaches a high enough internal temperature to kill the harmful bacteria that cause foodborne illness. It is important to use a food thermometer to measure the internal temperature of cooked foods. When cooking at home, keep hot foods hot ($\geq 60°C/140°F$) and cold foods cold ($\leq 4°C/40°F$). Harmful bacteria can grow rapidly in the danger zone between these temperatures. These temperatures are different from those identified in the food code and offer an added degree of safety in a home environment, which may not be as controlled as a food service or retail establishment. The following recommendations in relation to cooking are especially important to avoid infection with *L monocytogenes*. Reheat until steaming hot the following types of ready-to-eat foods: hot dogs, luncheon meats, cold cuts, fermented and dry sausage, and other deli-style meat and poultry products. Thoroughly reheating food can help kill any bacteria that might be present. If you cannot reheat these foods, do not eat them.

We all enjoy the benefits of using the microwave oven for cooking and reheating foods in minutes, even seconds. However, microwaves often cook food unevenly, thus creating hot and cold spots in the food. Bacteria can survive in the cold spots.

This uneven cooking occurs because the microwaves bounce around the oven irregularly. Microwaves also heat food elements like fats, sugars, and liquids more quickly than carbohydrates and proteins. Extra care must be taken to even out the cooking so that harmful bacteria are destroyed.

Chill: Refrigerate Promptly

Refrigerate food quickly because cold temperatures keep most harmful bacteria from multiplying. Do not overstuff the refrigerator. Cold air must circulate to help keep food safe. Keeping a constant refrigerator temperature of 4°C (40°F) or below is one of the most effective ways to reduce the risk of foodborne illness. Use an appliance thermometer to be sure the temperature is correct. The freezer temperature should be 18°C (0°F) or below.

Perishables, prepared food, and leftovers should be refrigerated or frozen within 2 hours, and large amounts of leftovers should be divided into shallow containers to allow for quick cooling in the refrigerator. At family outings or barbecues, use a cooler to keep perishable foods cold. Always use ice or cold packs, and fill the cooler with food. A full cooler maintains its cold temperatures longer than one that is partially filled. Foods must be kept at a safe temperature during thawing. The safe ways to defrost food are in the refrigerator, in cold water, and in the microwave oven. Food thawed in cold water or in the microwave oven should be cooked immediately.

As noted earlier, food safety guidelines are fundamental in controlling foodborne illnesses in all populations. Although general education is essential in reducing cases and outbreaks of foodborne illnesses among all consumers, it is of particular importance for high-risk populations, either because of food consumption practices or greater vulnerability to specific pathogens.

SUMMARY

The immune system is a highly complex and integrated mechanism that can readily be compromised, thus increasing the risk of a person acquiring a foodborne infection. With improved medical therapies and the lengthening of the life span, the number of individuals with compromised immune systems is increasing and will continue to do so into the future. There is a significant amount of research and information available on how and why foodborne pathogens cause illness and how to prevent it from occurring. In theory, all foodborne illness is preventable and everyone who handles food from the grower to the consumer has a responsibility to ensure its safety while in their custody. Despite this situation, foodborne illnesses and deaths continue to occur. All consumers, including the immunocompromised, have a right to assume that the food they buy is safe; however, certain types of food, such as raw meat, are to be expected to have foodborne pathogens present. Therefore, proper handling of foods in health care settings and in the home is also critical, and health professionals have a responsibility to advise their patients on behaviors to minimize the likelihood of foodborne infection. Protecting the vulnerable from foodborne infection is a team effort that includes the manufacturer, health professionals (including doctors, nurses, registered dieticians, and transplant coordinators), and the patient. Studies of education of vulnerable populations about foodborne illnesses have shown that this may be challenging (reviewed in Refs.[49–51]). However, there are many educational tools available to assist the busy health professional with this mission. Some of these resources, geared toward specific populations, can be obtained from http://www.cdc.gov/foodsafety/consumers.html#populations. Available there are food safety guides for pregnant women, older adults, people with cancer, people with diabetes, people with HIV/AIDS, and transplant recipients.

REFERENCES

1. Maury J, Nicoletti C, Guzzo-Chambraud L, et al. The filamentous brush border glycocalyx, a mucin-like marker of enterocyte hyper-polarization. Eur J Biochem 1995;228(2):323–31.
2. Ayabe T, Satchell DP, Wilson CL, et al. Secretion of microbicidal alpha-defensins by intestinal Paneth cells in response to bacteria. Nat Immunol 2000;1(2):113–8.
3. Muniz LR, Knosp C, Yeretssian G. Intestinal antimicrobial peptides during homeostasis, infection and disease. Front Immunol 2012;3:310–7.
4. Lamont JT. Mucus: the front line of intestinal mucosal defense. Ann N Y Acad Sci 1992;664:190–201.
5. Kraehenbuhl JP, Neutra MR. Epithelial M cells: differentiation and function. Annu Rev Cell Dev Biol 2000;16:301–32.
6. Cazac BB, Roes J. TGF-beta receptor controls B cell responsiveness and induction of IgA in vivo. Immunity 2000;13(4):443–51.
7. Mowat AM. Anatomical basis of tolerance and immunity to intestinal antigens. Nat Rev Immunol 2003;3(4):331–41.
8. Leon F, Roldan E, Sanchez L, et al. Human small-intestinal epithelium contains functional natural killer lymphocytes. Gastroenterology 2003;125(2): 345–56.
9. Rolfe RD. Colonization resistance. In: Mackie RI, White BA, Isaacson RE, editors. Gastrointestinal microbiology. New York: Chapman & Hall; 1997. p. 501–36.
10. Tannock GW. Modification of the normal microbiota by diet, stress, antimicrobial agents, and probiotics. In: Mackie RI, White BA, Isaacson RE, editors. Gastrointestinal microbiology. New York: Chapman & Hall; 1997. p. 434–65.
11. Sampson H. Food allergy. In: Middleton E, editor. Allergy: principles and practice. New York: Mosby-Year Book; 2003.
12. Sugiyama H, Mills DC. Intraintestinal toxin in infant mice challenged intragastrically with Clostridium botulinum spores. Infect Immun 1978;21(1):59–63.
13. Gaskins HR. Immunological aspects of host/microbiota interactions at the intestinal epithelium. In: Mackie RI, White BA, Isaacson RE, editors. Gastrointestinal microbiology. New York: Chapman & Hall; 1997. p. 537–87.
14. Berg RD. Bacterial translocation from the gastrointestinal tract. Adv Exp Med Biol 1999;473:11–30.
15. O'Boyle CJ, MacFie J, Mitchell CJ, et al. Microbiology of bacterial translocation in humans. Gut 1998;42(1):29–35.
16. Guarner C, Runyon BA, Young S, et al. Intestinal bacterial overgrowth and bacterial translocation in cirrhotic rats with ascites. J Hepatol 1997;26(6): 1372–8.
17. Smith JL. Long-term consequences of foodborne toxoplasmosis: effects on the unborn, the immunocompromised, the elderly and the immunocompetent. J Food Prot 1997;60:1595–611.
18. Gerber CP, Rose JB, Haas CN. Sensitive populations: who is at the greatest risk? Int J Food Microbiol 1996;30:112–23.
19. Kendall P, Medeiros LC, Hillers V, et al. Food handling behaviors of special importance for pregnant women, infants and young children, the elderly, and immune-compromised people. J Am Diet Assoc 2003;103:1646–9.

20. National Center for Health Statistics. Health, United States, 2003. Hyattsville (MD): US Department of Health and Human Services, Centers for Disease Control and Prevention; 2003.
21. Centers for Disease Control and Prevention. Public health and aging: trends in aging–United States and worldwide. MMWR Morb Mortal Wkly Rep 2003;52(06): 101–6.
22. Smith JL. Foodborne illness in the elderly. J Food Prot 1998;61:1229–39.
23. Meyers BR. Infectious diseases in the elderly: an overview. Geriatrics 1989;44: 4–6.
24. Lew JF, Glass R, Gangarosa RE, et al. Diarrhea1 deaths in the United States, 1979 through 1987. J Am Med Assoc 1991;265:3280–4.
25. Gordon SM, Oshiro LS, Jarvis WR, et al. Foodborne Snow Mountain agent gastroenteritis with secondary person-to-person spread in a retirement community. Am J Epidemiol 1990;131(4):702–10.
26. Ledner WM, Lemon SM, Kirkpatrick JW, et al. Frequency of illness associated with epidemic hepatitis A virus infections in adults. Am J Epidemiol 1985;122: 226–33.
27. Bowen GS, McCarthy MA. Hepatitis A associated with a hardware store water fountain and a contaminated well in Lancaster County, Pennsylvania 1980. Am J Epidemiol 1983;117:695–705.
28. Gust I. Design of hepatitis A vaccines. Br Med Bull 1990;46:319–28.
29. Gottschlich MM. Nutrition in the burned pediatric patient. In: Queen PM, Lang CE, editors. Handbook of pediatric nutrition. Gaithersburg (MD): Aspen Publishers; 1993. p. 537.
30. Buzby JC. Children and microbial foodborne illness. FoodReview 2001;24(2): 32–7.
31. Cunningham AL, Grohman GS, Hatkness J, et al. Gastrointestinal viral infections in homosexual men who were symptomatic and seropositive for immunodeficiency virus. J Infect Dis 1988;158:386–91.
32. Gorbach SL, Gorbach Bartlett JG, Backlow NR. Infectious disease. New York: WB Saunders; 1992.
33. Baine WB, Gangarosa EJ, Bennett JV. Institutional salmonellosis. J Infect Dis 1982;128:357–682.
34. Clifford CP, Crook DW, Conlon CP, et al. Impact of waterborne outbreak of cryptosporidiosis on AIDS and renal transplant patients. Lancet 1990;1: 1455–6.
35. Centers for Disease Control and Prevention (CDC). Guidelines for preventing opportunistic infections among hematopoietic stem cell transplant recipients. Recommendations of CDC, the Infectious Disease Society of America, and the American Society of Blood and Marrow Transplantation. MMWR Morb Mortal Wkly Rep 2000;49(RR10):1–128.
36. Lund BM, O'Brien SJ. The occurrence and prevention of foodborne disease in vulnerable people. Foodborne Pathog Dis 2011;8(9):961–73.
37. World Health Organization/Food and Agriculture Organization (WHO/FAO). Risk assessment of *Listeria monocytogenes* in RTE foods. MRA Series 5. Rome (Italy): World Health Organization/Food and Agriculture Organization (WHO/FAO); 2004.
38. Yolken RH, Bishop CA, Townsend TR, et al. Infectious gastroenteritis in bone marrow recipients. N Engl J Med 1982;306:1009–12.
39. Echavarria M. Adenoviruses in immunocompromised hosts. Clin Microbiol Rev 2008;21:704–15.

40. Lindemans CA, Leen AM, Boelens JJ. How I treat adenovirus in hemtapoietic stem cell transplant recipients. Blood 2010;116:5476–85.
41. Bok K, Green KY. Norovirus gastroenteritis in immunocompromised patients. N Engl J Med 2012;367:2126–32.
42. Hierholzer JC. Adenoviruses in the immunocompromised host. Clin Microbiol Rev 1992;5:262–74.
43. Townsend TR, Yolken RH, Bishop CA, et al. Outbreak of coxsackie Al gastroenteritis, a complication of bone-marrow transplantation. Lancet 1982;1: 820–3.
44. Silk BJ, Date KA, Jackson KA, et al. Invasive listeriosis in the Foodborne Diseases Active Surveillance Network (FoodNet), 2004-2009: further targeted prevention needed for higher-risk groups. Clin Infect Dis 2012;54(Suppl 5): S396–404.
45. Smith JL. Foodborne infections during pregnancy. J Food Prot 1999;62:818–29.
46. Goulet V, Jacquet C, Martin P, et al. Surveillance of human listeriosis in France, 2001-2003. Euro Surveill 2006;11(6):79–81.
47. Craske J. Hepatitis C and non-A non-B hepatitis revisited: hepatitis E, F and G. J Infect 1992;25:243–50.
48. Gust I, Purcell RH. Report of a workshop: waterborne non-A non-B hepatitis. J Infect Dis 1987;156:630–5.
49. Obayashi PA. Food safety for the solid organ transplant patient: preventing foodborne illness while on chronic immunosuppressive drugs. Nutr Clin Pract 2012;27(6):758–66.
50. Kaplan MH, Klein SW, McPhee J, et al. Group B coxsackievirus infections in infants younger than three months of age: a serious childhood illness. Rev Infect Dis 1983;5:1019–32.
51. Herringshaw D, Longo M. Healthy kids: germ free. J Nutr Educ 2000;32(233A): 22–3.

Shiga Toxin–Producing *Escherichia coli* O104:H4

An Emerging Pathogen with Enhanced Virulence

Dakshina M. Jandhyala, PhD[a],*, Vijay Vanguri, MD[b],
Erik J. Boll, PhD[c], YuShuan Lai[c], Beth A. McCormick, PhD[c],
John M. Leong, MD, PhD[d]

KEYWORDS

- EAEC • Shiga toxin • Hemolytic uremic syndrome • Bloody diarrhea
- Foodborne illness • O104:H4 • STEC

KEY POINTS

- Pathogenic *Escherichia coli* are genetically diverse and encompass a broad variety of pathotypes, such as Shiga toxin–producing *Escherichia coli* (STEC) or enteroaggregative *E coli* (EAEC), which cause distinct clinical syndromes.
- STEC is a major foodborne pathogen worldwide and can cause hemolytic uremic syndrome (HUS), the triad of anemia, thrombocytopenia, and renal failure.
- The STEC most commonly associated with disease is *E coli* serotype O157:H7, but there has been increasing awareness of the threat posed by non-O157 STEC strains.
- A major outbreak of STEC disease in Germany in 2011 was associated with an unusually high rate of HUS, with more than 900 cases, making it the single most severe recorded outbreak of STEC.
- The German outbreak strain, STEC O104:H4, is genetically similar to EAEC O104:H4, but is lysogenized by a lambdoid phage that encodes Shiga toxin.
- STEC O104:H4, likely derived in part by the acquisition of a Shiga toxin–encoding phage by an EAEC strain, represents an emerging foodborne pathogen with enhanced capacity to cause severe illness.

Disclosure: Support of our work was made through grants from the National Institute of Health, Bethesda, MA: AI088336-02 (D.M.J.), DK56754 and DK33506 (B.A.M.), and AI46454 (J.M.L.); the Carlsberg Foundation Post-Doctoral Scholarship (E.J.B.); and the Charlton Grant Research Program, Tufts University (D.M.J.).

[a] Division of Geographic Medicine and Infectious Diseases, Tufts Medical Center, 750 Washington Street, Boston, MA 02111, USA; [b] Department of Pathology, University of Massachusetts Medical School, One Innovation Drive, Biotech Three, Worcester, MA 01605, USA; [c] Department of Microbiology and Physiological Systems, University of Massachusetts Medical School, 55 Lake Avenue North, Worcester, MA 01655, USA; [d] Department of Molecular Biology and Microbiology, Tufts University School of Medicine, 136 Harrison Avenue, Boston, MA 02111, USA
* Corresponding author.
E-mail address: djandhyala@tuftsmedicalcenter.org

Infect Dis Clin N Am 27 (2013) 631–649
http://dx.doi.org/10.1016/j.idc.2013.05.002
0891-5520/13/$
id.theclinics.com

DIVERSE *ESCHERICHIA COLI* PATHOTYPES

Escherichia coli are largely commensal bacteria residing in the mucus layer of the mammalian colon. However, several strains have virulence attributes that give them the capacity to cause diarrheal, urogenic, or systemic illnesses. Pathogenic *E coli* have been categorized into several pathotypes, each causing illness with distinctive features, and 6 pathotypes, including enterohemorrhagic *E coli* (EHEC), enterotoxogenic *E coli* (ETEC), and enteroaggregative *E coli* (EAEC), are associated with intestinal disease.[1] These may also be subdivided into serogroups and serotypes based on their lipopolysaccharide (O) or flagellar (H) antigens.

SHIGA TOXIN–PRODUCING *E COLI*, INCLUDING EHEC

Shiga toxin-producing *E coli* (STEC) are a diverse group of bacteria that produce 1 or more types of Shiga toxin (Stx).[1,2] They comprise many serotypes, and virulence may differ between strains, with some having an estimated infectious dose in the range of 1 to 100 colony forming units.[2] EHEC are a subset of STEC that carry the locus of enterocyte effacement (LEE) pathogenicity island (described later) and are associated with disease in humans. A subset of EHEC, EHEC 1, includes serotype O157:H7 and is clinically the most important group, responsible for ~73,000 cases annually in the United States[3] and most STEC infections worldwide.[4,5] Recently, there has been an increasing awareness that non-O157 STEC strains represent a significant and growing health threat.[6]

STX-INDUCED DISEASE

Individuals of both sexes and all ages can suffer severe EHEC-mediated disease, but children and women seem to be at a higher risk, and elderly people often develop neurologic disease and have a higher mortality.[7,8] Hemorrhagic colitis is a serious local manifestation of Stx-mediated disease and can progress to gangrenous colitis, bowel perforation, as well as peritonitis or sepsis.[8] In the United States, approximately 5% to 10% of reported O157:H7 infections result in hemolytic uremic syndrome (HUS),[3,7] the triad of hemolytic anemia, thrombocytopenia, and renal failure.

HUS is characterized by a thrombotic microangiopathy that involves Stx-mediated dysregulation of the alternative complement pathway, damage to endothelium, and consumption of platelets.[9] The kidney is the most frequently affected organ, and HUS is a leading cause of renal failure in children, with a mortality of 3% to 5%.[10] The vasculopathy can be seen in extrarenal sites as well, including the mesenteric bed, lung, heart, and pancreas. Central nervous system involvement is also present in a subset of cases, and neurologic sequelae may be ominous and associated with significant rates of mortality.[7] Histologic lesions of HUS consist of endothelial damage and platelet-fibrin thrombi, frequently in the glomeruli of the kidney. Ultrastructural evaluation of kidney biopsies in patients with HUS shows glomerular endothelial swelling and loss of fenestrations, as well as separation of the endothelial cell from the basement membrane by an intervening accumulation of electron lucent debris. The endothelial damage precedes the development of the classic clinical triad of oliguric or anuric acute kidney injury, microangiopathic hemolytic anemia, and decreased platelet count.[11] Long-term chronic sequelae including chronic kidney disease, arterial hypertension, neurologic impairment, and diabetes mellitus have been reported to occur in 20% of patients with childhood HUS.[8]

The spectrum of tissue damage in HUS is likely caused by tissue distribution of the Stx receptor globotriaosyl ceramide (Gb$_3$).[12] Human glomerular epithelial cells, proximal tubular cells, and renal microvascular endothelial cells produce Gb_3 and are sensitive to Stx.[13–15] Similarly, microvascular and neural tissue of the central nervous system are Gb_3-positive, providing a plausible explanation for the neurologic manifestations of STEC-mediated disease.[16]

CLINICAL COURSE OF EHEC O157:H7 INFECTION

On EHEC O157:H7 ingestion, diarrhea typically begins after just a few days (although the range may span 2–12 days), and after 1 to 3 days the diarrhea becomes bloody in 80% to 90% of patients (**Fig. 1**).[11,17,18] Approximately a week after the onset of diarrhea, most patients begin to show signs of improvement, but 5% to 10% develop severe systemic disease, such as HUS. Given the seriousness of HUS, bloody diarrhea after 1 to 3 days of nonbloody diarrhea, especially in children, warrants concern for infection with EHEC.[19]

DIAGNOSIS OF EHEC O157:H7

In the United States, EHEC O157:H7, which can be identified on sorbitol MacConkey (SMAC) agar, is the only STEC for which screening is common (although not uniformly routine[20]). The SMAC agar assay does not specifically detect non-O157 STEC serogroups,[3] so measurement of stool-associated Stx by enzyme immune assay (EIA) is often advised to identify these infections.[3,21] However, Stx in stool may be at nondetectable concentrations, thereby requiring enrichment steps. Furthermore, EIAs can deliver false-positive results or detect STEC that are unlikely to cause HUS. Both SMAC and EIA detection methods require significant time, potentially

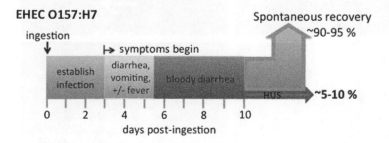

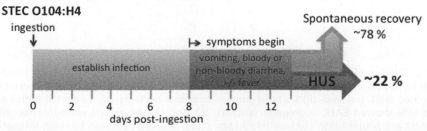

Fig. 1. The course of disease of EHEC O157:H7 infection differs from that of STEC O104:H4. Note the longer median incubation time before symptom onset for the STEC O104:H4 outbreak strain compared with EHEC O157:H7. (*Data from* Tarr PI, Gordon CA, Chandler WL. Shiga-toxin-producing *Escherichia coli* and haemolytic uraemic syndrome. Lancet 2005;365(9464):1073–86; and Frank C, Werber D, Cramer JP, et al. Epidemic profile of Shiga-toxin-producing *Escherichia coli* O104:H4 outbreak in Germany. N Engl J Med 2011;365(19):1771–80.)

delaying appropriate patient management, and therefore molecular diagnostics such as polymerase chain reaction are a potentially time-saving alternative.[22] However, no molecular diagnostics for STEC have been approved by the US Food and Drug Administration.[3]

VIRULENCE FEATURES OF EHEC

A key virulence feature of EHEC O157:H7 is its ability to form attaching and effacing (AE) lesions on the intestinal epithelium. These lesions are characterized by the intimate attachment of bacteria to the host cell, the effacement of epithelial microvilli, and formation of actin pedestallike structures beneath bound bacteria (**Fig. 2**) on the surface of epithelial cells. The formation of AE lesions depends on the LEE, a pathogenicity island that encodes proteins required for attachment, several effector proteins that act in the host cell cytoplasm, and a type 3 secretion system that mediates the injection of these effectors into the host cell cytoplasm.[23]

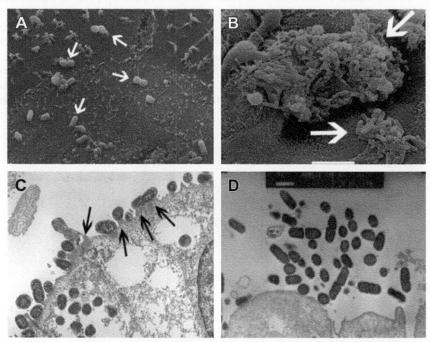

Fig. 2. EHEC and EAEC interact with host cells in distinct fashions. (*A*) CaCo-2a cells infected with EHEC derivative strain TUV-93[104] and scanning electron microscopy (SEM) showed cell-attached EHEC (*arrows*). (*B*) Cultured human intestinal explants were infected with EAEC and SEM showed EAEC aggregates (*arrows*). (*C*) Gnotobiotic piglets were infected with TUV-93 and transmission electron microscopy (TEM) showed pedestals beneath intimately attached EHEC (*arrows*). (*D*) Polarized T84 intestinal epithelial cells were infected with EAEC strain 042 and TEM indicated attached bacterial aggregates and effacement of the apical brush border. ([*B, D*] *Adapted from* Nataro JP, Hicks S, Phillips AD, et al. T84 cells in culture as a model for enteroaggregative *Escherichia coli* pathogenesis. Infect Immun 1996;64(11):4761–8, with permission; and Nataro JP, Steiner T, Guerrant RL. Enteroaggregative *Escherichia coli*. Emerg Infect Dis 1998;4(2):251–61; [*C*] *Courtesy of* A. Donohue-Rolfe and S. Tzipori.)

PROPERTIES OF STX

Although HUS as a clinical syndrome can occur outside bacterial infection (so-called atypical HUS), EHEC, by virtue of its production of Stxs, is responsible for most HUS cases.[24–26] Based on protein sequence and serotype, Stxs are grouped into 2 major types (Stx1 or Stx2),[27] and for reasons that are not clear, EHEC O157:H7 strains that produce only Stx2 are associated with a higher risk for HUS.[2] Stxs are potent cytotoxins consisting of a single enzymatically active A-subunit noncovalently associated with 5 B-subunits.[2] The Stx B-subunits bind a host cell surface glycosphingolipid receptor termed Gb_3. After receptor binding, the toxin is endocytosed and by a process termed retrotranslocation moves from the early endosome through the Golgi to the endoplasmic reticulum, where the A-subunit is translocated to the cytoplasm. The A-subunit depurinates a specific adenine residue of the 28S ribosomal RNA subunit,[28,29] resulting in the inhibition of protein synthesis and activation of proinflammatory and proapoptotic pathways.[30–32]

TREATMENT OF EHEC O157:H7 INFECTION

Data from EHEC O157:H7 outbreaks and experimental models suggest Stx upregulation on treatment with ciprofloxacin,[33–38] and antimicrobials, particularly fluoroquinolones, are generally withheld because of the concern that such therapy may precipitate HUS.[8,11,39] A potential explanation for the apparent increased risk of HUS after antibiotic treatment as observed in some studies is that activation of the SOS stress response by certain antibiotics such as fluoroquinolones can induce the lysogenic phage encoding Stx, resulting in the production and release of toxin.[40–42] In addition, released phage may infect other susceptible *E coli* present in the gut, further amplifying Stx production.[43] However, the response to some antibiotics may be strain dependent,[44,45] and some studies suggest that antibiotic treatment is not associated with a risk of HUS[46] or might reduce the risk of HUS.[47]

Given that no therapy has been conclusively shown to prevent the onset of HUS or reduce renal damage once HUS has occurred, treatment of EHEC-mediated disease is generally limited to supportive measures.[8,11,24,48] Treatments used for other forms of diarrhea or for diseases similar to HUS, such as thrombotic thrombocytopenia purpura (TTP) or atypical HUS, are either contraindicated for treating STEC-associated disease or have limited or conflicting evidence supporting efficacy. For example, the use of antimotility agents in patients with STEC infection has been associated with a greater risk of HUS and neurologic manifestations, or a sustained duration of bloody diarrhea in patients who do not have HUS.[46,49,50] The efficacy or safety of treatments such as plasma exchange, the use of glucocorticoids, and recently eculizumab (Soliris), which is used to treat atypical HUS, is undetermined.[51,52] In contrast, the supportive therapy for volume expansion beginning within the first 4 days after presentation of EHEC O157:H7-mediated diarrhea is associated with protection from oligoanuria, emphasizing the importance of early detection and hospitalization of patients with EHEC infection.[53,54]

EAEC

A second *E coli* pathotype is EAEC (also known as EAggEC), which was first described in the mid-1980s.[55,56] EAEC is a major cause of travelers' diarrhea,[57] persistent diarrhea amongst patients positive for the human immunodeficiency virus[58,59] and malnourished children,[60,61] acute diarrhea in adults and children in the United States,[62] and an agent of foodborne outbreaks.[63,64] EAEC can also persist subclinically.[65] A characteristic attribute of EAEC is its ability to form biofilms on abiotic surfaces and its corresponding aggregative adherence (AA) to mammalian cells, which has been described as resulting in a stacked-brick appearance.[66] EAEC encompass diverse serotypes, but notably with respect to the recent emergence of a new non-O157 STEC strain (see later discussion) include strains of serotype O104:H4.[67] Thus, clinical and phylogenetic features support the conclusion that EAEC represent a distinct but highly heterogeneous E coli pathotype.[68]

PATHOGENESIS OF EAEC

EAEC causes tissue damage, including local inflammation, on colonization of the intestinal mucosa (reviewed in Ref.[68]). Inflammation may be a result of the exuberant colonization of the mucosal surface, but EAEC also encodes toxins that can directly damage host cells (**Table 1**). Although few data are available concerning the segment(s) of the human intestine that are colonized by EAEC, infection of organ cultures/human intestinal biopsy cultures suggests that EAEC can adhere to the small and large bowel mucosa, although the relative specificity for each of these intestinal segments may differ between strains.[68,69] In gnotobiotic piglets, EAEC form a thick mucus gellike matrix containing stacked-brick bacterial aggregates on the epithelium of the distal small intestine and cecum, with concomitant hyperemia and diarrhea.[70] In intestinal loop models, EAEC strains induce villus shortening and hemorrhagic necrosis of the villus tips, edema, and submucosal mononuclear infiltration.[71]

VIRULENCE FEATURES OF EAEC

Given the signs and symptoms and intestinal pathology of EAEC infection, much of the effort to understand the pathogenesis of EAEC infection has centered on virulence factors that promote AA, mucosal damage, inflammation, or fluid secretion. The EAEC strain 042 and a few other strains have served as models for diarrheal EAEC in many studies, and 1 caveat to our understanding of EAEC is that a small group of strains may not reflect the full heterogeneity of this pathotype. The documented or putative EAEC virulence factors are summarized in **Table 1**.

AA fimbriae (AAF), as well as proteins that promote proper localization of fimbriae on the bacterial surface, facilitate adherence to the human intestinal mucosa and formation of a thick biofilm within the mucus layer covering the epithelium, thus promoting persistent mucosal colonization.[72] This process may also trigger host inflammatory responses[73,74] and disrupt epithelial barrier function.[75] The serine protease autotransporters of Enterobacteriaceae (SPATEs), which are commonly found in EAEC as well as other diarrheagenic E coli, modulate immune responses,[76] alter the intestinal epithelial cytoskeleton,[77] and in some studies, are strongly associated with clinical illness.[78] The putative virulence factor EAEC heat-stabile enterotoxin 1 shares amino acid similarity with the heat-stabile enterotoxin of ETEC and shows enterotoxic activity in vitro.[79] AggR is a transcriptional regulator that controls several genes, including those associated with AAF and at least 2 pathogenicity islands.[80,81]

TREATMENT OF EAEC

EAEC-associated diarrhea lasted a mean of 17 days in an early cohort study, indicating that this pathogen can cause a persistent infection that might lead to malnutrition in children, and providing a potential rationale for antibiotic-mediated eradication or nutritional supplementation.[82,83] Early eradication of EAEC using antibiotics may also prevent person-to-person transmission, particularly during outbreaks. Treatment

Table 1
Virulence factors of EAEC

EAEC Virulence Factors	Clinical Attributes and Biological Characteristics	2011 Outbreak Strain[a]
Adhesins and Colonization Factors		
AAF	Contributes to the characteristic AA phenotype and facilitates adherence, epithelial barrier disruption, and inflammation. AAF I, II, III, and IV are plasmid encoded[73–75,105,106]	+ (AAF/I)
Other non-AAF adhesins (eg, Hda)	Contributes to the characteristic stacked-brick phenotype[107]	
Dispersin (*aap*)	Promotes penetration of intestinal mucus and may promote colonization of the epithelium[108,109]	+
Enterotoxins and Hemolysins		
Enteroaggregative heat-stabile toxin 1 (EAST1, *astA*)	Similar to the heat-stabile enterotoxin of ETEC[79]	
Shigella enterotoxin-1 (ShET-1)	Enterotoxin that induces secretion[110]	
Hemolysin E (*hlyE*)	A pore-forming hemolysin; the role in pathogenesis has not been determined, and it is present in pathogenic and nonpathogenic EAEC[111]	
Member of SPATE (Serine Protease Autotransporters of Enterobacteriaceae)		
Pet (plasmid encoded toxin)	Enterotoxin with protease and cytoskeletal altering activities[112,113]	
Pic (protein involved in colonization)	Modulates immune responses and induces the secretion and degradation of mucin; may contribute to the mucus-rich biofilm that is characteristic of EAEC mucosal colonization[76,114]	+
SigA	The *Shigella flexneri* homolog alters the cytoskeleton in intestinal epithelial cells, similar to Pet[77]	+
SepA	Associated with illness, and the *Shigella flexneri* homolog has been shown to contribute to intestinal inflammation and mucosal atrophy[78,115]	+
Transcription Factor		
Transcriptional regulator AggR (*aggR*)	Global regulator of EAEC virulence genes, including the AAF operons and *aap*; common to most EAEC; not absolutely required for virulence[80,116]	+
Other		
Flagellin	Highly conserved bacterial protein required for motility; interaction with basolaterally expressed toll-like receptor 5 on intestinal epithelial cells results in induction of the neutrophil chemoattractant interleukin-8[117,118]	+

Abbreviation: AAF, AA fimbriae.
[a] + indicates that the German STEC O104:H4 outbreak strain encodes the virulence factor.

of EAEC can be limited by the ubiquitous presence of antibiotic resistance genes. Ninety percent of diarrheal EAEC isolates were found to be resistant or partially resistant to several antibiotics, including β-lactams, chloramphenicol, streptomycin, kanamycin, tetracycline, sulfamethoxazole, and trimethoprim.[84] Resistance to carbapenems and quinolones was absent or rare among the isolates analyzed. Ciprofloxacin resistance has been noted rarely, and the drug has been used successfully to treat EAEC infection.[83] In general, fluoroquinolones, amoxicillin/clavulanic acid, azithromycin, rifaximin, and nalidixic acid may be effective treatments for EAEC.[85–87]

GERMAN STEC O104:H4 OUTBREAK OF 2011, ASSOCIATED WITH A HIGH RATE OF HUS

Between early May and late July 2011, a cluster of STEC outbreaks took place in Europe, resulting in 4075 infections, 908 cases of HUS, and more than 50 deaths, 34 of which were associated with HUS.[88,89] This episode represents the largest recorded outbreak of HUS. Although persons from 16 countries were affected, cases in Germany represented more than 95% of the reported infections. The causative agent in this outbreak was STEC O104:H4, which was traced to contaminated fenugreek sprouts.[90] The O104:H4 serotype has been associated with non–Stx-producing EAEC isolates[67] as well as with rare STEC-mediated disease in humans,[91–95] with only 5 reported cases in the last 12 years. The nature of the German outbreak differed from previous EHEC O157 outbreaks in several other ways. First, the incidence of bloody diarrhea or HUS was higher in adults than in children,[89] in contrast to the more commonly observed increased risk of serious disease among children and the elderly. Although it is hard to assess to what extent the different epidemiologic features reflect the differences in the mode of acquisition, they may reflect (unidentified) differences in fundamental aspects of pathogenesis. Consistent with the latter suggestion, the median time of incubation before the development of symptoms (8 days) was greater than the 3-day to 4-day incubation period typically reported for EHEC O157:H7 (see **Fig. 1**).[89] In addition, the percentage of HUS cases among infected individuals (22%) was higher than the 5% to 10% rate, typically reported for HUS from large EHEC O157:H7 outbreaks, suggesting that the outbreak strain was particularly virulent.[3,7]

PATHOGENESIS OF STEC O104:H4

Although the German outbreak is too recent to permit extensive exploration of the pathogenesis of STEC O104:H4, it is clear that this strain causes a disease distinct from that caused by EHEC O157:H7. For example, whereas EHEC O157:H7 forms AE lesions on the epithelial surface (see **Fig. 2**), the O104:H4 strain forms aggregates closely associated with the mucus layer in germ-free mice[96] or on monkey colonic explants (**Fig. 3**). Germ-free mice infected with EHEC O157:H7 developed acute renal tubular necrosis (ATN) 5 days after infection, whereas animals infected with STEC O104:H4 did not develop ATN until 13 to 15 days after infection, consistent with the longer incubation period for human disease (see **Fig. 1**).[89,96] Ampicilin-treated mice infected with STEC O104:H4 lost weight, developed ATN, and died, whereas the disease in mice infected with Stx2-negative O104:H4 strains was less severe. These findings were recapitulated in a rabbit model, emphasizing a role of Stx2 in the virulence of STEC O104:H4.[97]

STEC O104:H4, A HYBRID PATHOGEN

Consistent with its unique features, the STEC O104:H4 strain responsible for the German outbreak differs in 2 main aspects from most other clinically important

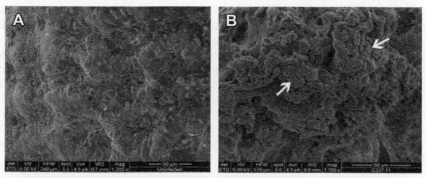

Fig. 3. STEC O104:H4 strain C227-11 forms aggregates on colonic mucosa. Uninfected monkey colonic explants (*A*) or those infected with the German outbreak strain C227-11 (*B*) were subjected to SEM. Arrow indicates bacterial aggregates. (*Courtesy of* N. Boisen and J. Nataro, University of Virginia School of Medicine, VA. Processed at the Core Imaging Facility at the University of Maryland, Baltimore, MD.)

STEC strains. First, it lacks the LEE pathogenicity island that encodes the type III translocation system. Second, the STEC O104:H4 outbreak strain encodes many virulence factors commonly produced by EAEC, including AAF (specifically AAF/I), SPATE proteases, and the AggR global regulator (**Fig. 4**).[67,98]

In contrast to EAEC strains, STEC O104:H4 encodes Stx2, consistent with the ability to induce HUS. As mentioned earlier, EHEC O157:H7 strains expressing Stx2 alone

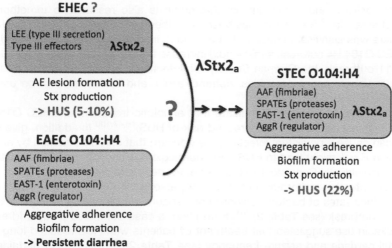

Fig. 4. Possible derivation of the 2011 German outbreak strain STEC O104:H4. EHEC and EAEC encode distinct sets of virulence factors and are associated with different modes of pathogenesis. EAEC O104:H4 may have acquired the lambdoid $Stx2_a$ phage from a hypothetical EHEC donor to generate STEC O104:H4. This strain, which encodes a combination of EAEC and EHEC virulence factors, is associated with an increased rate of HUS. (*Data from* Rasko DA, Webster DR, Sahl JW, et al. Origins of the *E. coli* strain causing an outbreak of hemolytic-uremic syndrome in Germany. N Engl J Med 2011;365(8):709–17; and Brzuszkiewicz E, Thurmer A, Schuldes J, et al. Genome sequence analyses of two isolates from the recent *Escherichia coli* outbreak in Germany reveal the emergence of a new pathotype: entero-aggregative-haemorrhagic *Escherichia coli* (EAHEC). Arch Microbiol 2011;193(12):883–91.)

(rather than Stx1 alone or both Stx1 and Stx2) are associated with a greater risk of HUS.[2] Genomic sequencing showed that, similar to EHEC, the German STEC O104:H4 strain encodes $Stx2_a$ within a lysogenized lambdoid bacteriophage.[67] A phylogenetic comparison of outbreak isolates with several EAEC O104:H4 strains showed that only the outbreak isolates are lysogenic for the $Stx2_a$ phage.[67] In addition, the outbreak strain carries a plasmid that encodes an extended-spectrum β-lactamase CTX-M-15, a β-lactamase that is uncommon amongst other O104:H4 isolates.[67] These observations support the hypothesis that the recent acquisition of the phage-encoded virulence factor $Stx2_a$, as well as an antibiotic resistance determinant, has given rise to the exceptionally virulent STEC O104:H4 German outbreak strain (see **Fig. 4**).

TREATMENT OF STEC O104:H4 INFECTION

The enormity of the 2011 STEC O104:H4 outbreak in Germany resulted in many patients undergoing different treatments throughout the country, and allowed for a multicenter case-controlled study concerning the efficacy of different strategies to treat STEC O104:H4-associated HUS.[52] Treatments reported include the use of antibiotics, therapeutic plasma exchange (TPE), TPE with glucocorticoids, immunoadsorption, and the use of the alternative complement pathway inhibitor eculizumab (summarized in **Table 2**).

Whether or not to treat diarrheal infections with antimicrobials during the German STEC O104:H4 outbreak strain was not straightforward. This strain was shown to be resistant to all penicillins and cephalosporins, consistent with the presence of a β-lactamase–producing plasmid.[95,98] Although susceptible to fluoroquinolones, aminoglycosides, and carbapenems, this strain is also resistant to trimethoprim-sulfamethoxazole.[98] Second, as has been described earlier for EHEC O157:H7 infection, there was significant concern that antibiotic treatment of patients infected with the STEC O104:H4 outbreak strain would increase the risk of HUS. As a result, during the 2011 outbreak, the German Society for Infectious Disease recommended that fluoroquinolones, aminoglycosides, cotrimoxazole, and fosfomycin not be used to treat patients with STEC infection.[99]

Nevertheless, not all studies indicate that antibiotic treatment of EHEC O157:H7 infection is associated with an increased risk of HUS.[46,47,100] In addition, given that EAEC can cause a persistent infection, the concern that chronic infection by an Stx-producing E coli might lead to HUS and neurologic dysfunction motivated treatment of some individuals. Consistent with the effectiveness of antibiotic treatment of non–Stx-EAEC infection, azithromycin therapy in persons with HUS appeared to significantly reduce rates of bacterial colonization, seizure, and mortality during the STEC O104:H4 outbreak (see **Table 2**).[101] In addition, a case-controlled study addressing ciprofloxacin use suggested that treatment of patients with HUS reduced long-term intestinal carriage and seizure frequency (see **Table 2**).[52] This finding pertained to treatment during but not before HUS. Although the current data are inconclusive as to the risk or benefit of antibiotic treatment of STEC O104:H4 infection, it is tempting to speculate that antibiotics incapable of inducing Stx phage could be beneficial.

TPE is a cornerstone of therapy for TTP,[102] which, like HUS, is a thrombotic microangiopathy. Nevertheless, rather than a manifestation of toxemia, TTP seems in many cases to be caused by a self-reactive antibody to the metalloproteinase ADAMTS13, resulting in lower rates of cleavage of von Willebrand factor multimers and a subsequent procoagulant state. TPE decreases levels of the pathogenic antibody in TTP. Stx-mediated HUS does not seem to respond to this treatment,[9] a finding that could

Table 2
Studies of treatment efficacy for STEC O104:H4 infection

Treatment	Notes/Results	Reference(s)
Meropenam/ciprofloxacin (intensive care unit: + rifaximin)[a]	A significant decrease in mortality, duration of STEC excretion in stools (ie, 8 days shorter), and incidence of seizures in treated patients, who presented with HUS before antibiotic treatment	52
Azithromycin[b]	Used for meningococcal prophylaxis in patients with HUS being treated with eculizumab. Treatment was associated with a decrease in the frequency of long-term O104:H4 carriage	101
Various antibiotics	Study of 24 patients, of whom 7 were treated with various antibiotics, including ciprofloxacin. 57% of antibiotic-treated patients compared with 88% of controls developed HUS.	119
TPE	No benefit among 251 patients with HUS who underwent TPE vs 47 patients not given TPE, but who also had milder disease	52
TPE	5 patients with HUS with progressive neurologic dysfunction who underwent TPE recovered. Justification of TPE has been questioned	120,121
Prednisone + TPE	No benefit detected in patients pretreated with prednisone before TPE vs TPE alone	52
Immunoadsorption	12 patients with HUS who developed neurologic signs a median of 8 days after enteritis onset were treated with multiple courses of immunoadsorption. All patients survived and 10 recovered completely. The rationale for treatment was that the late onset of neurologic symptoms indicated an autoimmune response, but autoantibodies were not immunologically validated	102
Eculizumab	One report of 3 children with HUS who underwent TPE and eculizumab treatment who were reported to have improved dramatically	103
Eculizumab	No benefit was conferred to 67 adult HUS patients who were treated with eculizumab and TPE vs a control group of patients with HUS with similar disease severity who were treated with TPE but not eculizumab	52

[a] Some patients who were admitted to the intensive care unit were also treated with rifaximin.
[b] Short-course azithromycin was recently shown to be associated with sudden cardiac death.[122] Because ~10% of HUS mortality may result from cardiac arrhythmias, it has been argued that azithromycin should not be used to treat patients with HUS.[123]

be caused by the short half-life of Stx in circulation or to irreversible endothelial injury that may occur before clinical manifestations and initiation of apheresis.[52] Nevertheless, depletion of the immunoglobulin fraction followed by intravenous immunoglobulin repletion was suggested to improve short-term neurologic status in a small cohort of STEC O104:H4–infected individuals who developed HUS.[102]

Eculizumab, a novel monoclonal antibody directed against the C5 complement component, is a therapeutic option in atypical (non–Stx-associated) HUS, in which dysfunctional complement regulatory proteins result in unchecked activation of the alternative complement pathway. Coinciding with the early weeks of the 2011 outbreak, eculizumab had been reported to be effective in decreasing neurologic impairment in the days after infusion in 3 children with severe EHEC-Stx HUS.[103] However, trials of eculizumab in affected adults appeared to show no short-term benefit.[51]

SUMMARY

Because STEC strains vary greatly in their capacity to cause human disease, virulence determinants in addition to the simple production of Stx are likely to function as key factors in the ability of a given STEC strain to induce serious systemic disease. In recent years, there has been an increased awareness of the clinical importance of non-O157 STEC. Genomic analysis suggests that the particularly virulent German STEC strain, one that caused HUS at an increased rate and in a population not typically associated with HUS, is a hybrid E coli strain of serotype O104:H4. This strain encodes several virulence factors associated with EAEC and forms aggregates on the intestinal mucosa similarly to EAEC, but has acquired an $Stx2_a$-producing phage. The EAEC-like features of STEC O104:H4 may have contributed to the high rate of HUS and the unique epidemiology witnessed during the 2011 STEC O104:H4 outbreak, indicating that the dynamic evolution of pathogens can give rise to highly virulent strains. Given that specific therapies to treat or prevent HUS are not yet clearly defined, the early and specific detection of both O157 and non-O157 STEC is critical to ensure the best possible prognosis for an infected individual.

ACKNOWLEDGMENTS

We would like to give special thanks to Nadia Boisen and James Nataro for providing the scanning electron microscope images in **Fig. 3** and to S. Tzipori and A. Donohue-Rolfe for providing the transmission electron microscope images in **Fig. 2**.

REFERENCES

1. Kaper JB, Nataro JP, Mobley HL. Pathogenic Escherichia coli. Nat Rev Microbiol 2004;2(2):123–40.
2. Paton JC, Paton AW. Pathogenesis and diagnosis of Shiga toxin-producing Escherichia coli infections. Clin Microbiol Rev 1998;11(3):450–79.
3. Gould LH, Bopp C, Strockbine N, et al. Recommendations for diagnosis of Shiga toxin–producing Escherichia coli infections by clinical laboratories. MMWR Recomm Rep 2009;58(RR-12):1–14.
4. Whittam TS. Evolution of Escherichia coli O157:H7 and other Shiga toxin-producing E. coli strains. In: Kaper JB, O'Brien AD, editors. Escherichia coli O157:H7 and other Shiga toxin-producing E. coli strains. Washington, DC: American Society for Microbiology; 1998. p. 195–212.
5. Karmali MA, Gannon V, Sargeant JM. Verocytotoxin-producing Escherichia coli (VTEC). Vet Microbiol 2010;140(3–4):360–70.
6. Johnson KE, Thorpe CM, Sears CL. The emerging clinical importance of non-O157 Shiga toxin-producing Escherichia coli. Clin Infect Dis 2006;43(12):1587–95.
7. Gould LH, Demma L, Jones TF, et al. Hemolytic uremic syndrome and death in persons with Escherichia coli O157:H7 infection, foodborne diseases active surveillance network sites, 2000-2006. Clin Infect Dis 2009;49(10):1480–5.

8. Bitzan M, Schaefer F, Reymond D. Treatment of typical (enteropathic) hemolytic uremic syndrome. Semin Thromb Hemost 2010;36(6):594–610.

9. Trachtman H, Austin C, Lewinski M, et al. Renal and neurological involvement in typical Shiga toxin-associated HUS. Nat Rev Nephrol 2012;8(11):658–69.

10. Scheiring J, Andreoli SP, Zimmerhackl LB. Treatment and outcome of Shiga-toxin-associated hemolytic uremic syndrome (HUS). Pediatr Nephrol 2008; 23(10):1749–60.

11. Tarr PI, Gordon CA, Chandler WL. Shiga-toxin-producing *Escherichia coli* and haemolytic uraemic syndrome. Lancet 2005;365(9464):1073–86.

12. Obrig TG. *Escherichia coli* Shiga toxin mechanisms of action in renal disease. Toxins (Basel) 2010;2(12):2769–94.

13. Hughes AK, Stricklett PK, Schmid D, et al. Cytotoxic effect of Shiga toxin-1 on human glomerular epithelial cells. Kidney Int 2000;57(6):2350–9.

14. Hughes AK, Stricklett PK, Kohan DE. Cytotoxic effect of Shiga toxin-1 on human proximal tubule cells. Kidney Int 1998;54(2):426–37.

15. Obrig TG, Louise CB, Lingwood CA, et al. Endothelial heterogeneity in Shiga toxin receptors and responses. J Biol Chem 1993;268(21):15484–8.

16. Obata F, Tohyama K, Bonev AD, et al. Shiga toxin 2 affects the central nervous system through receptor globotriaosylceramide localized to neurons. J Infect Dis 2008;198(9):1398–406.

17. Appleman SS, Ascher D, Park C. Clinical spectrum of Shiga toxin-producing *Escherichia coli* (STEC) in adults and children. Clin Pediatr (Phila) 2009;48(1): 99–102.

18. Tarr PI. Shiga toxin-associated hemolytic uremic syndrome and thrombotic thrombocytopenic purpura: distinct mechanisms of pathogenesis. Kidney Int Suppl 2009;(112):S29–32.

19. Holtz LR, Neill MA, Tarr PI. Acute bloody diarrhea: a medical emergency for patients of all ages. Gastroenterology 2009;136(6):1887–98.

20. Tarr PI, Neill MA. *Escherichia coli* O157:H7. Gastroenterol Clin North Am 2001; 30(3):735–51.

21. Klein EJ, Stapp JR, Clausen CR, et al. Shiga toxin-producing *Escherichia coli* in children with diarrhea: a prospective point-of-care study. J Pediatr 2002;141(2): 172–7.

22. Gerritzen A, Wittke JW, von Ahsen N, et al. Direct faecal PCR for diagnosis of Shiga-toxin-producing *Escherichia coli*. Lancet Infect Dis 2012;12(2):102.

23. Melton-Celsa A, Mohawk K, Teel L, et al. Pathogenesis of Shiga-toxin producing *Escherichia coli*. Curr Top Microbiol Immunol 2012;357:67–103.

24. Loirat C, Saland J, Bitzan M. Management of hemolytic uremic syndrome. Presse Med 2012;41(3 Pt 2):e115–35.

25. Karmali MA, Petric M, Lim C, et al. *Escherichia coli* cytotoxin, haemolytic-uraemic syndrome, and haemorrhagic colitis. Lancet 1983;2(8362):1299–300.

26. Thorpe CM, Ritchie JM, Acheson DW. Enterohemorrhagic and other Shiga toxin-producing *Escherichia coli*. In: Donnenberg MS, editor. *Escherichia coli*: virulence mechanisms of a versatile pathogen. San Diego (CA): Elsevier; 2002. p. 119–54.

27. Scheutz F, Teel LD, Beutin L, et al. Multicenter evaluation of a sequence-based protocol for subtyping Shiga toxins and standardizing Stx nomenclature. J Clin Microbiol 2012;50(9):2951–63.

28. Obrig TG, Moran TP, Brown JE. The mode of action of Shiga toxin on peptide elongation of eukaryotic protein synthesis. Biochem J 1987;244(2): 287–94.

29. Endo Y, Tsurugi K, Yutsudo T, et al. Site of action of a Vero toxin (VT2) from *Escherichia coli* O157:H7 and of Shiga toxin on eukaryotic ribosomes. RNA N-glycosidase activity of the toxins. Eur J Biochem 1988;171(1–2):45–50.

30. Tesh VL. The induction of apoptosis by Shiga toxins and ricin. Curr Top Microbiol Immunol 2012;357:137–78.

31. Roche JK, Keepers TR, Gross LK, et al. CXCL1/KC and CXCL2/MIP-2 are critical effectors and potential targets for therapy of *Escherichia coli* O157:H7-associated renal inflammation. Am J Pathol 2007;170(2):526–37.

32. Thorpe CM, Smith WE, Hurley BP, et al. Shiga toxins induce, superinduce, and stabilize a variety of C-X-C chemokine mRNAs in intestinal epithelial cells, resulting in increased chemokine expression. Infect Immun 2001;69(10):6140–7.

33. Carter AO, Borczyk AA, Carlson JA, et al. A severe outbreak of *Escherichia coli* O157:H7–associated hemorrhagic colitis in a nursing home. N Engl J Med 1987; 317(24):1496–500.

34. Riley LW, Remis RS, Helgerson SD, et al. Hemorrhagic colitis associated with a rare *Escherichia coli* serotype. N Engl J Med 1983;308(12):681–5.

35. Pavia AT, Nichols CR, Green DP, et al. Hemolytic-uremic syndrome during an outbreak of *Escherichia coli* O157:H7 infections in institutions for mentally retarded persons: clinical and epidemiologic observations. J Pediatr 1990;116(4):544–51.

36. Ostroff SM, Kobayashi JM, Lewis JH. Infections with *Escherichia coli* O157:H7 in Washington State. The first year of statewide disease surveillance. JAMA 1989; 262(3):355–9.

37. Wong CS, Jelacic S, Habeeb RL, et al. The risk of the hemolytic-uremic syndrome after antibiotic treatment of *Escherichia coli* O157:H7 infections. N Engl J Med 2000;342(26):1930–6.

38. Smith KE, Wilker PR, Reiter PL, et al. Antibiotic treatment of *Escherichia coli* O157 infection and the risk of hemolytic uremic syndrome, Minnesota. Pediatr Infect Dis J 2012;31(1):37–41.

39. Seifert ME, Tarr PI. Therapy: azithromycin and decolonization after HUS. Nat Rev Nephrol 2012;8(6):317–8.

40. Kimmitt PT, Harwood CR, Barer MR. Toxin gene expression by shiga toxin-producing *Escherichia coli*: the role of antibiotics and the bacterial SOS response. Emerg Infect Dis 2000;6(5):458–65.

41. Zhang X, McDaniel AD, Wolf LE, et al. Quinolone antibiotics induce Shiga toxin-encoding bacteriophages, toxin production, and death in mice. J Infect Dis 2000;181(2):664–70.

42. Gamage SD, Patton AK, Strasser JE, et al. Commensal bacteria influence *Escherichia coli* O157:H7 persistence and Shiga toxin production in the mouse intestine. Infect Immun 2006;74(3):1977–83.

43. McGannon CM, Fuller CA, Weiss AA. Different classes of antibiotics differentially influence Shiga toxin production. Antimicrob Agents Chemother 2010;54(9): 3790–8.

44. Grif K, Dierich MP, Karch H, et al. Strain-specific differences in the amount of Shiga toxin released from enterohemorrhagic *Escherichia coli* O157 following exposure to subinhibitory concentrations of antimicrobial agents. Eur J Clin Microbiol Infect Dis 1998;17(11):761–6.

45. Walterspiel JN, Ashkenazi S, Morrow AL, et al. Effect of subinhibitory concentrations of antibiotics on extracellular Shiga-like toxin I. Infection 1992;20(1):25–9.

46. Bell BP, Griffin PM, Lozano P, et al. Predictors of hemolytic uremic syndrome in children during a large outbreak of *Escherichia coli* O157:H7 infections. Pediatrics 1997;100(1):E12.

47. Ikeda K, Ida O, Kimoto K, et al. Effect of early fosfomycin treatment on prevention of hemolytic uremic syndrome accompanying *Escherichia coli* O157:H7 infection. Clin Nephrol 1999;52(6):357–62.
48. Noris M, Remuzzi G. Hemolytic uremic syndrome. J Am Soc Nephrol 2005; 16(4):1035–50.
49. Cimolai N, Basalyga S, Mah DG, et al. A continuing assessment of risk factors for the development of *Escherichia coli* O157:H7-associated hemolytic uremic syndrome. Clin Nephrol 1994;42(2):85–9.
50. Cimolai N, Morrison BJ, Carter JE. Risk factors for the central nervous system manifestations of gastroenteritis-associated hemolytic-uremic syndrome. Pediatrics 1992;90(4):616–21.
51. Kielstein JT, Beutel G, Fleig S, et al. Best supportive care and therapeutic plasma exchange with or without eculizumab in Shiga-toxin-producing *E. coli* O104:H4 induced haemolytic-uraemic syndrome: an analysis of the German STEC-HUS registry. Nephrol Dial Transplant 2012;27(10):3807–15.
52. Menne J, Nitschke M, Stingele R, et al. Validation of treatment strategies for enterohaemorrhagic *Escherichia coli* O104:H4 induced haemolytic uraemic syndrome: case-control study. BMJ 2012;345:e4565.
53. Hickey CA, Beattie TJ, Cowieson J, et al. Early volume expansion during diarrhea and relative nephroprotection during subsequent hemolytic uremic syndrome. Arch Pediatr Adolesc Med 2011;165(10):884–9.
54. Ake JA, Jelacic S, Ciol MA, et al. Relative nephroprotection during *Escherichia coli* O157:H7 infections: association with intravenous volume expansion. Pediatrics 2005;115(6):e673–80.
55. Scaletsky IC, Silva ML, Trabulsi LR. Distinctive patterns of adherence of enteropathogenic *Escherichia coli* to HeLa cells. Infect Immun 1984;45(2):534–6.
56. Nataro JP, Kaper JB, Robins-Browne R, et al. Patterns of adherence of diarrheagenic *Escherichia coli* to HEp-2 cells. Pediatr Infect Dis J 1987;6(9): 829–31.
57. Taylor DN, Bourgeois AL, Ericsson CD, et al. A randomized, double-blind, multicenter study of rifaximin compared with placebo and with ciprofloxacin in the treatment of travelers' diarrhea. Am J Trop Med Hyg 2006;74(6):1060–6.
58. Mossoro C, Glaziou P, Yassibanda S, et al. Chronic diarrhea, hemorrhagic colitis, and hemolytic-uremic syndrome associated with HEp-2 adherent *Escherichia coli* in adults infected with human immunodeficiency virus in Bangui, Central African Republic. J Clin Microbiol 2002;40(8):3086–8.
59. Wanke CA, Mayer H, Weber R, et al. Enteroaggregative *Escherichia coli* as a potential cause of diarrheal disease in adults infected with human immunodeficiency virus. J Infect Dis 1998;178(1):185–90.
60. Wanke CA, Schorling JB, Barrett LJ, et al. Potential role of adherence traits of *Escherichia coli* in persistent diarrhea in an urban Brazilian slum. Pediatr Infect Dis J 1991;10(10):746–51.
61. Bhatnagar S, Bhan MK, Singh KD, et al. Prognostic factors in hospitalized children with persistent diarrhea: implications for diet therapy. J Pediatr Gastroenterol Nutr 1996;23(2):151–8.
62. Nataro JP, Mai V, Johnson J, et al. Diarrheagenic *Escherichia coli* infection in Baltimore, Maryland, and New Haven, Connecticut. Clin Infect Dis 2006;43(4): 402–7.
63. Itoh Y, Nagano I, Kunishima M, et al. Laboratory investigation of enteroaggregative *Escherichia coli* O untypeable:H10 associated with a massive outbreak of gastrointestinal illness. J Clin Microbiol 1997;35(10):2546–50.

64. Scavia G, Staffolani M, Fisichella S, et al. Enteroaggregative *Escherichia coli* associated with a foodborne outbreak of gastroenteritis. J Med Microbiol 2008;57(Pt 9):1141–6.

65. Nataro JP, Steiner T, Guerrant RL. Enteroaggregative *Escherichia coli*. Emerg Infect Dis 1998;4(2):251–61.

66. Nataro JP, Steiner T. Enteroaggregative and diffusely adherent *Escherichia coli*. In: Donnenberg MS, editor. *Escherichia coli*: virulence mechanisms of a versatile pathogen. San Diego (CA): Elsevier; 2002. p. 189–207.

67. Rasko DA, Webster DR, Sahl JW, et al. Origins of the *E. coli* strain causing an outbreak of hemolytic-uremic syndrome in Germany. N Engl J Med 2011; 365(8):709–17.

68. Estrada-Garcia T, Navarro-Garcia F. Enteroaggregative *Escherichia coli* pathotype: a genetically heterogeneous emerging foodborne enteropathogen. FEMS Immunol Med Microbiol 2012;66(3):281–98.

69. Hicks S, Candy DC, Phillips AD. Adhesion of enteroaggregative *Escherichia coli* to pediatric intestinal mucosa in vitro. Infect Immun 1996;64(11):4751–60.

70. Tzipori S, Montanaro J, Robins-Browne RM, et al. Studies with enteroaggregative *Escherichia coli* in the gnotobiotic piglet gastroenteritis model. Infect Immun 1992;60(12):5302–6.

71. Vial PA, Robins-Browne R, Lior H, et al. Characterization of enteroadherent-aggregative *Escherichia coli*, a putative agent of diarrheal disease. J Infect Dis 1988;158(1):70–9.

72. Nataro JP. Enteroaggregative *Escherichia coli* pathogenesis. Curr Opin Gastroenterol 2005;21(1):4–8.

73. Boll EJ, Struve C, Sander A, et al. The fimbriae of enteroaggregative *Escherichia coli* induce epithelial inflammation in vitro and in a human intestinal xenograft model. J Infect Dis 2012;206(5):714–22.

74. Harrington SM, Strauman MC, Abe CM, et al. Aggregative adherence fimbriae contribute to the inflammatory response of epithelial cells infected with enteroaggregative *Escherichia coli*. Cell Microbiol 2005;7(11):1565–78.

75. Strauman MC, Harper JM, Harrington SM, et al. Enteroaggregative *Escherichia coli* disrupts epithelial cell tight junctions. Infect Immun 2010;78(11): 4958–64.

76. Ruiz-Perez F, Wahid R, Faherty CS, et al. Serine protease autotransporters from *Shigella flexneri* and pathogenic *Escherichia coli* target a broad range of leukocyte glycoproteins. Proc Natl Acad Sci U S A 2011;108(31):12881–6.

77. Al-Hasani K, Navarro-Garcia F, Huerta J, et al. The immunogenic SigA enterotoxin of *Shigella flexneri* 2a binds to HEp-2 cells and induces fodrin redistribution in intoxicated epithelial cells. PLoS One 2009;4(12):e8223.

78. Boisen N, Scheutz F, Rasko DA, et al. Genomic characterization of enteroaggregative *Escherichia coli* from children in Mali. J Infect Dis 2012;205(3): 431–44.

79. Savarino SJ, Fasano A, Watson J, et al. Enteroaggregative *Escherichia coli* heat-stable enterotoxin 1 represents another subfamily of *E. coli* heat-stable toxin. Proc Natl Acad Sci U S A 1993;90(7):3093–7.

80. Dudley EG, Thomson NR, Parkhill J, et al. Proteomic and microarray characterization of the AggR regulon identifies a pheU pathogenicity island in enteroaggregative *Escherichia coli*. Mol Microbiol 2006;61(5):1267–82.

81. Nataro JP, Yikang D, Yingkang D, et al. AggR, a transcriptional activator of aggregative adherence fimbria I expression in enteroaggregative *Escherichia coli*. J Bacteriol 1994;176(15):4691–9.

82. Bhan MK, Raj P, Levine MM, et al. Enteroaggregative *Escherichia coli* associated with persistent diarrhea in a cohort of rural children in India. J Infect Dis 1989;159(6):1061–4.
83. Okeke IN, Nataro JP. Enteroaggregative *Escherichia coli*. Lancet Infect Dis 2001;1(5):304–13.
84. Yamamoto T, Echeverria P, Yokota T. Drug resistance and adherence to human intestines of enteroaggregative *Escherichia coli*. J Infect Dis 1992;165(4):744–9.
85. Kaur P, Chakraborti A, Asea A. Enteroaggregative *Escherichia coli*: an emerging enteric food borne pathogen. Interdiscip Perspect Infect Dis 2010;2010:254159.
86. Glandt M, Adachi JA, Mathewson JJ, et al. Enteroaggregative *Escherichia coli* as a cause of traveler's diarrhea: clinical response to ciprofloxacin. Clin Infect Dis 1999;29(2):335–8.
87. Infante RM, Ericsson CD, Jiang ZD, et al. Enteroaggregative *Escherichia coli* diarrhea in travelers: response to rifaximin therapy. Clin Gastroenterol Hepatol 2004;2(2):135–8.
88. World Health Organization. Outbreaks of *E. coli* O104:H4 infection: update 30. 2011. Available at: http://www.euro.who.int/en/what-we-do/health-topics/emergencies/international-health-regulations/news/news/2011/07/outbreaks-of-e.-coli-o104h4-infection-update-30. Accessed June 22, 2013.
89. Frank C, Werber D, Cramer JP, et al. Epidemic profile of Shiga-toxin-producing *Escherichia coli* O104:H4 outbreak in Germany. N Engl J Med 2011;365(19): 1771–80.
90. Buchholz U, Bernard H, Werber D, et al. German outbreak of *Escherichia coli* O104:H4 associated with sprouts. N Engl J Med 2011;365(19):1763–70.
91. Scavia G, Morabito S, Tozzoli R, et al. Similarity of Shiga toxin-producing *Escherichia coli* O104:H4 strains from Italy and Germany. Emerg Infect Dis 2011; 17(10):1957–8.
92. Bae WK, Lee YK, Cho MS, et al. A case of hemolytic uremic syndrome caused by *Escherichia coli* O104:H4. Yonsei Med J 2006;47(3):437–9.
93. Monecke S, Mariani-Kurkdjian P, Bingen E, et al. Presence of enterohemorrhagic *Escherichia coli* ST678/O104:H4 in France prior to 2011. Appl Environ Microbiol 2011;77(24):8784–6.
94. Mellmann A, Bielaszewska M, Kock R, et al. Analysis of collection of hemolytic uremic syndrome-associated enterohemorrhagic *Escherichia coli*. Emerg Infect Dis 2008;14(8):1287–90.
95. Mellmann A, Harmsen D, Cummings CA, et al. Prospective genomic characterization of the German enterohemorrhagic *Escherichia coli* O104:H4 outbreak by rapid next generation sequencing technology. PLoS One 2011;6(7):e22751.
96. Al Safadi R, Abu-Ali GS, Sloup RE, et al. Correlation between in vivo biofilm formation and virulence gene expression in *Escherichia coli* O104:H4. PLoS One 2012;7(7):e41628.
97. Zangari T, Melton-Celsa AR, Panda A, et al. Virulence of the Shiga toxin type 2-expressing *Escherichia coli* O104:H4 German outbreak isolate in two animal models. Infect Immun 2013;81(5):1562–74.
98. Bielaszewska M, Mellmann A, Zhang W, et al. Characterisation of the *Escherichia coli* strain associated with an outbreak of haemolytic uraemic syndrome in Germany, 2011: a microbiological study. Lancet Infect Dis 2011;11(9):671–6.
99. DGI. EHEC infection and antibiotic therapy. 2011. Available at: http://www.dgi-net.de/images/stories/DGI-position_paper_EHECantibiotics_English_version_plus_references_20110604.pdf. Accessed June 22, 2013.

100. Neill MA. Treatment of disease due to Shiga toxin-producing *Escherichia coli*: infectious disease management. In: Kaper JB, Obrien AD, editors. *Escherichia coli* O157:H7 and other Shiga toxin-producing *E. coli* strains. Washington, DC: ASM Press; 1998. p. 357–63.

101. Nitschke M, Sayk F, Hartel C, et al. Association between azithromycin therapy and duration of bacterial shedding among patients with Shiga toxin-producing enteroaggregative *Escherichia coli* O104:H4. JAMA 2012;307(10):1046–52.

102. Greinacher A, Friesecke S, Abel P, et al. Treatment of severe neurological deficits with IgG depletion through immunoadsorption in patients with *Escherichia coli* O104:H4-associated haemolytic uraemic syndrome: a prospective trial. Lancet 2011;378(9797):1166–73.

103. Lapeyraque AL, Malina M, Fremeaux-Bacchi V, et al. Eculizumab in severe Shiga-toxin-associated HUS. N Engl J Med 2011;364(26):2561–3.

104. Campellone KG, Giese A, Tipper DJ, et al. A tyrosine-phosphorylated 12-amino-acid sequence of enteropathogenic *Escherichia coli* Tir binds the host adaptor protein Nck and is required for Nck localization to actin pedestals. Mol Microbiol 2002;43(5):1227–41.

105. Czeczulin JR, Balepur S, Hicks S, et al. Aggregative adherence fimbria II, a second fimbrial antigen mediating aggregative adherence in enteroaggregative *Escherichia coli*. Infect Immun 1997;65(10):4135–45.

106. Dudley EG, Abe C, Ghigo JM, et al. An IncI1 plasmid contributes to the adherence of the atypical enteroaggregative *Escherichia coli* strain C1096 to cultured cells and abiotic surfaces. Infect Immun 2006;74(4):2102–14.

107. Boisen N, Struve C, Scheutz F, et al. New adhesin of enteroaggregative *Escherichia coli* related to the Afa/Dr/AAF family. Infect Immun 2008;76(7):3281–92.

108. Velarde JJ, Varney KM, Inman KG, et al. Solution structure of the novel dispersin protein of enteroaggregative *Escherichia coli*. Mol Microbiol 2007;66(5): 1123–35.

109. Sheikh J, Czeczulin JR, Harrington S, et al. A novel dispersin protein in enteroaggregative *Escherichia coli*. J Clin Invest 2002;110(9):1329–37.

110. Fasano A, Noriega FR, Liao FM, et al. Effect of shigella enterotoxin 1 (ShET1) on rabbit intestine in vitro and in vivo. Gut 1997;40(4):505–11.

111. Navarro-Garcia F, Elias WP. Autotransporters and virulence of enteroaggregative E. coli. Gut Microbes 2011;2(1):13–24.

112. Navarro-Garcia F, Sears C, Eslava C, et al. Cytoskeletal effects induced by pet, the serine protease enterotoxin of enteroaggregative *Escherichia coli*. Infect Immun 1999;67(5):2184–92.

113. Eslava C, Navarro-Garcia F, Czeczulin JR, et al. Pet, an autotransporter enterotoxin from enteroaggregative *Escherichia coli*. Infect Immun 1998;66(7): 3155–63.

114. Navarro-Garcia F, Gutierrez-Jimenez J, Garcia-Tovar C, et al. Pic, an autotransporter protein secreted by different pathogens in the Enterobacteriaceae family, is a potent mucus secretagogue. Infect Immun 2010;78(10):4101–9.

115. Benjelloun-Touimi Z, Sansonetti PJ, Parsot C. SepA, the major extracellular protein of *Shigella flexneri*: autonomous secretion and involvement in tissue invasion. Mol Microbiol 1995;17(1):123–35.

116. Morin N, Santiago AE, Ernst RK, et al. Characterization of the AggR regulon in enteroaggregative *Escherichia coli*. Infect Immun 2013;81(1):122–32.

117. Steiner TS, Nataro JP, Poteet-Smith CE, et al. Enteroaggregative *Escherichia coli* expresses a novel flagellin that causes IL-8 release from intestinal epithelial cells. J Clin Invest 2000;105(12):1769–77.

118. Gewirtz AT, Navas TA, Lyons S, et al. Cutting edge: bacterial flagellin activates basolaterally expressed TLR5 to induce epithelial proinflammatory gene expression. J Immunol 2001;167(4):1882–5.
119. Geerdes-Fenge HF, Lobermann M, Nurnberg M, et al. Ciprofloxacin reduces the risk of hemolytic uremic syndrome in patients with *Escherichia coli* O104:H4-associated diarrhea. Infection 2013;41:669–73.
120. Colic E, Dieperink H, Titlestad K, et al. Management of an acute outbreak of diarrhoea-associated haemolytic uraemic syndrome with early plasma exchange in adults from southern Denmark: an observational study. Lancet 2011;378(9796):1089–93.
121. Tarr PI, Sadler JE, Chandler WL, et al. Should all adult patients with diarrhoea-associated HUS receive plasma exchange? Lancet 2012;379(9815):516 [author reply: 7].
122. Ray WA, Murray KT, Hall K, et al. Azithromycin and the risk of cardiovascular death. N Engl J Med 2012;366(20):1881–90.
123. Seifert ME, Tarr PI. Azithromycin decolonization of STEC–a new risk emerges. Nat Rev Nephrol 2012;8(7):429.

Epidemiology, Prevention, and Control of the Number One Foodborne Illness: Human Norovirus

Erin DiCaprio, MS[a], Yuanmei Ma, PhD[a], John Hughes, PhD[b],
Jianrong Li, PhD, DVM[a,c],*

KEYWORDS

- Human norovirus • Foodborne illness • Acute gastroenteritis • Epidemiology
- Detection methods • Prevention and control strategies • Vaccine development

KEY POINTS

- Human norovirus (NoV) is the number 1 cause of foodborne disease outbreaks worldwide, accounting for more than 60% of foodborne illness and 95% of nonbacterial acute gastroenteritis.
- Human NoV is highly stable, contagious, and only a few virus particles can cause illness. Symptoms of human NoV infection include diarrhea, vomiting, nausea, abdominal cramping, chills, headache, dehydration, and a high-grade fever.
- Human NoV is difficult to study, because it cannot be grown in cell culture system and lacks a small animal model.
- It has been technically challenging to develop rapid, accurate, and sensitive detection methods for human NoV in foods and environment. Most detection methods focus on genomic RNA-based assays.

Continued

Disclosure: This study was supported by a special emphasis grant (2010-01498) from the National Integrated Food Safety Initiative (NIFSI) of the USDA and a food safety challenge grant (2011-68003-30005) from the Agriculture and Food Research Initiative (AFRI) of the USDA National Institute of Food and Agriculture.

[a] Department of Food Science and Technology, College of Food, Agricultural, and Environmental Sciences, The Ohio State University, 110 Parker Food Science and Technology Building, 2015 Fyffe Road, Columbus, OH 43210, USA; [b] Department of Molecular Virology, Immunology, and Molecular Genetics, College of Medicine, The Ohio State University, 370 West 9th Avenue, Columbus, OH 43210, USA; [c] Division of Environmental Health Sciences, College of Public Health, The Ohio State University, 250 Cunz Hall, 1841 Neil Avenue, Columbus, OH 43210, USA
* Corresponding author. Department of Food Science and Technology, College of Food, Agricultural, and Environmental Sciences, The Ohio State University, 233 Parker Food Science Building, 2015 Fyffe Road, Columbus, OH 43210.
E-mail address: li.926@osu.edu

Infect Dis Clin N Am 27 (2013) 651–674
http://dx.doi.org/10.1016/j.idc.2013.05.009
0891-5520/13/$ – see front matter © 2013 Elsevier Inc. All rights reserved.

id.theclinics.com

Continued

- There is no effective measure to control human NoV. Commonly used sanitizers are not effective against human NoV. High-pressure processing is promising to inactivate human NoV in foods.
- No vaccine or antiviral drug for human NoV has been approved by the US Food and Drug Administration. Human NoV VLP–based vaccines and live vectored vaccines have been developed and tested in animal models or human clinical trials.

INTRODUCTION

The most recent data from the Centers of Disease Control (CDC) estimate that human norovirus (NoV) is responsible for more than 21 million total cases of illness annually, causing 95% of all nonbacterial gastroenteritis reported each year.[1] Human NoV is highly infectious, resistant to common disinfectants, and causes debilitating illness; for these reasons, the virus is considered a category B biodefense agent by the National Institute of Allergies and Infectious Disease. In recent years, the importance of viruses as a cause of foodborne disease has been increasingly appreciated. Of the viruses commonly associated with foodborne disease, human NoV is the most important and is estimated to account for 58% of all foodborne illness reported every year.[2] Based on data available in 2011, more than 5 million cases of food-related illness caused by human NoV are estimated to occur each year, leading to 15,000 hospitalizations and nearly 150 deaths.[3,4] The estimated annual cost of human NoV foodborne disease, based on hospitalizations and lost wages, reaches nearly 2 billion US dollars.[3,5] Despite the considerable impact of human NoV on public health, there are no approved antiviral drugs or vaccines to combat the virus.

Human NoV causes severe gastroenteritis, characterized by vomiting, diarrhea, and stomach cramps. Vomiting is seen more commonly in infants and children, whereas adults usually present with diarrhea. The diarrhea associated with the disease is free of blood, mucus, and leukocytes.[6] This characteristic differentiates NoV-associated diarrhea from diarrhea caused by bacterial pathogens such as *E coli* O157:H7, in which blood appears in the stools. The incubation period for the disease is usually 10 to 51 hours and the duration of the disease is 28 to 60 hours.[7,8] NoV affects people of all ages and usually does not require hospitalization. However, severe disease may be observed in infants, children, the elderly, or immunocompromised individuals, all of whom may require supportive care. In immunocompromised patients, chronic NoV infections have been documented, leading to increased morbidity and mortality compared with the general population.[9] NoV outbreaks seem to have no clear seasonality, but more cases are reported in the winter months. After infection, individuals may shed virus in the stool for 20 to 40 days at titers as high as 10^8 to 10^9 genome copies per gram of stool.[10] Human NoV is highly stable in the environment and is resistant to common disinfectants, such as alcohol-based sanitizers and phenolic compounds, so the propagation of disease after a point source outbreak commonly occurs.

HUMAN NOV CLASSIFICATION AND HOST SUSCEPTIBILITY

The first documented human NoV outbreak occurred in 1968 in the town of Norwalk, Ohio. In 1972, the virus was officially identified using immune electron microscopy

(IEM).[11] Human NoV is commonly called the stomach flu or winter vomiting disease because of its symptoms and the increase in disease occurrence during the winter months. Human NoV is a member of the genus *Norovirus* within the family Caliciviridae. The *Norovirus* genus is subdivided into 5 genogroups: GI to GV, with GI, GII, and GIV causing human disease.[12] GIII are bovine NoVs, and GV includes murine NoV. The genogroups are further divided into genotypes, and at least 21 genotypes are assigned to the GII genogroup alone.[13] The most prevalent human NoV strains circulating in the human population belong to genogroup II, genotype 4 (GII.4). In the past 10 years, more than 3 global pandemics have occurred, all of which were caused by strains of GII.4.[14] The GII.4-2009 New Orleans strain, was identified in the winter of 2009 to 2010 and was the prevalent strain identified in outbreaks in the United States in 2010, displacing the GII.4-2006 Minerva strain.[15] More recently a new emerging strain has been identified, the GII.4-2012 Sydney strain, which accounted for more than half of the human NoV outbreaks reported between September and December, 2012.[16]

It has long been debated whether long-term immunity is acquired after human NoV infection. Data are limited to a few volunteer studies involving just a few human NoV strains. It is believed that the diversity between strains of human NoV plays an integral part in its evasion of the immune system. Even closely related strains of human NoV show major antigenic and receptor binding differences. Host susceptibility also plays an important role in human NoV infections. Early volunteer studies with human NoV strain GI.1 found that some individuals did not show symptoms of disease after exposure to the virus.[17] Recent studies have shown that individuals with blood type O are more susceptible to GI.1 strain infections than people with other blood types. Human NoVs use the histoblood group antigens (HBGAs), a family of glycans found on many cell types, as functional receptors.[18] HGBAs are found on erythrocytes and on epithelial cells, as well as in some body secretions such as saliva and breast milk. Different strains of human NoV may have different binding affinity to different HBGAs, which include A, B, H, and Lewis antigens.[19] The α-1, 3/4 fucosyl transferase *(FUT3)* and α-1,2-fucosyltransferase *(FUT2)* genes determine an individual's status as either a secretor or nonsecretor. Individuals with the *FUT3* allele alone are considered nonsecretor, whereas individuals with both the *FUT3* and *FUT2* alleles are considered secretor. The *FUT3* gene encodes the Lewis enzyme, which adds fucose to either the α-1,3 or α-2,4 linkage of the HBGA precursor disaccharide, leading to the synthesis of the trisaccharide required for the Lewis A phenotype. The Lewis A phenotype is also referred to as the nonsecretor phenotype. The *FUT2* gene encodes a fucosyltransferase, which adds fucose to α-1,2 linkages of the precursor, creating the H type 1 antigen. Further glycosylation by the Lewis, A, and B enzymes occurs, leading to the expression of other HBGA and the secretor phenotypes.[17] An individual's blood type and secretor/nonsecretor status have been shown to play a role in susceptibility to infection with particular human NoV strains.[20]

VIRAL STRUCTURE, GENOME ORGANIZATION, AND VIRAL PROTEINS

Under electron microscopy (EM), human NoVs look like small round particles ranging from 27 to 38 nm in diameter. It is a nonenveloped virus. The outer shell of the virus particle is a highly stable protein capsid, which carries 32 shallow, cuplike circular indentations and shows icosahedral symmetry. Inside the capsid is the genetic material, which is a single-stranded positive-sense RNA genome. The genome of human NoV is approximately 7.7 kb long and is divided into 3 open reading frames (ORF).[21] ORF1 encodes the nonstructural polyprotein, ORF2 encodes the major capsid protein VP1, and ORF3 encodes the minor capsid protein VP2. The polyprotein encoded by

ORF1 is further proteolytically cleaved into 6 nonstructural proteins in the order of p48, nucleoside-triphosphatase, p22, VPg, 3CL^pro, and RNA dependent RNA polymerase (RdRp).[22] The functions of many of these proteins have been deciphered by homologies found in cultivable surrogate viruses such as murine NoV and feline calicivirus.[22] During the replication and gene expression, the virus produces subgenomic RNA which only encodes VP1 and VP2. A virally encoded protein, VPg, covalently links to the 5' end of human NoV genomic and subgenomic RNAs.[23] The function of VPg may be involved in the initiation of viral protein translation by recruiting translational machinery.

The capsid of human NoV is made up of 90 dimers of the major capsid protein VP1 and 1 or 2 copies of the minor capsid protein VP2. VP1 is composed of ~530 to 555 amino acids with a molecular weight that ranges from 58 to 60 kDa. Expression of VP1 protein alone can form empty noninfectious viruslike particles (VLPs), which are antigenically and morphologically similar to the native human NoV virions.[21] VP1 is vital for the determination of antigenicity, receptor binding activity, immunogenicity, strain specificity, and the classification of NoV genogroups and genotypes.[18,21] VP1 folds to form 2 domains, shell (S) and protrusion (P), linked by a flexible hinge region (**Fig. 1**).[24] The S domain is involved in the formation of the continuous shell surface, and the P domain forms the prominent protrusion emanating from the shell.[24] The P domain is further divided into 2 subdomains: P1 and P2 (see **Fig. 1**). The P domain is the primary site of antibody recognition and receptor binding, which plays an important role in human NoV infection and determines the host susceptibility.[18]

CHALLENGES IN HUMAN NOV RESEARCH

The study of human NoV has been hindered by the absence of a cell culture system and the lack of a small animal model. Therefore, many aspects of human NoV such as molecular biology, gene expression, replication, pathogenesis, and immunology are poorly understood. The survival of human NoV and the effectiveness of measures to inactivate human NoV cannot be accurately evaluated. Because human NoV cannot be grown in cell culture, most laboratory efforts to study the virus use cultivable surrogates.[25,26] These surrogates include viruses that are closely related to human NoV in terms of genetic makeup, size, receptor binding, pathogenicity, and environmental stability. Examples of these surrogate viruses include murine NoV, feline calicivirus, porcine sapovirus, and Tulane virus. The major disadvantage of the use of murine NoV and feline calicivirus as surrogates is that both viruses do not cause gastroenteritis. Murine NoV causes systemic infection in mice, whereas feline calicivirus causes respiratory tract infection in cats.[25,26] It has been proposed that porcine sapovirus and Tulane virus may be better surrogates, because they cause symptoms of gastroenteritis in animals.[27] Particularly, Tulane virus recognizes the type A and B HBGAs, similar to human NoV. Other surrogates used for the study of human NoV include VLPs and P domain particles (P-particles).[28,29] These particles resemble portions of the human NoV protein capsid, which are important for receptor binding of the virus to the host cell and antigenic recognition of the virus by the immune system. The particles are noninfectious, because they are composed only of protein and lack the viral

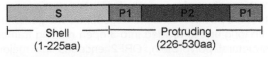

Fig. 1. Domain organization in NoV capsid (VP1) protein.

genome component of the native virus. Although the use of surrogates has aided in the understanding of human NoV, there are limitations in comparing data generated from the use of surrogates with human NoV.

EPIDEMIOLOGY AND TRANSMISSION OF HUMAN NOV

The mode of transmission of human NoV is typically the fecal-oral route, with direct transmission from person to person; however, indirect transmission can occur through contaminated food, water, surfaces, and fomites. There is also evidence of direct transmission via aerosolized vomitus.[30] The infectious dose of human NoV is very low, usually reported as fewer than 10 viral particles. A recent publication[31] based on human volunteer studies and mathematical modeling estimated a high risk of infection (49%) caused by exposure to 1 human NoV particle. Human NoV is shed in the stool of infected individuals, and viral shedding peaks 1 to 3 days after infection. Viral shedding typically lasts 20 to 40 days in immunocompetent individuals; however, in immunocompromised individuals, viral shedding has been reported up to 56 days after infection, and in chronic cases, viral shedding can occur for years.[9] From 10^5 to 10^{11} viral copies per gram of feces can typically be shed by an infected individual.[31–33] Approximately one-third of human NoV–infected individuals are asymptomatic but actively shed the virus, leading to further propagation of disease.[13]

As mentioned previously, in immunocompromised patients, human NoV infections can be more severe or even chronic. Increased duration of NoV illness has been documented in immunosuppressed patients as a result of congenital immunodeficiency, chemotherapy, immunosuppressive therapy, and human immunodeficiency virus (HIV) infection.[34–38] Complications from human NoV infections in the immunocompromised include dehydration, malnutrition, and dysfunction of the intestinal barrier, which contributes to the higher mortality observed for these individuals.[9] Viral shedding is also increased in these patients and can last from weeks to years.[39,40] In addition, in contrast to the general population, who are normally infected by just a few stable variants of human NoV, the clinical samples of immunocompromised patients have tested positive for an array of human NoV variants not normally observed in healthy individuals.[40] For these patients, proper hand hygiene should be used to limit human NoV exposure as well as isolation from visitors or staff showing the symptoms of gastroenteritis.

Outbreaks of human NoV have been popularized in the lay press in association with cruise ships, but they can occur in any area where people are in close contact. Human NoV outbreaks have been reported in restaurants, retirement communities, schools, hospitals, nursing homes, hotels, stadia, and military installations.[41] Recent outbreak data from the CDC indicate that more than half of the confirmed outbreaks of human NoV in 2010 to 2011 occurred in long-term care facilities.[1] Of 1518 confirmed outbreaks in 2010 to 2011, 889 (59%) were attributed to long-term care facilities, 123 (8%) were traced to restaurants, 99 (7%) were sourced to parties or events, 65 (4%) were from hospitals, 64 (4%) from schools, 55 (4%) from cruise ships, and 223 (14%) were from other or unknown sources. The high density of individuals in each of these settings, paired with the fact that food consumed at these locations is normally prepared by others, contributes to the high instance of human NoV outbreaks in these locations.

Human NoV is highly stable in the environment, which makes it difficult to eradicate after primary infections have occurred. It has been estimated that the stool of an individual with an active NoV infection may shed up to 100 billion virus particles per gram of feces.[33] This fact, paired with the low infectious dose of human NoV, accounts for the rapid spread of the virus in a closed community as a result of poor hygiene. Because approximately 30% of human NoV infections are asymptomatic,[33,42,43] consequently, asymptomatic carriers can pass human NoV to other people or to foods that they handle.

Human NoV foodborne disease is commonly associated with foods that undergo little or no processing before consumption, such as fresh produce and raw shellfish, or prepared foods to which a food handler can unknowingly transfer the virus during preparation. Human NoV outbreaks have been associated with many types of food, including fresh cut fruit, lettuce, tomatoes, melons, salads, green onions, strawberries, blueberries, raspberries, salsa, oysters, clams, and other shellfish.[44,45]

In the confirmed NoV foodborne outbreaks from 2001 to 2008 that could be traced to a single food commodity, leafy vegetables contributed to 33% of the outbreaks, fruits/nuts were associated with 16% of outbreaks, and mollusks were responsible for 13% of these outbreaks.[3] However, complex foods were implicated in 41% of the 2001 to 2008 outbreaks, whereas only 28% was attributed to a simple food.[3] Evidence suggests that most of these foods may have become contaminated through the poor hygiene of food handlers, but viral contamination can occur upstream in the food production process. An outbreak of human NoV associated with raspberries was linked to sewage in irrigation water.[46–48] Outbreaks of human NoV have also been associated with oysters that were grown in water contaminated with human waste.[49,50] Hence, prevention measures for production, processing, handling, and preparation should be considered to help minimize human NoV contamination at all steps from farm to fork.

RECENT OUTBREAKS OF HUMAN NOV

Investigations of human NoV outbreaks are complicated. Outbreaks associated with foods, water, fomites, and person-to-person contact are presented in **Table 1** to show the many ways in which this virus can be transmitted. Determining human NoV as the cause of outbreaks is often hampered by the limited modes of detection of the virus and the genetic diversity found within the genus *Norovirus*. The determination of human NoV as the cause of an outbreak is often determined by a combination of symptomatology and the exclusion of other enteric pathogens as the culprit.

However, important advances in the surveillance of human NoV outbreaks have been made in recent years. In March 2009, CaliciNet, an outbreak surveillance network for human NoV, was launched by the CDC partnering with state health departments. CaliciNet participants can electronically enter epidemiologic and sequence data for NoV outbreaks, allowing for linking of multistate or common source outbreaks and the identification of emerging virus strains. As of 2011, 20 local and state health departments had been certified to upload laboratory results to CaliciNet.[15] The enhanced capacity of health departments to test for human NoV and the database of epidemiologic data will undoubtedly improve the accuracy and efficacy of outbreak investigations.

In the winter of 2009 to 2010, CaliciNet identified the emergence of a prevalent strain of human NoV circulating in the United States, the GII.4-2009 New Orleans strain. In January 2013, the CDC released the CaliciNet surveillance data for September to December 2012, which indicated a new predominant human NoV strain circulating in the United States, the GII.4-2012 Sydney strain, displacing the GII.4-2009 New Orleans strain. This human NoV variant accounted for 141 (53%) of the 266 total outbreaks during the 4-month period. The remaining outbreaks were caused by 10 other GI and GII strains.[16] Of the outbreaks associated with GII.4-2012 Sydney in the United

Table 1
Recent NoV outbreaks by various transmission routes

Dates	Location	Transmission	Description	Genotype(s)	Reference
November–December, 2010	United States	Person to person	Players and staff from 13 separate National Basketball Association franchises; direct player-to-player transmission	GII.1	Desai et al,[114] 2011
October, 2010	United States	Fomites	An open-top laminated woven bag; aerosolized vomit	GII.2	Repp & Keene,[115] 2012
January–February, 2010	England	Foodborne	Oysters harvested from category A waters in Europe	Unspecified	Dore et al,[116] 2010
February, 2009	Guatemala	Waterborne	Students and chaperones on a school trip at a resort; water	GI.7, GII.12, GII.17	Arvelo et al,[117] 2012
January, 2009	Germany	Foodborne	Outbreak in a military installment; prepared salad	GII.4	Wadl et al,[118] 2010
January, 2008	Korea	Waterborne	Individuals swimming at a water park; groundwater	GI.4	Koh et al,[119] 2011
July, 2005	Spain	Foodborne	Campers at a summer camp; meal, asymptomatic food handler	GII.4	Barrabeig et al,[120] 2010
August–September, 2005	United States	Unknown	Residents of New Orleans displaced after Hurricane Katrina were housed in the Reliant Park Complex in Houston, TX	Multiple strains	Yee et al,[121] 2007
September, 1998	United States	Foodborne; person to person	Football players from North Carolina and Florida; a box lunch, person to person	GI.1	Becker et al,[122] 2000

States, 72 (51%) were transmitted by direct person-to-person contact, 29 (20%) were foodborne, 1 (1%) was waterborne, and 39 (28%) were transmitted by an unknown route.[16] In previous seasons, there has been a peak in human NoV outbreaks in the month of January, so the impact on morbidity and mortality of the GII.2-2012 Sydney strain may not be fully understood until after this threshold.

The GII.4-2012 Sydney strain was first identified in Australia in March 2012 and has been correlated with increased outbreaks in Europe and Japan compared with previous seasons.[16,51] New GII.4 variants have emerged every 2 to 3 years since 1995, which is believed to be caused by population immunity and genetic drift.[16,51] Gene and protein sequence analysis identified GII.4-2012 Sydney as phylogenetically distinct from the GII.4-2009 New Orleans and the GII.4-2007 Apeldoorn strains. GII.4-2012 Sydney had amino acid changes in the P2 domain of VP1 in the major epitopes involved in cell receptor binding.[51] These changes to the P2 domain could explain the high incidence of outbreaks associated with the new variant.

DETECTION METHODS FOR HUMAN NOV

Clinically, diagnosis of human NoV infection is usually based on the symptoms, such as acute onset of vomiting; watery, nonbloody diarrhea with abdominal cramps; nausea; low-grade fever; and headaches. However, to confirm the cause, we must rely on laboratory diagnostic tools, particularly because many human NoV infections are asymptomatic. Because human NoVs cannot be grown in cell culture, viral RNA, viral proteins, or viral particles are targets for detection. Limitations for NoV detection are low concentration of viruses in a sample and extreme genetic and antigenic diversity seen within the genus *Norovirus*. There are no cross-reactive antibodies that can detect all circulating strains using enzyme immunoassays (EIAs). Likewise, nucleic acid detection assays are also hampered by low sequence homology because of genetic diversity. Thus, a single primer pair is insufficient for detecting all NoV strains and yet be free of false-positive reactions. For viral particle detection, EM, IEM, and solid-phase IEM (SPIEM) are expensive, require a highly trained observer to distinguish NoVs from other enteric viruses, and a large number of outbreak specimens cannot be rapidly examined.

Detection of human NoV in implicated foods is complicated by the complexity of the food matrix and low levels of viruses.[52] In general, determination of foodborne outbreaks associated with human NoV relies on epidemiologic investigations or laboratory testing. The virus must be isolated from people who have become ill after consumption of the same food items. Sometimes, an outbreak may be traced to a food handler who also harbors human NoV. The recent trend in food microbiology to focus on viruses will certainly lead to improved molecular detection methods for human NoV in foods.

A summary of detection methods can be found in **Table 2**. Initially, RNA detection methods for NoVs were reverse-transcriptase polymerase chain reaction (RT-PCR) assays.[53,54] RT quantitative PCR (RT-qPCR) assays are considered to be the gold standard for NoV detection and are used in many public health, clinical, food, environmental, and research laboratories.[55–57] In addition to RT-PCR and RT-qPCR, other amplification variations, such as RT multiplex PCR,[55,58,59] RT-nested PCR,[60,61] direct RT-PCR,[62] RT-nested, real-time PCR,[63] RT-booster PCR,[64] and nucleic acid sequence-based amplifications[50,51] have been used for the detection of NoVs in various specimens. Recently, a reverse transcription loop-mediated isothermal amplification approach has also been used for the rapid detection of NoVs.[65–67] To have a

Table 2
Detection methods for human NoV

Detection Methods	Comments/Issues
Reverse-transcriptase polymerase chain reaction (RT-PCR)	Early amplification method for NoV detection; amplicons useful for confirming NoVs by sequencing or probes; risk for carryover contamination resulting in false-positive results; enzyme inhibitors result in false-negative results; primers determine specificity but can lead to false-negative results
RT quantitative PCR	Gold standard for NoV detection; faster detection than RT-PCR; less chance for carryover contamination (single closed vessel format); generally more sensitive; quantitative assay; more expensive equipment and reagents
RT multiplex PCR	Detects >1 target (eg, genogroup); similar annealing temperatures suggested for primer sets; potential false-negative results for targets with low initial sample copy number
RT-nested PCR	Risk for carryover contamination; enhanced sensitivity (compared with RT-PCR), up to 10,000 increase in sensitivity
Direct RT-PCR	Eliminates RNA extraction and purification; more rapid throughput; potential for less operator carryover contamination
RT-nested, real-time PCR	Risk for carryover contamination
RT-booster PCR	Double-round PCR; enhanced sensitivity; greater contamination risk
Nucleic acid sequence-based amplification	Isothermal amplification; excellent sensitivity; rapid assay; can be multiplexed
Reverse transcription loop-mediated isothermal amplification	Simple to use NoV genogroup assay; excellent sensitivity and specificity; reduced assay time; no carryover contamination (single-step format)
EIA	Low cost; fairly rapid assay (4 h); excellent sensitivity and specificity when homologous NoVs or antigens are used, lower sensitivity and specificity with heterologous sporadic and outbreak specimens; not recommended for diagnosing sporadic cases; false-positive results in neonates; RIDASCREEN third-generation FDA-approved test has higher sensitivity and specificity
Immunochromatographic	Useful for screening and point-of-care testing (POCT); easy to use; simple sample preparation; extremely rapid test (15–30 min); reduced sensitivity; applicable for outbreak cases; negative results should be confirmed
EM, IEM, and SPIEM	Useful for detecting new viruses when primers repeatedly fail (ie, outbreaks or cases negative by molecular approaches should be screened by EM); pooling and concentrating samples may enhance detection when other methods are negative; direct EM has limited sensitivity for NoV detection; specific antisera needed for immune aggregation with IEM and SPIEM; useful for determining NoV antigenic types; reduced throughput rate for specimen examination; excellent for detecting new viruses; used to detect or confirm NoV outbreaks

90% probability for detecting an NoV as a cause for an outbreak, at least 3 samples from the same patient need to be tested using a standard RT-PCR assay.[68]

Because NoV molecular detection methods, like RT-qPCR, are not always cost-effective or adaptable to some health care settings (eg, physician offices, local health departments, small laboratories, off-site clinics, nursing homes, field sites) commercial EIAs have been developed for testing human specimens.[69–73] Immunologic detection of NoVs has shown limited application of early-generation EIAs/enzyme-linked immunosorbent assays (ELISAs). A review of 10 EIA/ELISA studies indicated that the sensitivity for NoV detection ranged from 31% to 90% and specificity ranged from 65% to 100%.[74] The evaluation of third-generation EIAs has shown vast improvement in both sensitivity and specificity.[59,60] Consequently, some commercial EIA kits offer an improvement for rapid diagnosis of sporadic infections and also are more applicable for outbreak screenings. To have a 90% probability for detecting an NoV as a cause for an outbreak, a minimum of 6 specimens from the same patient have to be tested when using earlier-generation ELISAs.[68]

Immunochromatographic (ICGs) assays have been developed and could be helpful, especially for screening specimens from sporadic and outbreak cases.[75–79] In addition, simple, sensitive, specific, rapid, and inexpensive point-of-care tests (POCTs) would be a helpful medical and public health asset. The best POCTs for NoVs are ICG assays. POCT kits for human NoVs have the potential to be improved in sensitivity and specificity as a result of recent developments in fluorescence immunochromatography.[80]

Human NoVs have been detected by EM procedures.[11,69,74] Although direct EM has limited sensitivity, in any outbreak in which human NoV is the suspected cause and molecular detection results are repeatedly negative for human NoV, patient specimens should be examined by direct EM for a potential viral pathogens. Because of the low specificity of many of the human NoV molecular assays, a correct diagnosis may be missed by these techniques and direct EM would elucidate human NoV as the cause. Also, other nonspecified viral agents may be identified using direct EM and may not be detected by clinical laboratory assays. Because many diagnostic laboratories may not have the capacity for direct EM analysis of viruses causing gastroenteritis, a partnering with the public health system would be required for this type of identification. In addition, pooling outbreak specimens and concentrating specimen pools would speed the detection of any cause. Once a potential cause has been detected in a pool, then more time can be taken to examine individual specimens for an agent that matches any agent found in a concentrated pool.

It is difficult to predict future trends for the detection of human NoVs. However, there is a high probability that the current RT-qPCR approach for detecting NoVs in clinical specimens will be modified by using nanoparticle probes. A nucleic acid, multiplexed test, based on nanosphere and microarray technology, is already available for the detection of respiratory viruses.[81] The complete process, from sample to final results, takes approximately 2.5 hours.[81] With this technology, it should be feasible to detect in clinical specimens a wide variety of NoV genogroups, genotypes, and new genetic variants all in the same specimen on a real-time basis. The future is bright for the rapid and accurate point-of-care detection of NoVs.

PREVENTION METHODS FOR HUMAN NOV CONTAMINATION AND INFECTION

Human NoV has high environmental stability and a low infectious dose, which makes controlling the transmission of the virus challenging. The CDC has published guidelines for disinfection procedures after a human NoV outbreak, and the recommended disinfectant for surface disinfection is 1000 to 5000 ppm of household bleach (sodium hypochlorite).[13] However, because human NoV cannot be cultivated, the efficacy of this treatment and other disinfectants approved by the US Environmental Protection Agency for human NoV has been established using surrogate viruses.[82–84] These surrogate viruses may not accurately represent the disinfection kinetics of human NoV, but they remain the most suitable representation. The CDC recommends increasing cleaning wards to twice daily and contact surfaces to 3 times daily with 1000 to 5000 ppm chlorine or an EPA-approved disinfectant during a human NoV outbreak, to increase the efficacy of decontamination. A summary of current data on the efficacy of sanitizers against human NoV clinical isolates can be found in **Table 3**.[85] Most of these data have relied solely on RT-qPCR assessment of genomic RNA copies; however, a method coupling genomic RNA detection with human NoV binding ability to HBGAs has recently been used to more accurately determine viral inactivation.[86]

Although sanitizers can be used on human NoV–contaminated surfaces, most are not approved for food use. According to the US Food and Drug Administration (FDA), sodium hypochlorite at the concentration of less than 200 ppm may be used for food sanitization purposes (FDA CFR 178.1010, 2011). This concentration of chlorine is not effective (1–2 log virus reduction) in removing viral contaminants.[87–91] The food matrix and organic material also affect the ability of the sanitizers to inactive viruses. Thermal treatment is an effective means for inactivation of most pathogens; however, appropriate D values (the temperature and time required to eliminate 1 log of a pathogen) have not been established for human NoV. Recent data on the thermal inactivation of human NoV are presented in **Table 3**. However, the highest-risk foods for human NoV contamination (fresh produce and shellfish) are normally minimally processed, eaten raw, or mildly heated.

Several nonthermal processing options exist for the treatment of fresh produce and shellfish, including: high-pressure processing (HPP), γ irradiation, ultraviolet irradiation, ozone, and pulsed electric field. Many of these technologies have been evaluated for efficacy against human NoV using surrogates (such as murine NoV and feline calicivirus).[29,92,93] Research in nonthermal processing on human NoV clinical isolates is summarized in **Table 3**. The most promising human NoV inactivation technology seems to be HPP. Human NoV–inoculated oysters treated with 600 MPa for 5 minutes were subsequently fed to human volunteers and these oysters did not cause infection in humans, indicating virus inactivation.[94] Similarly, pressures of 700 MPa for 45 minutes could inhibit the binding of human NoV VLPs to their HBGA receptors.[28] Another study using high-pressure treatment of 600 MPa for 5 minutes to treat GI.1 and GII.4 NoV isolates significantly decreased the ability of the virus to bind to HBGA receptors.[95] These studies of HPP are promising; however, further research using human NoV isolates is required to substantiate these findings, as well as to more appropriately evaluate other nonthermal processes for viral inactivation.

POTENTIAL VACCINE CANDIDATES AGAINST HUMAN NOV
The Need to Develop a Vaccine for Human NoV

Vaccination is the most effective strategy to protect humans from infectious diseases. There is no FDA-approved vaccine for human NoV. Although human NoV causes self-limiting illness, it causes significant health, economical, and emotional burdens. Recent epidemiologic studies found that severe clinical outcomes including death are often associated with high-risk populations such as the elderly, children, and immunocompromised individuals. The CDC estimates that 900,000 clinic visits by children in the developed world occur annually as a result of NoV infections, leading to an

Table 3
Methods for the inactivation of human NoVs

Treatment	Effectiveness	References
Sanitizers		
Chlorine (1000 ppm)	Surface wiping; 1 log reduction in GI.4 RNA and 1.5 log reduction in GII.4 RNA	Tuladhar et al,[123] 2012
Sodium hypochlorite (160 ppm)	Surface treatment for 30 s; 5 log reduction in GI.1 RNA	Liu et al,[124] 2010
Alcohol or isopropanol (50%–75%)	Not efficient for GII.4 RNA	Nowak et al,[125] 2011
Alcohol or isopropanol (90%)	<2 log reduction in GII.4 RNA	Park et al,[126] 2010
Alcohol (95%)	Ineffective in reducing GI.1 RNA	Liu et al,[124] 2010
Quaternary ammonium compounds	Not efficient for GII.4 RNA	Nowak et al,[125] 2011
Chlorine dioxide (200 ppm)	Not efficient for GII.4 RNA	Nowak et al,[125] 2011
Hydrogen peroxide (2.1%)	Treatment for 5 min; 2 log reduction in GI.8 RNA and 1 log reduction in GII.4 RNA	Li et al,[127] 2011
Thermal Processing		
64°C	64°C for 1 min; 0.9 logs reduction of GI.1 in binding to gastric mucin–coated beads	Dancho et al,[95] 2012
73°C	73°C for 2 min; 3.1 logs reduction of GI.1 in binding to gastric mucin–coated beads	Dancho et al,[95] 2012
70°C	70°C for 3 min; 1 log reduction in GI.8 RNA, but no reduction in GII.4 RNA	Li et al,[127] 2011
Nonthermal Processing		
HPP (600 MPa at 6°C for 5 min)	Oysters seeded with GI.1 strain treated by HPP; no infection (0/10) in human volunteers consuming oysters; complete inactivation	Leon et al,[94] 2011
HPP (400 MPa at 25° for 5 min)	60% (3/5) infection in human volunteers consuming HPP-treated oysters; incomplete inactivation	Leon et al,[94] 2011
HPP (400 MPa at 6° for 5 min)	21% (3/14) infection in human volunteers consuming HPP-treated oysters; incomplete inactivation	Leon et al,[94] 2011
HPP (600 MPa at 6°C for 5 min)	GI.1 and GII.4 strains reduced binding to gastric mucin–coated beads to 0.3% and 4.0%; 4.7-log RNA reduction	Dancho et al,[95] 2012
Ultraviolet light	2.0 J/cm^2 treatment; 3.8 log reduction in GI.1 RNA	Dancho et al,[95] 2012
Gaseous ozone	1 log reduction for NoV RNA on surfaces	Hudson et al,[128] 2007

estimated 64,000 hospitalizations.[96] From 1999 to 2007, human NoV caused, on average, 797 deaths per year in the United States; however, this estimate has been reduced in recent years.[96] Mortality of NoV-associated infection increases during the epidemic seasons, and the burden of human NoV is greater in the developing world. The CDC estimates that NoV causes the death of 200,000 children younger than 5 years every year in developing countries.[97] An effective vaccine would be highly beneficial. The increasing clinical significance of human NoV infections suggests that there is an urgent need for an efficacious vaccine against human NoV, particularly for the populations at high risk, such as food handlers, military personnel, elderly, infants, children, and immunocompromised individuals. An effective vaccine would not only prevent acute gastroenteritis caused by this virus but also block transmission routes and thus improve food safety, public health, and biodefense.

Protein-Based Subunit Vaccine Candidates

Because human NoV is not cultivable, most vaccine studies have been focused on a subunit vaccine using VP1 as the antigen. The VP1 protein has been expressed in many expression systems, including yeast, *Escherichia coli*, insect cells, mammalian cell lines, tobacco, and potatoes.[21,98,99] In most expression systems, VP1 can self-assemble into VLPs that are structurally and antigenically similar to native virions. These VLPs contain optimal epitopes that can trigger human NoV–specific immune responses in hosts. A baculovirus-insect cell expression system has been shown to be the most efficient expression system for VLPs.[100] Mice immunized with VLP-based vaccine candidates stimulated a variable level of antibody, T-cell, and intestinal and vaginal mucosal immunities, which were dependent on vaccination dosage, route, and type of adjuvants.[99,100] However, it is not known whether these immunities are protective, because mice are not susceptible to human NoV infection. Recently, it was found that gnotobiotic pigs inoculated with human NoV developed symptoms of gastroenteritis, including mild diarrhea, viral shedding in feces, and pathologic changes in the small intestine.[101] Subsequently, it was found that gnotobiotic pigs vaccinated with VLPs and mucosal adjuvants (immunostimulating complexes [ISCOM] or mutant *E coli* LT toxin [mLT, R192G]) triggered NoV-specific antibody responses, thyroxine 1 (Th_1)/Th_2 serum cytokines and cytokine-secreting cells, and mucosal immune responses.[102] Both vaccine candidates induced increased protection rates against viral shedding and diarrhea compared with unvaccinated controls.[102] These data suggest that the VLP-based vaccine is protective in gnotobiotic pigs.

The VLP-based vaccine candidate has been tested in human clinical trials (**Table 4**). In 1999, Ball and colleagues[103] performed the first clinical study to show that baculovirus-expressed human NoV VLPs were safe and immunogenic in humans when administered orally. El-Kamary and colleagues[104] and Tacket and colleagues[105] (2003) performed a human volunteer study using Norwalk VLPs as antigens. Thirty-six healthy adult volunteers received 250 µg (n = 10), 500 µg (n = 10), or 2000 µg (n = 10) of orally administered VLPs (without adjuvant) or placebo (n = 6). All vaccinees developed significant increases in IgA anti-VLP antibody-secreting cells. Ninety percent who received 250 µg developed increases in serum anti-VLP IgG. However, neither the rates of seroconversion nor antibody titers increased at the higher vaccination doses. Later, the effects of VLP (containing chitosan) vaccination dose on immune responses were further compared in human volunteers. Only 20% of individuals developed serum IgG and 40% of individuals developed serum IgA when receiving 15 µg of VLPs. The rate of IgG and IgA was increased to 56% and 72%, respectively, when the vaccination dose increased to 50 µg. Although these studies showed that VLP-based vaccine candidates are safe and immunogenic, it was not determined whether they can protect humans from human NoV–induced gastroenteritis. Recently, a human study was conducted in healthy adults to assess the protection efficacy of a VLP vaccine candidate (with chitosan and monophosphoryl lipid A [MPL] as adjuvants) to

Table 4
Vaccine candidates against human NoV

Vaccine Candidates	Dosage (µg)	Adjuvants	Vaccination Routes and Numbers of Dose	Animal Model or Human Subject	Immune Response and Protection Efficacy	References
Baculovirus-derived VLPs	100	Liquid water, no adjuvant	Two doses, orally (days 1 and 21)	5 human subjects	60% subjects developed serum IgG, 80% serum IgA, no fecal IgA	Ball et al,[103] 1999
Baculovirus-derived VLPs	250	Liquid water, no adjuvant	Two doses, orally (days 1 and 21)	15 human subjects	100% subjects developed serum IgG, 80% serum IgA, 10% fecal IgA	Ball et al,[103] 1999
Baculovirus-derived VLPs	250	Liquid water, no adjuvant	Two doses, orally (days 0 and 21)	10 human subjects	90% subjects developed serum IgG, 90% serum IgA, 40% salivary IgA, 28.5% fecal IgA, 80% vaginal IgA	Tacket et al,[129] 2003
Baculovirus-derived VLPs	500	Liquid water, no adjuvant	Two doses, orally (days 0 and 21)	10 human subjects	70% subjects developed serum IgG, 60% serum IgA, 30% salivary IgA, 42.9% fecal IgA, 66.7% vaginal IgA	Tacket et al,[129] 2003
Baculovirus-derived VLPs	2000	Liquid water, no adjuvant	Two doses, orally (days 0 and 21)	10 human subjects	80% subjects developed serum IgG, 100% serum IgA, 50% salivary IgA, 30% fecal IgA	Tacket et al,[129] 2003
Baculovirus-derived VLPs	250	Liquid containing ISCOM or mutant E coli LT toxin	Three doses (1 oral and 2 intranasal) (days 0, 10, 21)	8 gnotobiotic piglets	100 seroconversion, Th$_1$/Th$_2$ serum cytokines and cytokine-secreting cells, increased IgM, IgA, and IgG antibody-secreting cells; protection against viral shedding and diarrhea (75%–100%)	Souza et al,[102] 2007

Vaccine	Dose (µg)	Formulation	Administration	Subjects	Results	Reference
Baculovirus-derived VLPs	15	Dry powder containing chitosan (MPL at 25 µg)	Two doses, intranasally (days 0 and 21)	5 human subjects	20% subjects developed serum IgG; and 40% developed serum IgA	El-Kamary et al,[104] 2007; Tacket et al,[105] 2009
Baculovirus-derived VLPs	50	Dry powder containing chitosan (MPL at 25 µg)	Two doses, intranasally (days 0 and 21)	20 human subjects	56% subjects developed serum IgG; and 72% developed serum IgA	Tacket et al,[105] 2009
Baculovirus-derived VLPs	100	Dry powder containing chitosan (MPL at 25 µg)	Two doses, intranasally (days 0 and 21)	20 human subjects	63% subjects developed serum IgG; and 79% developed serum IgA	Tacket et al,[105] 2009
Baculovirus-derived VLPs	100	Lyophilized, containing MPL and chitosan	Two doses, intranasally, (3 wk apart)	50 human subjects	70% of vaccine recipients developed IgA seroresponse; significantly reduced gastroenteritis (69% of placebo recipients vs 37% of vaccine recipients) and NoV infection (82% of placebo recipients vs 61% of vaccine recipients)	Atmar et al,[96] 2011
Baculovirus-derived VLPs (VP1 + VP2)	50	Liquid containing alhydrogel	Two doses, intramuscularly (days 0 and 30)	2 chimpanzees	No cross-protection. Chimpanzees vaccinated with GI VLPs, but not GII VLPs, were protected from Norwalk virus (GI.1) infection	Bok et al,[106] 2011
VSV vectored Vaccine	10^6 PFU	Liquid Dulbecco's modified Eagle's medium, no adjuvant	One dose, intranasally (day 3)	5 gnotobiotic piglets	100% serum IgG, fecal, nasal, and vaginal IgA; protection against intestinal pathologic changes	Ma et al,[130] 2011

prevent acute viral gastroenteritis after challenge with a homologous viral strain, Norwalk virus (genotype GI.1).[96] Within 98 human subjects, 50 participants received the VLP vaccine, 48 participants received placebo, and 90 received both doses (47 participants in the vaccine group and 43 in the placebo group). Norwalk virus-specific IgA antibody was detected in 70% of vaccine recipients. After challenge with Norwalk virus, vaccination significantly reduced the frequency of Norwalk virus gastroenteritis. Sixty-nine percent of placebo recipients developed gastroenteritis, whereas only 37% of vaccine recipients had symptoms. In addition, 82% of placebo recipients had Norwalk virus infection, whereas only 61% of vaccine recipients had infection. It was concluded that the VLP vaccine candidate provided protection against illness and infection after challenge with a homologous virus (see **Table 4**).[96]

The advantage of a VLP-based vaccine candidate is that it is safe and immunogenic in humans. However, the duration of the immune response may be limited because VLPs are nonreplicating proteins. It is unknown whether it can provide cross-protection against heterogeneous strains of human NoV; however, as discussed earlier, no long-term immunity is acquired after human NoV infection because of strain diversity, so cross-protection against heterogeneous strains is unlikely. For example, chimpanzees vaccinated with VLPs derived from GII.4 strains failed to protect Norwalk virus (GI.1 strain), providing evidence that VLPs may not provide cross-protection against different genotype of NoV.[106] In addition, production of VLPs in vitro is time consuming and expensive. Immunization usually requires a high dosage of VLPs and multiple booster immunizations. The efficacy of VLP-based vaccines relies on the addition of mucosal adjuvants such as cholera toxin, E coli toxin, ISCOM, chitosan, and MPL.

Live Vectored Vaccine Candidates

The first live-virus vector vaccine was reported by Smith and colleagues in 1983.[107] A recombinant vaccinia virus expressing hepatitis B surface antigen–induced hepatitis B–specific antibodies in rabbits. This discovery has inspired the development of many other live-virus vectors, DNA viruses (adenoviruses and herpesviruses); positive-strand RNA viruses (alphaviruses and flaviviruses); negative-sense RNA viruses (vesicular stomatitis virus [VSV], and Newcastle disease virus). In general, a live vectored vaccine may be suitable for the following 3 conditions: viruses that cause persistent infections, such as HIV and hepatitis C virus (HCV); viruses that are highly lethal such as severe acute respiratory syndrome, Ebola, and Marburg viruses; and viruses that cannot be grown in cell culture, such as human NoV.

Three live vectored vaccine candidates have been developed for human NoV. Harrington and colleagues[108] first developed a Venezuelan equine encephalitis (VEE) vectored human NoV vaccine candidate. VEE replicons expressing Norwalk VLPs induced systemic, mucosal, and heterotypic immunities against NoV. Recently, adenovirus expressing capsid protein of human NoV has been constructed.[109] Mice vaccinated by the adenovirus-vectored human NoV vaccine produced systemic, mucosal, and cellular Th_1/Th_2 immune responses. A combination of an adenovirus-vectored vaccine and a VLP-based subunit vaccine can enhance human NoV–specific immunity.[110] Recently, Ma and Li[111] generated a recombinant VSV vectored human NoV vaccine candidate (rVSV-VP1). Mice inoculated with a single dose (10^6 PFU) of rVSV-VP1 through intranasal and oral routes stimulated a significantly stronger humoral and cellular immune response than baculovirus-expressed VLP vaccination. Furthermore, recombinant rVSV-VP1 triggered strong human NoV–specific immunity in gnotobiotic piglets and protected pigs from the challenge of a human NoV GII.4 strain, showing that live vectored human NoV vaccine is protective in an animal model.[112]

Although live vectored vaccine candidates are promising, it may be challenging to implement their use in human clinical trials. For example, the biosafety of VEE may be an issue, because VEE is a biodefense pathogen and the use of functional VEE genes is restricted. Delivery of the adenovirus-vectored vaccine may be hampered because a large portion of the global population has preexisting immunities against the adenovirus vector.[113] Although VSV is not a human pathogen, there is little experience with VSV administration in humans. At least 3 independent phase I human clinical trials are being performed to test the safety, immune response, and effectiveness of the VSV-based HIV vaccines and oncolytic therapy in humans. It seems clear that detailed information on safety and efficacy of VSV-based vaccines in humans will be forthcoming. The outcomes of these studies will facilitate future clinical trials of VSV vectored NoV vaccine candidates in humans.

SUMMARY

Human NoV is the number 1 cause of foodborne illness. Despite the research efforts, human NoV is still poorly understood and understudied. There is no effective measure to eliminate this virus from food and the environment. Future research efforts should focus on developing: (1) an efficient cell culture system and a small animal model, (2) rapid and sensitive detection methods, (3) novel sanitizers and control interventions, and (4) vaccines and antiviral drugs. Furthermore, there is an urgent need to build multidisciplinary and multi-institutional teams to combat this important biodefense agent.

REFERENCES

1. Norovirus: Trends and outbreaks. Centers for Disease Control and Prevention. Available at: http://www.cdc.gov/norovirus/trends-outbreaks.html. Accessed March 19, 2012.
2. Scallan E, Hoekstra RM, Angulo FJ, et al. Foodborne illness acquired in the United States–major pathogens. Emerg Infect Dis 2011;17(1):7–15.
3. Hall AJ, Eisenbart VG, Etingue AL, et al. Epidemiology of foodborne norovirus outbreaks, United States, 2001-2008. Emerg Infect Dis 2012;18(10):1566–73.
4. Batz MB, Hoffmann S, Morris JG Jr. Ranking the disease burden of 14 pathogens in food sources in the United States using attribution data from outbreak investigations and expert elicitation. J Food Prot 2012;75(7):1278–91.
5. Hoffmann S, Batz MB, Morris JG Jr. Annual cost of illness and quality-adjusted life year losses in the United States due to 14 foodborne pathogens. J Food Prot 2012;75(7):1292–302.
6. Glass PJ, White LJ, Ball JM, et al. Norwalk virus open reading frame 3 encodes a minor structural protein. J Virol 2000;74(14):6581.
7. Lopman BA, Reacher MH, Vipond IB, et al. Clinical manifestation of norovirus gastroenteritis in health care settings. Clin Infect Dis 2004;39(3):318–24.
8. Rockx B, De Wit M, Vennema H, et al. Natural history of human calicivirus infection: a prospective cohort study. Clin Infect Dis 2002;35(3):246–53.
9. Bok K, Green KY. Norovirus gastroenteritis in immunocompromised patients. N Engl J Med 2012;367(22):2126–32.
10. Glass RI, Parashar UD, Estes MK. Norovirus gastroenteritis. N Engl J Med 2009; 361(18):1776–85.
11. Kapikian AZ, Wyatt RG, Dolin R, et al. Visualization by immune electron-microscopy of a 27-nm particle associated with acute infectious nonbacterial gastroenteritis. J Virol 1972;10(5):1075–81.

12. Zheng DP, Ando T, Fankhauser RL, et al. Norovirus classification and proposed strain nomenclature. Virology 2006;346(2):312–23.
13. Division of Viral Diseases, National Center for Immunization and Respiratory Diseases, Centers for Disease Control and Prevention. Updated norovirus outbreak management and disease prevention guidelines. MMWR Recomm Rep 2011; 60(RR-3):1–18.
14. Siebenga JJ, Vennema H, Zheng DP, et al. Norovirus illness is a global problem: emergence and spread of norovirus GII.4 variants, 2001-2007. J Infect Dis 2009;200(5):802–12.
15. Vega E, Barclay L, Gregoricus N, et al. Novel surveillance network for norovirus gastroenteritis outbreaks, United States. Emerg Infect Dis 2011;17(8): 1389–95.
16. Centers for Disease Control and Prevention (CDC). Notes from the field: emergence of new norovirus strain GII.4 Sydney–United States, 2012. MMWR Morb Mortal Wkly Rep 2013;62:55.
17. Donaldson EF, Lindesmith LC, Lobue AD, et al. Norovirus pathogenesis: mechanisms of persistence and immune evasion in human populations. Immunol Rev 2008;225(1):190.
18. Tan M, Jiang X. Norovirus and its histo-blood group antigen receptors: an answer to a historical puzzle. Trends Microbiol 2005;13(6):285–93.
19. de Rougemont A, Ruvoen-Clouet N, Simon B, et al. Qualitative and quantitative analysis of the binding of GII.4 norovirus variants onto human blood group antigens. J Virol 2011;85(9):4057–70.
20. Le Pendu J, Ruvoen-Clouet N, Kindberg E, et al. Mendelian resistance to human norovirus infections. Semin Immunol 2006;18(6):375–86.
21. Jiang X, Wang M, Graham DY, et al. Expression, self-assembly, and antigenicity of the Norwalk virus capsid protein. J Virol 1992;66(11):6527.
22. Hardy ME. Norovirus protein structure and function. FEMS Microbiol Lett 2005; 253(1):1–8.
23. Daughenbaugh KF, Fraser CS, Hershey JW, et al. The genome-linked protein VPg of the Norwalk virus binds eIF3, suggesting its role in translation initiation complex recruitment. EMBO J 2003;22(11):2852–9.
24. Prasad BV, Hardy ME, Dokland T, et al. X-ray crystallographic structure of the Norwalk virus capsid. Science 1999;286(5438):287.
25. Wobus CE, Thackray LB, Virgin HW 4th. Murine norovirus: a model system to study norovirus biology and pathogenesis. J Virol 2006;80(11):5104–12.
26. Doultree JC, Druce JD, Birch CJ, et al. Inactivation of feline calicivirus, a Norwalk virus surrogate. J Hosp Infect 1999;41(1):51–7.
27. Farkas T, Sestak K, Wei C, et al. Characterization of a rhesus monkey calicivirus representing a new genus of Caliciviridae. J Virol 2008;82(11):5408–16.
28. Lou F, Huang P, Neetoo H, et al. High-pressure inactivation of human norovirus virus-like particles provides evidence that the capsid of human norovirus is highly pressure resistant. Appl Environ Microbiol 2012;78(15):5320–7.
29. Feng K, Divers E, Ma Y, et al. Inactivation of a human norovirus surrogate, human norovirus virus-like particles, and vesicular stomatitis virus by gamma irradiation. Appl Environ Microbiol 2011;77(10):3507–17.
30. Marks PJ, Vipond IB, Regan FM, et al. A school outbreak of Norwalk-like virus: evidence for airborne transmission. Epidemiol Infect 2003;131(1): 727–36.
31. Teunis PF, Moe CL, Liu P, et al. Norwalk virus: how infectious is it? J Med Virol 2008;80(8):1468–76.

32. Aoki Y, Suto A, Mizuta K, et al. Duration of norovirus excretion and the longitudinal course of viral load in norovirus-infected elderly patients. J Hosp Infect 2010;75(1):42–6.
33. Atmar RL, Opekun AR, Gilger MA, et al. Norwalk virus shedding after experimental human infection. Emerg Infect Dis 2008;14(10):1553–7.
34. Armbrust S, Kramer A, Olbertz D, et al. Norovirus infections in preterm infants: wide variety of clinical courses. BMC Res Notes 2009;2:96.
35. Ludwig A, Adams O, Laws HJ, et al. Quantitative detection of norovirus excretion in pediatric patients with cancer and prolonged gastroenteritis and shedding of norovirus. J Med Virol 2008;80(8):1461–7.
36. Fishman JA. Infections in immunocompromised hosts and organ transplant recipients: essentials. Liver Transpl 2011;17(Suppl 3):S34–7.
37. Koo HL, DuPont HL. Noroviruses as a potential cause of protracted and lethal disease in immunocompromised patients. Clin Infect Dis 2009;49(7):1069–71.
38. Wingfield T, Gallimore CI, Xerry J, et al. Chronic norovirus infection in an HIV-positive patient with persistent diarrhoea: a novel cause. J Clin Virol 2010; 49(3):219–22.
39. Sukhrie FH, Siebenga JJ, Beersma MF, et al. Chronic shedders as reservoir for nosocomial transmission of norovirus. J Clin Microbiol 2010;48(11):4303–5.
40. Siebenga JJ, Beersma MF, Vennema H, et al. High prevalence of prolonged norovirus shedding and illness among hospitalized patients: a model for in vivo molecular evolution. J Infect Dis 2008;198(7):994–1001.
41. Seymour IJ, Appleton H. Foodborne viruses and fresh produce. J Appl Microbiol 2001;91(5):759–73.
42. Graham DY, Jiang X, Tanaka T, et al. Norwalk virus infection of volunteers: new insights based on improved assays. J Infect Dis 1994;170(1):34–43.
43. Phillips G, Lopman B, Tam CC, et al. Diagnosing norovirus-associated infectious intestinal disease using viral load. BMC Infect Dis 2009;9:63.
44. Herwaldt BL, Lew JF, Moe CL, et al. Characterization of a variant strain of Norwalk virus from a food-borne outbreak of gastroenteritis on a cruise ship in Hawaii. J Clin Microbiol 1994;32(4):861–6.
45. Hjertqvist M, Johansson A, Svensson N, et al. Four outbreaks of norovirus gastroenteritis after consuming raspberries, Sweden, June-August 2006. Euro Surveill 2006;11(9):E060907.1.
46. Falkenhorst G, Krusell L, Lisby M, et al. Imported frozen raspberries cause a series of norovirus outbreaks in Denmark, 2005. Euro Surveill 2005;10(9): E050922.2.
47. Gaulin CD, Ramsay D, Cardinal P, et al. Epidemic of gastroenteritis of viral origin associated with eating imported raspberries. Can J Public Health 1999;90(1):37–40.
48. Le Guyader FS, Mittelholzer C, Haugarreau L, et al. Detection of noroviruses in raspberries associated with a gastroenteritis outbreak. Int J Food Microbiol 2004;97(2):179–86.
49. Dowell SF, Groves C, Kirkland KB, et al. A multistate outbreak of oyster-associated gastroenteritis: implications for interstate tracing of contaminated shellfish. J Infect Dis 1995;171(6):1497–503.
50. Morse DL, Guzewich JJ, Hanrahan JP, et al. Widespread outbreaks of clam- and oyster-associated gastroenteritis. Role of Norwalk virus. N Engl J Med 1986; 314(11):678–81.
51. van Beek J, Ambert-Balay K, Botteldoorn N, et al. Indications for worldwide increased norovirus activity associated with emergence of a new variant of genotype II.4, late 2012. Euro Surveill 2013;18(1):8–9.

52. Le Guyader FS, Neill FH, Dubois E, et al. A semiquantitative approach to esti-
    mate Norwalk-like virus contamination of oysters implicated in an outbreak. Int
    J Food Microbiol 2003;87(1–2):107–12.
53. Atmar RL, Estes MK. Diagnosis of noncultivatable gastroenteritis viruses, the hu-
    man caliciviruses. Clin Microbiol Rev 2001;14(1):15–37.
54. Green J, Norcott JP, Lewis D, et al. Norwalk-like viruses: demonstration of
    genomic diversity by polymerase chain reaction. J Clin Microbiol 1993;31(11):
    3007–12.
55. Antonishyn NA, Crozier NA, McDonald RR, et al. Rapid detection of norovirus
    based on an automated extraction protocol and a real-time multiplexed
    single-step RT-PCR. J Clin Virol 2006;37(3):156–61.
56. Kageyama T, Kojima S, Shinohara M, et al. Broadly reactive and highly sensitive
    assay for Norwalk-like viruses based on real-time quantitative reverse transcrip-
    tion-PCR. J Clin Microbiol 2003;41(4):1548–57.
57. Richards GP, Watson MA, Fankhauser RL, et al. Genogroup I and II norovi-
    ruses detected in stool samples by real-time reverse transcription-PCR using
    highly degenerate universal primers. Appl Environ Microbiol 2004;70(12):
    7179–84.
58. Hoehne M, Schreier E. Detection of norovirus genogroup I and II by multiplex
    real-time RT-PCR using a 3'-minor groove binder-DNA probe. BMC Infect Dis
    2006;6:69.
59. Pang XL, Preiksaitis JK, Lee B. Multiplex real time RT-PCR for the detection and
    quantitation of norovirus genogroups I and II in patients with acute gastroenter-
    itis. J Clin Virol 2005;33(2):168–71.
60. Green J, Henshilwood K, Gallimore CI, et al. A nested reverse transcriptase
    PCR assay for detection of small round-structured viruses in environmentally
    contaminated molluscan shellfish. Appl Environ Microbiol 1998;64(3):
    858–63.
61. O'Neill HJ, McCaughey C, Wyatt DE, et al. Gastroenteritis outbreaks associated
    with Norwalk-like viruses and their investigation by nested RT-PCR. BMC Micro-
    biol 2001;1:14.
62. Nishimura N, Nakayama H, Yoshizumi S, et al. Detection of noroviruses in fecal
    specimens by direct RT-PCR without RNA purification. J Virol Methods 2010;
    163(2):282–6.
63. Boxman IL, Verhoef L, Dijkman R, et al. Year-round prevalence of norovirus in the
    environment of catering companies without a recently reported outbreak of
    gastroenteritis. Appl Environ Microbiol 2011;77(9):2968–74.
64. De Medici D, Suffredini E, Crudeli S, et al. Effectiveness of an RT-booster-PCR
    method for detection of noroviruses in stools collected after an outbreak of
    gastroenteritis. J Virol Methods 2007;144(1–2):161–4.
65. Fukuda S, Takao S, Kuwayama M, et al. Rapid detection of norovirus from fecal
    specimens by real-time reverse transcription-loop-mediated isothermal amplifi-
    cation assay. J Clin Microbiol 2006;44(4):1376–81.
66. Iturriza-Gomara M, Xerry J, Gallimore CI, et al. Evaluation of the Loopamp (loop-
    mediated isothermal amplification) kit for detecting norovirus RNA in faecal sam-
    ples. J Clin Virol 2008;42(4):389–93.
67. Yoda T, Suzuki Y, Yamazaki K, et al. Application of a modified loop-mediated
    isothermal amplification kit for detecting norovirus genogroups I and II. J Med
    Virol 2009;81(12):2072–8.
68. Duizer E, Pielaat A, Vennema H, et al. Probabilities in norovirus outbreak diag-
    nosis. J Clin Virol 2007;40(1):38–42.

69. Castriciano S, Luinstra K, Petrich A, et al. Comparison of the RIDASCREEN norovirus enzyme immunoassay to IDEIA NLV GI/GII by testing stools also assayed by RT-PCR and electron microscopy. J Virol Methods 2007;141(2):216–9.

70. Costantini V, Grenz L, Fritzinger A, et al. Diagnostic accuracy and analytical sensitivity of IDEIA norovirus assay for routine screening of human norovirus. J Clin Microbiol 2010;48(8):2770–8.

71. Gray JJ, Kohli E, Ruggeri FM, et al. European multicenter evaluation of commercial enzyme immunoassays for detecting norovirus antigen in fecal samples. Clin Vaccine Immunol 2007;14(10):1349–55.

72. Morillo SG, Luchs A, Cilli A, et al. Norovirus 3rd generation kit: an improvement for rapid diagnosis of sporadic gastroenteritis cases and valuable for outbreak detection. J Virol Methods 2011;173(1):13–6.

73. Siqueira JA, Linhares Ada C, Oliveira Dde S, et al. Evaluation of third-generation RIDASCREEN enzyme immunoassay for the detection of norovirus antigens in stool samples of hospitalized children in Belem, Para, Brazil. Diagn Microbiol Infect Dis 2011;71(4):391–5.

74. MacCannell T, Umscheid CA, Agarwal RK, et al. Guideline for the prevention and control of norovirus gastroenteritis outbreaks in healthcare settings. Infect Control Hosp Epidemiol 2011;32(10):939–69.

75. Bruggink LD, Witlox KJ, Sameer R, et al. Evaluation of the RIDA(®)QUICK immunochromatographic norovirus detection assay using specimens from Australian gastroenteritis incidents. J Virol Methods 2011;173(1):121–6.

76. Bruins MJ, Wolfhagen MJ, Schirm J, et al. Evaluation of a rapid immunochromatographic test for the detection of norovirus in stool samples. Eur J Clin Microbiol Infect Dis 2010;29(6):741–3.

77. Kirby A, Gurgel RQ, Dove W, et al. An evaluation of the RIDASCREEN and IDEIA enzyme immunoassays and the RIDAQUICK immunochromatographic test for the detection of norovirus in faecal specimens. J Clin Virol 2010;49(4):254–7.

78. Park KS, Baek KA, Kim DU, et al. Evaluation of a new immunochromatographic assay kit for the rapid detection of norovirus in fecal specimens. Ann Lab Med 2012;32(1):79–81.

79. Thongprachum A, Khamrin P, Tran DN, et al. Evaluation and comparison of the efficiency of immunochromatography methods for norovirus detection. Clin Lab 2012;58(5–6):489–93.

80. Pyo D, Yoo J. New trends in fluorescence immunochromatography. J Immunoassay Immunochem 2012;33(2):203–22.

81. Buchan B, Anderson N, Jannetto P, et al. Simultaneous detection of influenza A and its subtypes (H1, H3, 2009 H1N1), influenza B, and RSV A and B in respiratory specimens on an automated, random access, molecular platform. 21st European Congress of Clinical Microbiology and Infectious Diseases (ECCMID). Milan, May 7, 2011.

82. Predmore A, Li J. Enhanced removal of a human norovirus surrogate from fresh vegetables and fruits by a combination of surfactants and sanitizers. Appl Environ Microbiol 2011;77(14):4829–38.

83. Feliciano L, Li J, Lee J, et al. Efficacies of sodium hypochlorite and quaternary ammonium sanitizers for reduction of norovirus and selected bacteria during ware-washing operations. PLoS One 2012;7(12):e50273.

84. Li J, Predmore A, Divers E, et al. New interventions against human norovirus: progress, opportunities, and challenges. Annu Rev Food Sci Technol 2012;3:331–52.

85. Norovirus in healthcare facilities fact sheet. Centers for Disease Control and Prevention. Available at: http://www.cdc.gov/hai/pdfs/norovirus/229110-ANoroCaseFactSheet508.pdf. Accessed March 19, 2013.

86. Tian P, Yang D, Jiang X, et al. Specificity and kinetics of norovirus binding to magnetic bead-conjugated histo-blood group antigens. J Appl Microbiol 2010;109(5):1753–62.

87. Bae J, Schwab KJ. Evaluation of murine norovirus, feline calicivirus, poliovirus, and MS2 as surrogates for human norovirus in a model of viral persistence in surface water and groundwater. Appl Environ Microbiol 2008;74(2):477–84.

88. Baert L, Vandekinderen I, Devlieghere F, et al. Efficacy of sodium hypochlorite and peroxyacetic acid to reduce murine norovirus 1, b40-8, *Listeria monocytogenes*, and *Escherichia coli* o157:H7 on shredded iceberg lettuce and in residual wash water. J Food Prot 2009;72(5):1047–54.

89. Baert L, Uyttendaele M, Vermeersch M, et al. Survival and transfer of murine norovirus 1, a surrogate for human noroviruses, during the production process of deep-frozen onions and spinach. J Food Prot 2008;71(8):1590–7.

90. Gulati BR, Allwood PB, Hedberg CW, et al. Efficacy of commonly used disinfectants for the inactivation of calicivirus on strawberry, lettuce, and a food-contact surface. J Food Prot 2001;64(9):1430–4.

91. Dawson DJ, Paish A, Staffell LM, et al. Survival of viruses on fresh produce, using MS2 as a surrogate for norovirus. J Appl Microbiol 2005;98(1):203–9.

92. Lou F, Neetoo H, Chen H, et al. Inactivation of a human norovirus surrogate by high-pressure processing: effectiveness, mechanism, and potential application in the fresh produce industry. Appl Environ Microbiol 2011;77(5):1862–71.

93. Lou F, Neetoo H, Li J, et al. Lack of correlation between virus barosensitivity and the presence of a viral envelope during inactivation of human rotavirus, vesicular stomatitis virus, and avian metapneumovirus by high-pressure processing. Appl Environ Microbiol 2011;77(24):8538–47.

94. Leon JS, Kingsley DH, Montes JS, et al. Randomized, double-blinded clinical trial for human norovirus inactivation in oysters by high hydrostatic pressure processing. Appl Environ Microbiol 2011;77(15):5476–82.

95. Dancho BA, Chen H, Kingsley DH. Discrimination between infectious and noninfectious human norovirus using porcine gastric mucin. Int J Food Microbiol 2012;155(3):222–6.

96. Atmar RL, Bernstein DI, Harro CD, et al. Norovirus vaccine against experimental human Norwalk virus illness. N Engl J Med 2011;365(23):2178–87.

97. Patel MM, Widdowson MA, Glass RI, et al. Systematic literature review of role of noroviruses in sporadic gastroenteritis. Emerg Infect Dis 2008;14(8):1224–31.

98. Mason HS, Ball JM, Shi JJ, et al. Expression of Norwalk virus capsid protein in transgenic tobacco and potato and its oral immunogenicity in mice. Proc Natl Acad Sci U S A 1996;93(11):5335–40.

99. Zhang XR, Buehner NA, Hutson AM, et al. Tomato is a highly effective vehicle for expression and oral immunization with Norwalk virus capsid protein. Plant Biotechnol J 2006;4(4):419–32.

100. Ball JM, Hardy ME, Atmar RL, et al. Oral immunization with recombinant Norwalk virus-like particles induces a systemic and mucosal immune response in mice. J Virol 1998;72(2):1345.

101. Souza M, Cheetham SM, Azevedo MS, et al. Cytokine and antibody responses in gnotobiotic pigs after infection with human norovirus genogroup II.4 (HS66 strain). J Virol 2007;81(17):9183–92.

102. Souza M, Costantini V, Azevedo MS, et al. A human norovirus-like particle vaccine adjuvanted with ISCOM or MLT induces cytokine and antibody responses and protection to the homologous GII.4 human norovirus in a gnotobiotic pig disease model. Vaccine 2007;25(50):8448.
103. Ball JM, Graham DY, Opekun AR, et al. Recombinant Norwalk virus-like particles given orally to volunteers: phase I study. Gastroenterology 1999;117(1): 40–8.
104. El-Kamary S, Pasetti M, Tacket C, et al. Phase 1 dose escalation, safety and immunogenicity of intranasal dry powder norovirus vaccine. 3rd International Calicivirus Conference. Cancun, November 10, 2007.
105. Tacket C, Frey S, Bernstein D, et al. Phase 1 dose-comparison, safety and immunogenicity of intranasal dry powder Norwalk VLP vaccine. 5th International Conference on Vaccines for Enteric Diseases. Malaga, September 9, 2009.
106. Bok K, Parra GI, Mitra T, et al. Chimpanzees as an animal model for human norovirus infection and vaccine development. Proc Natl Acad Sci U S A 2011; 108(1):325–30.
107. Smith GL, Mackett M, Moss B. Infectious vaccinia virus recombinants that express hepatitis B virus surface antigen. Nature 1983;302(5908):490–5.
108. Harrington PR, Yount B, Johnston RE, et al. Systemic, mucosal, and heterotypic immune induction in mice inoculated with Venezuelan equine encephalitis replicons expressing Norwalk virus-like particles. J Virol 2002;76(2):730–42.
109. Guo L, Wang J, Zhou H, et al. Intranasal administration of a recombinant adenovirus expressing the norovirus capsid protein stimulates specific humoral, mucosal, and cellular immune responses in mice. Vaccine 2008;26(4):460–8.
110. Guo L, Zhou H, Wang M, et al. A recombinant adenovirus prime-virus-like particle boost regimen elicits effective and specific immunities against norovirus in mice. Vaccine 2009;27(38):5233–8.
111. Ma Y, Li J. Vesicular stomatitis virus as a vector to deliver virus-like particles of human norovirus: a new vaccine candidate against an important noncultivable virus. J Virol 2011;85(6):2942.
112. Duan Y, Ma Y, Hughes J, et al. A vesicular stomatitis virus (VSV)-based human norovirus vaccine provides protection against norovirus challenge in a gnotobiotic pig model. Madison (WI): American Society for Virology; 2012.
113. Sekaly RP. The failed HIV Merck vaccine study: a step back or a launching point for future vaccine development? J Exp Med 2008;205(1):7–12.
114. Desai R, Yen C, Wikswo M, et al. Transmission of norovirus among NBA players and staff, winter 2010–2011. Clin Infect Dis 2011;53(11):1115–7.
115. Repp KK, Keene WE. A point-source norovirus outbreak caused by exposure to fomites. J Infect Dis 2012;205(11):1639–41.
116. Dore B, Keaveney S, Flannery J, et al. Management of health risks associated with oysters harvested from a norovirus contaminated area, Ireland, February-March 2010. Euro Surveill 2010;15(19):pii/19567.
117. Arvelo W, Sosa SM, Juliao P, et al. Norovirus outbreak of probable waterborne transmission with high attack rate in a Guatemalan resort. J Clin Virol 2012 Sep;55(1):8–11.
118. Wadl M, Scherer K, Nielsen S, et al. Food-borne norovirus-outbreak at a military base, Germany, 2009. BMC Infect Dis 2010;10(30). http://dx.doi.org/10.1186/1471-2334-10-30.
119. Koh SJ, Cho HG, Kim BH, et al. An outbreak of gastroenteritis caused by norovirus-contaminated groundwater at a waterpark in Korea. J Korean Med Sci 2011;26(1):28–32.

120. Barrabeig I, Rovira A, Buesa J, et al. Foodborne norovirus outbreak: The role of an asymptomatic food handler. BMC Infect Dis 2010;10(269). http://dx.doi.org/10.1186/1471-2334-10-269.

121. Yee EL, Palacio H, Atmar RL, et al. Widespread outbreak of norovirus gastroenteritis among evacuees of hurricane katrina residing in a large "Megashelter" In Houston, Texas: Lessons learned for prevention. Clin Infect Dis 2007;44(8):1032-9.

122. Becker KM, Moe CL, Southwick KL, et al. Transmission of norwalk virus during football game. N Engl J Med 2000;343(17):1223-7.

123. Tuladhar E, Hazeleger WC, Koopmans M, et al. Residual viral and bacterial contamination of surfaces after cleaning and disinfection. Appl Environ Microbiol 2012;78(21):7769-75.

124. Liu P, Yuen Y, Hsiao HM, et al. Effectiveness of liquid soap and hand sanitizer against norwalk virus on contaminated hands. Appl Environ Microbiol 2009;76(2):394-9.

125. Nowak P, Topping JR, Fotheringham V, et al. Measurement of the virolysis of human gii.4 norovirus in response to disinfectants and sanitisers. J Virol Methods 2011;174(1-2):7-11.

126. Park GW, Barclay L, Macinga D, et al. Comparative efficacy of seven hand sanitizers against murine norovirus, feline calicivirus, and gii.4 norovirus. J Food Prot 2011;73(12):2232-8.

127. Li D, Baert L, Van Coillie E, Uyttendaele M. Critical studies on binding-based rt-pcr detection of infectious noroviruses. J Virol Methods 2011;177(2):153-9.

128. Hudson JB, Sharma M, Petric M. Inactivation of norovirus by ozone gas in conditions relevant to healthcare. J Hosp Infect 2007;66(1):40-5.

129. Tacket CO, Sztein MB, Losonsky GA, et al. Humoral, mucosal, and cellular immune responses to oral Norwalk virus-like particles in volunteers. Clin Immunol 2003;108(3):241-7.

130. Ma Y, Li J. Vesicular stomatitis virus as a vector to deliver virus like particles of human norovirus: a new vaccine candidate against an important noncultivable virus. J Virol 2011;85(6):2942-52.

Transmission of *Clostridium difficile* in Foods

Dallas G. Hoover, PhD[a],*,
Alexander Rodriguez-Palacios, DVM, DVSc, PhD, Diplomate ACVIM, Diplomate ACVM[b]

KEYWORDS

- *Clostridium difficile* • Foods • Zoonosis • Pseudomembranous colitis
- Antibiotic treatment

KEY POINTS

- *Clostridium difficile* causes diarrheal illness, often following the administration of antibiotics.
- The infective dose for *C difficile* infections (CDIs) is unknown.
- A contagious spore-forming organism, its spores are resistant to inactivation.
- CDI can progress to more protracted and threatening diseases such as pseudomembranous colitis, toxic megacolon, and perforated bowel.
- Long considered a nosocomial disease, increasing levels of community-associated CDI and growing evidence of limited person-to-person transmission raise questions of foodborne transmission of *C difficile* in light of its isolation from foods.

INTRODUCTION

Since 2005, epidemic and nonepidemic strains of *Clostridium difficile* have been repeatedly isolated from various foods in the Americas and Europe. Because the isolated strains have repeatedly resembled the genetic and virulent features of strains associated with severe *C difficile* infections (CDIs) in humans, there are increasing concerns that *C difficile* is a foodborne (and zoonotic) pathogen.[1]

Once an organism relatively obscure to the general public, *C difficile* now has established recognition as a highly contagious intestinal microorganism capable of causing protracted hospital-associated diarrheal illnesses, usually in situations when antibiotics are administered in patient care.[2] Contributing factors to this greater awareness are:

- A corresponding nationwide increase in the incidence of CDI
- A heightened severity of disease symptoms with higher reoccurrence rates
- A notable increase in antimicrobial resistance[3,4]

[a] Department of Animal & Food Sciences, University of Delaware, 531 South College Avenue, Newark, DE 19716-2150, USA; [b] Division of Gastroenterology and Liver Disease, Digestive Health Research Center, Case Western Reserve University School of Medicine, 2109 Adelbert Road, Cleveland, OH 44106, USA
* Corresponding author.
E-mail address: dgh@udel.edu

Infect Dis Clin N Am 27 (2013) 675–685
http://dx.doi.org/10.1016/j.idc.2013.05.004
0891-5520/13/$ – see front matter © 2013 Elsevier Inc. All rights reserved.

id.theclinics.com

PERSON-TO-PERSON TRANSMISSION

C difficile is an enteric pathogen that produces spores. Until very recently, CDIs were believed to be almost exclusively nosocomial, mostly attributable to transmission from infected patients to uninfected patients through the ingestion of spores present in shared rooms and on equipment surfaces, or on the hands or clothing of health care professionals; however, the importance of nosocomial (person-to-person) transmission has been recently questioned by whole-genome sequencing of isolates deemed to be epidemiologically linked by transmission in assumed cases of hospital outbreaks.[5] In contrast to methicillin-resistant *Staphylococcus aureus* infections, genome sequencing showed that patients in CDI outbreaks were not consistently affected by clonal transmission of *C difficile* strains. In some cases the strains were diverse and did not match strains from concurrent inpatients; in one case the strain matched a strain from a patient sampled 3 years earlier. Single-nucleotide polymorphisms indicated that a significant fraction of nosocomial CDIs are due to strains originating from sources outside hospitals. A large multilocus sequence typing (MLST) study, with data from 1276 *C difficile* gathered over 2.5 years, also found a low proportion of CDI cases linked to clonal strains; on average only 1 in every 4 new CDI cases had molecular evidence of a ward-based inpatient source.[6] The majority of CDIs (>75%) cannot be explained by nosocomial (person-to-person) transmission. There is a need to investigate other potential forms of CDI transmission, including foods and animals.[1,5,6] The possibility exists that most infections that are thought to be nosocomial actually represent asymptomatic importation of *C difficile* from the community into the hospital with subsequent development of the disease from disruption of the gut biota, such as the administration of antibiotics. Confirming evidence of a linkage between ingestion of contaminated foods and CDI is necessary before stating that *C difficile* causes foodborne disease; nonetheless, it is important to educate public health and food professionals about this possibility.

THE BACTERIUM

Like *Clostridium botulinum*, *C difficile* is a mesophilic, spore-forming bacterium requiring anaerobic conditions for growth, but unlike *C botulinum*, *C difficile* does not produce paralytic neurotoxins nor does it replicate opportunistically in moist, low-acid foods.[7] The major reservoir of *C difficile* is the gastrointestinal tract of humans and warm-blooded animals. In the gut it is a relatively slow-growing bacterium compared with other intestinal bacteria.[7] Phenotypically, *C difficile* closely resembles *Clostridium sporogenes*; however, unlike *C sporogenes*, *C difficile* cannot digest meat or milk, and produces no lipases.[7]

PHYSIOLOGY: BACTERIAL RESPONSE TO TEMPERATURES

Reported growth temperatures range from 25° to 45°C with optima between 30° and 37°C; however, some strains grow faster at higher temperatures. Similar to other pathogenic spore formers and mesophilic clostridia, spores of *C difficile* are relatively unaffected by exposures to cooking temperatures approaching 72°C.[8] Kept at 85°C for 15 minutes, or at 96°C for 3 minutes, spores can be reduced by 5 to 6 $\log_{10}$. Higher temperatures are needed to ensure consistent elimination of spores.[9]

Sublethal heating promotes germination so that subsequent growth under anaerobic conditions would be theoretically possible.[9] It is also reasonable to expect that even relatively low levels of spores of *C difficile* (eg, 10^1 spores/g) will be able to survive exposure to light cooking, such as sautéing. There are end-point cooking-temperature recommendations from the United States Department of Agriculture (USDA), according to the type of meal, to promote the consumption of safe foods, but these recommendations primarily address the destruction of vegetative bacterial cells (eg, *Salmonella*) and not spores. To date there are no official recommendations regarding the control of *C difficile* spores in foods.

MECHANISMS OF DISEASE

The components that enable *C difficile* to cause disease are called toxins A and B.[10] Not all strains of *C difficile* produce these toxins. Toxins A and B are among the largest polypeptide toxins known (400–600 kDa). Toxin A is a potent enterotoxin with slight cytotoxic activity while toxin B is an extremely potent cytotoxin.[10] Both toxins damage the gut lining by inactivation of Rho guanosine triphosphatases via glucosylation by disrupting cell cytoskeletons, causing cell rounding, impaired function, and death; however, the toxins may differ in their tropism toward different regions of the cell surface. Most strains associated with CDIs produce both toxins A and B; however, strains capable of producing only toxin B can be equally deleterious in clinical settings. Strains producing only toxin A appear not to be common in nature. Toxin B appears to be essential for disease to occur. Some *C difficile* also produce a third, unrelated toxin, called the binary toxin or *C difficile* transferase (CDT); however, CDT appears significantly less of a contributing disease-causing factor than toxins A and B, although CDT has been associated with epidemic strains. CDT acts on G-actin by adenosine diphosphate ribosylation to inhibit actin polymerization.[11] It may facilitate colonization by inducing the formation of cell protrusions, but its contribution to disease in humans is not well understood.[12]

ASYMPTOMATIC CARRIERS AND GUT BIOTA

Although *C difficile* is regarded as an environmental microorganism that is acquired via the oral route, the role of the environment in the epidemiology of CDI is unclear. Three percent to 5% of healthy adults are believed to be asymptomatic carriers of toxigenic *C difficile*. In hospitalized adults the estimation increases to 20%; in infants younger than 1 year the number dramatically increases to a range of 60% to 70% harboring toxigenic *C difficile* intestinally. Most infants have toxigenic *C difficile*, yet they are completely asymptomatic for diarrheal disease. *C difficile* colonization in infancy seems to confer protection against the disease as children mature.[13] Nontoxigenic strains are protective against colonization with toxigenic strains, and as such have been proposed as a probiotic strategy.[14] It is known that asymptomatic individuals can carry *C difficile* into hospitals; however, it is unclear how people become colonized and infected in the community.

A mechanism that is protective against intestinal colonization by *C difficile* depends on the integrity of the gut biota (or flora). Microbiome studies have shown that more diverse gut floras prevent colonization and CDIs, whereas less flora diversity correlates with disease susceptibility and lesser response to treatment.[15] Simultaneous studies have shown that the administration of fecal transplants can be highly therapeutic, with treatment outcomes in patients with multiple relapses of CDI surpassing standard antibiotic therapy.[16]

DISEASE SEVERITY HAS INCREASED OVER TIME

Initially it was thought that *C difficile* was asymptomatically acquired from other humans. First isolated from the stools of healthy newborns in 1935, *C difficile* was overlooked as a disease-causing agent until the mid-1970s, when the association of *C difficile* to pseudomembranous colitis (PMC) was realized. Once the relationship was determined, the epidemiology of CDIs was studied in detail.

It is now known that elderly and immune-compromised people stand the highest risk of contracting CDI and PMC; disease severity has also increased. PMC gets its name from characteristic patchy lesions that appear on the lining of the large intestine. The severity of symptoms of PMC is highly variable. Toxins produced by *C difficile* kill the tissues lining the bowel that can progress to life-threatening conditions such as toxic megacolon and bowel perforation. Ulcerative colitis and Crohn disease, other forms of patchy inflammatory bowel disease in chronically immune-compromised individuals, are now increasingly associated with concurrent CDIs (up to 10% of cases), which worsens long-term outcomes and complications.[17] Recurrence of CDI occurs, and has also increased to nearly 36% in some studies.

In recent years, disease severity has increased not only in the United States but also in other regions, including Europe and Australia. From a foodborne perspective, only *Campylobacter jejuni* is believed to cause more cases of bacterial diarrhea, but this may change if the numbers of CDIs continue to increase. Measures to control infection have helped reduce CDIs but, with few exceptions, the rising trend remains alongside the aging human population.[18]

ANTIBIOTICS AND INDIVIDUAL SUSCEPTIBILITY

Early on in the characterization of the disease, the association of PMC (linked to CDI in more than 95% of cases) with use of clindamycin was recognized, so that one of the original labels given to PMC was clindamycin colitis[19]; however, virtually any antibiotic that disturbs the intestinal biota can predispose to CDI. CDIs seldom occur without prior antibiotic therapy, and CDI can be observed in up to 30% of all cases of diarrhea induced by antibiotics. CDI can even occur after the use of metronidazole and vancomycin, which are first-choice anti–*C difficile* antibiotics. Intestinal biota imbalances in susceptible people that can lead to CDI are caused by antimicrobials, but they can also be due to other factors, such as:

- Nasogastric tube insertion
- Enteral feeding
- Enema administration
- Surgery
- Inflammatory bowel diseases
- Cancer
- Chemotherapy
- Antacids

ANIMAL RESERVOIRS, THE ZOONOTIC POTENTIAL

An exposure risk may be a problem of not only food exposure but also direct and indirect animal contact. For the most part, CDI is still considered a disease acquired from exposure to contaminated environments, primarily health care settings; however, there is increasing evidence suggesting that environments outside hospitals, and particularly animals and foods, could be unrecognized sources for exposure to *C difficile* by the fecal-oral route, at least in the community (**Box 1**). There is increasing molecular evidence that isolates of *C difficile* from animals and humans are shared, indicating zoonotic transmission.[20]

Box 1
Isolation sources of *Clostridium difficile*

Biological: Humans (bowel and genital tract), camels, horses, donkeys, dogs, cats, birds, swine, chickens, cattle, deer and other wildlife, root vegetables, meats

Environmental: Marine water and sediments, soil, sand, fresh water, rivers, estuaries, hospital facilities, sewage

Data from Refs.[7,21–24]

Zoonosis

A traditional organic fertilizer for crops is horse manure, which serves here as an example of a zoonotic concern for CDI. Horse manure can contain spores of *C difficile*, and these spores remain viable for years; about 7% of healthy horses carry *C difficile*,[25] making spore transfer to foods via fertilizer a realistic probability even if good agricultural practices are followed. Other livestock are of similar concern for CDI by manure or meat vectors; however, it should be noted that young poultry, cattle, and swine are colonized intestinally by *C difficile* more frequently than older animals. For poultry, more than 60% carry *C difficile* early in production, but by the time of slaughter incidence rates decline to a range between 6% and 12%.[26] Despite the low carriage prevalence as food animals reach harvest time, retail foods appear to be variably, yet more commonly contaminated with *C difficile*. Examples are given later in the article.

OCCURRENCE IN FOOD PRODUCTS

Bacterial endospores can persist for many years even in very harsh environments.[27] As one might expect, given the nature of bacteria spores and their presence in the intestinal tracts of livestock, a range of different foods, from vegetables to seafood, have been found to carry spores of *C difficile*, especially foods derived from animal tissue.[28] Spoiled gas-blown packages of raw ground beef and pork were the first foods found positive for *C difficile*.[29] The spoilage population was described as psychrotrophic clostridia; further testing isolated *C difficile* that proved negative for gas production, suggesting that the isolated *C difficile* was not active in spoilage of the product, but rather was associated with other gas-producing clostridia that were possibly all derived from host animals.

Meat Isolates

Since 2006, epidemic toxigenic strains of *C difficile* responsible for disease in humans have been found in various retail meats. Toxigenic strains of *C difficile* were found in 20% of sampled retail ground meats.[30] The occurrence of *C difficile* ranges widely from 0% to 42% in various categories of packaged meats, with most studies reporting a prevalence of less than 7%. In a sampling study at the retail store level, 6% of establishments across 3 provinces of Canada had at least 1 product positive for *C difficile*.[31] A seasonal pattern of food contamination that follows the pattern of CDI seasonality has also been documented since 2007 in North America.[1,31]

Poultry Isolates

Toxigenic strains have also been isolated from poultry.[32] The frequency of *C difficile* contamination oscillates between 3% and 18%, with variability across different parts of the chicken. For example, there were 7 positive samples for *C difficile* in 300 fecal

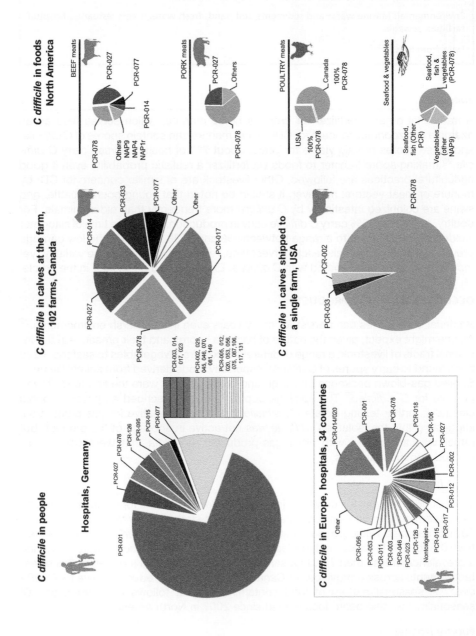

samples from live broiler chickens, and in poultry meat there were a total of 7 positive samples found in 32 samples of meat.[33] These isolates were characterized as toxin-type V, and pulsed-field gel electrophoresis gel type NAP7 or NAP7 variants. Susceptibilities to 11 antimicrobial agents suggested more modestly reduced resistances than reported for other toxin-type V isolates.

Ready-to-Eat Foods and Others

In a 2007 study in Arizona,[34] more than 40% of ready-to-eat meats tested positive for *C difficile*. There was a wide range of contamination based on food groups with *C difficile* found in both uncooked and cooked products. In addition, *C difficile* can also be isolated from vegetables, seafood and fish in North America.[35,36]

Virulent Types Found in Foods

After 2000, several *C difficile* strains associated with severe forms of CDIs appeared to be more virulent, resistant to a wider range of antibiotics, and capable of synthesizing up to 20-fold higher levels of toxins compared with isolates before 2000.[37] Such strains of *C difficile* were later found in food animals and retail foods.[30,31,38]

Polymerase chain reaction (PCR) ribotype 078 now predominates in foods in the United States and Canada. It is discomforting that the largest number of *C difficile* serotypes isolated from foods in the past 10 years are hypervirulent strains, such as PCR ribotypes 027 and 078.[39] It is unclear as to what factors are affecting this apparently undesirable trend.

Based on PCR ribotyping, the *C difficile* strains that have affected people in recent years can also be found in food animals and foods (**Fig. 1**), but not all strains found in foods are present in CDIs, and vice versa. Regional differences determine strain diversity and which strains predominate.[1]

C difficile in Hospital Meals

Physicians are now increasingly examining the role of foods in CDI hospital epidemiology. Two of the studies in the United States illustrate the need for intervention strategies to reduce the risk of pathogen exposure. One study in Pittsburgh showed the repeated isolation of *C difficile* from retail pork sausages sold nationally, after emphasizing no possibility of laboratory cross-contamination.[40] These findings highlight food-processing facilities as a potential critical control point.

Preventive interventions could also be beneficial at the consumer level, especially in patients at risk. Ongoing studies in Texas have shown that on average, 20% to 25% of meat meals served to patients (cold and warm, below 38°C) in hospital settings were contaminated with *C difficile* even though the foods were cooked at 74°C for 15 minutes as per hospital protocols.[41,42] Changes in food-preparation protocols inside and outside health care settings, with nutritional balancing of diets, deserve attention, especially to protect patients at risk during periods of high risk.

◀──────────────────────────────────────

Fig. 1. Overview of the most prevalent polymerase chain reaction (PCR) ribotypes of *Clostridium difficile* strains that have been isolated from humans with CDIs, foods, and animals. (*Reprinted from* Rodriguez-Palacios A, Borgmann S, Kline TR, et al. *Clostridium difficile* in foods and animals: history and measures to reduce exposure. Anim Health Res Rev 2013;14(1):11–29. Copyright © Cambridge University Press, 2013; with permission.)

Table 1
Summary of *Clostridium difficile* in foods

CDI Factors	Response
C difficile can cause disease in susceptible people if the bacterial strain can produce toxins, if the person has imbalanced gut flora, especially if the individual is elderly, or if the person has increased susceptibility to infections or has immune-debilitating conditions	It is advisable to reinforce preventive measures at the community level, because recent studies based on whole-genome sequencing and epidemiologic investigations are showing that person-to-person transmission is a questionable contributor in new CDIs
Regardless of the level of patient vulnerability, if there is no exposure to *C difficile*, there will not be CDI, because *C difficile* is a necessary factor for CDI to occur	Advise susceptible individuals to practice sound food safety measures, restrict visits to recreational waters, and limit their exposure to animal waste
When found in foods, *C difficile* is present in concentrations that are low in comparison with other pathogens (<10^4/g). Unfortunately, CDI hospital epidemiology indicates that only a few spores may induce disease in susceptible people	It is important to reduce the potential load of *C difficile* in the food supply because it remains difficult to predict the people and conditions linked to CDI. Host immunity and gut flora appear to be involved in CDI susceptibility
C difficile requires anaerobic conditions to grow well; however, growth is still possible in 1% oxygen. Minimum cooking-temperature recommendations by most food safety organizations are ineffective in inactivating spores of *C difficile*	Improve food safety and handling practices to ensure that foods are thoroughly cooked and properly handled and stored after cooking with regard to *C difficile*
Nontoxigenic *C difficile* isolates do not cause disease. Unfortunately, nontoxigenic strains are in a minority of *C difficile* isolates from foods in comparison with toxigenic isolates. Nontoxigenic isolates are more frequently present in food animals at processing facilities before harvest, and may be protective in probiotic applications	Research groups and policy makers should continue to work together to identify factors explaining how *C difficile* reaches the food supply and to reduce the presence of *C difficile* in foods. Probiotic strategies based on the use of nontoxigenic *C difficile* strains are under clinical and veterinary development

For a historical overview of the potential for foodborne and zoonotic transmission since the 1980s, see Ref.[1]

SUGGESTIONS TO ADDRESS FOODBORNE CDI CONCERNS

Clinical predictors, experience, and judgment could be empirically sufficient to deem whether a person could have a qualitative high or low risk of contracting CDI, especially if immune-compromising diseases and the administration of antimicrobial therapies are at play, and to suggest educational preventive measures. Foods seem to be a plausible route by which *C difficile* could access susceptible individuals; however, it seems that most of us are exposed to this pathogen and remain asymptomatic. Preventive measures that may be beneficial include the following.

1. Raise awareness among medical trainees about the presence of *C difficile* in foods and animals, and the potential for foodborne and zoonotic transmission.[43]
2. Increase educational efforts to reach primary health practitioners, food professionals, veterinarians, and pharmacists to work together to design and promote

educational preventive measures to involve and protect individuals most suscepti- ble to CDI.

3. Create an evidence-based system to establish criteria for public education related to foods, hygiene, and CDI. It has been 30 years since the first study in the early 1980s reported the presence of *C difficile* in vegetables, recreational waters, and animals.
4. Compose a list of recommendations to address aspects that have been identified as targets for preventive education. Emphasize disinfection measures in household settings, and promote thorough cooking practices during periods deemed to be of high patient susceptibility (**Table 1**).
5. Implement educational programs for food and kitchen professionals to highlight that susceptible patients should not be served foods that could contain *C difficile* if prepared following minimum food safety guidelines, or if eaten raw. Emphasize hygiene, the risk of fecal-oral transmission, and that safe end-point cooking tem- peratures currently recommended by food safety agencies are ineffective against *C difficile* (eg, 71°C for a few seconds).
6. Conduct appropriate studies to determine human infective dose and risk analysis for foodborne CDI.

FUTURE ASPECTS: COMPARISONS WITH ESTABLISHED FOODBORNE PATHOGENS

Given our current knowledge base, it is difficult, if not impossible, to accurately assess the risk or probability that food represents as a vector for CDI. Although there have been no confirmed cases of any foodborne disease caused by *C difficile*,[40,44] certainly all the known factors about *C difficile*, namely its human pathology and epidemiology, its reservoirs, the resistances and distribution of its spores, and its occurrence in foods, suggest that contaminated food products could and may be contributing to community-associated and hospital-associated CDIs. The conservative estimate for CDI cases acquired by community contact (ie, not nosocomial) is 20%, and exactly which community sources cause these cases remains unclear.

ACKNOWLEDGMENTS

Special thanks to Dr Lydia Medeiros, Professor of Human Nutrition at Ohio State University, for insightful comments about food safety education for high-risk populations.

REFERENCES

1. Rodriguez-Palacios A, Borgmann S, Kline TR, et al. *Clostridium difficile* in foods and animals: history and measures to reduce exposure. Anim Health Res Rev 2013;14(1):11–29.
2. Taubes G. Collateral damage: the rise of resistant *Clostridium difficile*. Science 2008;321(5887):360.
3. Wiegand PN, Nathwani D, Wilcox MH, et al. Clinical and economic burden of *Clostridium difficile* infection in Europe: a systematic review of healthcare- facility-acquired infection. J Hosp Infect 2012;81:h1–14.
4. Limbago B, Long C, Thompson A, et al. *Clostridium difficile* strains from community-associated infections. J Clin Microbiol 2009;47:3004–7.
5. Eyre DW, Golubchik T, Gordon NC, et al. A pilot study of rapid benchtop sequencing of Staphylococcus aureus and *Clostridium difficile* for outbreak detection and surveillance. BMJ Open 2012;2(3). pii:e001124.

6. Walker AS, Eyre DW, Wyllie DH, et al. Characterization of *Clostridium difficile* hospital ward-based transmission using extensive epidemiological data and molecular typing. PLoS Med 2012;9(2):e1001172.

7. Cato EP, George WL, Finegold SM. Genus *Clostridium*. In: Sneath PH, Mair NS, Sharpe ME, et al, editors. Bergey's manual of systematic bacteriology, vol. 2. Baltimore (MD): Williams & Wilkins; 1986. p. 1141–200.

8. Rodriguez-Palacios A, Reid-Smith RJ, Staempfli HR, et al. *Clostridium difficile* survives minimal temperature recommended for cooking ground meats. Anaerobe 2010;16:540–2.

9. Rodriguez-Palacios A, LeJeune JT. Moist-heat resistance, spore aging, and superdormancy in *Clostridium difficile*. Appl Environ Microbiol 2011;77:3085–91.

10. Kuehne SA, Cartman ST, Heap JT, et al. The role of toxin A and toxin B in *Clostridium difficile* infection. Nature 2010;467(7316):711–3.

11. Schwan C, Stecher BR, Tzivelekidis T, et al. *Clostridium difficile* toxin CDT induces formation of microtubule-based protrusions and increases adherence of bacteria. PLoS Pathog 2009;5:e1000626.

12. Papatheodorou P, Carette JE, Bell GW, et al. Lipolysis-stimulated lipoprotein receptor (LSR) is the host receptor for the binary toxin *Clostridium difficile* transferase (CDT). Proc Natl Acad Sci U S A 2011;108(39):16422–7.

13. Jangi S, Lamont JT. Asymptomatic colonization by *Clostridium difficile* in infants: implications for disease in later life. J Pediatr Gastroenterol Nutr 2010;51:2–7.

14. Wilson KH, Sheagren JN. Antagonism of toxigenic *Clostridium difficile* by nontoxigenic *C. difficile*. J Infect Dis 1983;147:733–6.

15. Shahinas D, Silverman M, Sittler T, et al. Toward an understanding of changes in diversity associated with fecal microbiome transplantation based on 16s rRNA gene deep sequencing. MBio 2012;3(5). http://dx.doi.org/10.1128/mBio.00338–12.

16. van Nood E, Vrieze A, Nieuwdorp M, et al. Duodenal infusion of donor feces for recurrent *Clostridium difficile*. N Engl J Med 2013;368:407–15.

17. Ananthakrishnan AN, Guzman-Perez R, Gainer V, et al. Predictors of severe outcomes associated with *Clostridium difficile* infection in patients with inflammatory bowel disease. Aliment Pharmacol Ther 2012;35(7):789–95.

18. Bartlett JG. Historical perspectives on studies of *Clostridium difficile* and *C. difficile* infection. Clin Infect Dis 2008;46(Suppl 1):S4–11.

19. Tadesco FJ, Stanley RJ, Alpers DH. Diagnostic features of clindamycin-associated pseudomembranous colitis. N Engl J Med 1971;290:841–3.

20. Arroyo LG, Kruth SA, Willey BM, et al. PCR ribotyping of *Clostridium difficile* isolates originating from human and animal sources. J Med Microbiol 2005;54: 163–6.

21. Borriello SP, Honour P, Turner T, et al. Household pets as a potential reservoir for *Clostridium difficile* infection. J Clin Pathol 1983;36:84–7.

22. Janezic S, Ocepek M, Zidaric V, et al. *Clostridium difficile* genotypes other than ribotype 078 that are prevalent among human, animal and environmental isolates. BMC Microbiol 2012. http://dx.doi.org/10.1186/1471-2180-12-48.

23. French E, Rodriguez-Palacios A, LeJeune JT. Enteric bacterial pathogens with zoonotic potential isolated from farm-raised deer. Foodborne Pathog Dis 2010; 7(9):1031–7.

24. Thakur S, Sandfoss M, Kennedy-Stoskopf S, et al. Detection of *Clostridium difficile* and *Salmonella* in feral swine populations in North Carolina. J Wildl Dis 2011; 47:774–6.

25. Medina-Torres CF, Weese JS, Staempfli HR. Prevalence of *Clostridium difficile* in horses. Vet Microbiol 2011;152:212–5.

26. Zidaric V, Zemljic M, Janezic S, et al. High diversity of *Clostridium difficile* genotypes isolated from a single poultry farm producing replacement laying hens. Anaerobe 2008;14:325–7.
27. Baverud V, Gustafsson A, Franklin A, et al. *Clostridium difficile*: prevalence in horses and environment, and antimicrobial susceptibility. Equine Vet J 2003;35: 465–71.
28. Gould LH, Limbago B. *Clostridium difficile* in food and domestic animals: a new foodborne pathogen? Clin Infect Dis 2010;51:577–82.
29. Broda DM, DeLacy KM, Bell RG, et al. Psychrotrophic *Clostridium* sp. associated with 'blown pack' spoilage of chilled vacuum-packed red meats and dog rolls in gas-impermeable plastic casings. Int J Food Microbiol 1996;29:335–52.
30. Rodriguez-Palacios A, Staempfli HR, Duffield T, et al. *Clostridium difficile* in retail ground meat in Canada. Emerg Infect Dis 2007;13:485–7.
31. Rodriguez-Palacios A, Reid-Smith RJ, Staempfli HR, et al. Possible seasonality of *Clostridium difficile* in retail meat in Canada. Emerg Infect Dis 2009;15:802–5.
32. Weese JS, Reid-Smith RJ, Avery BP, et al. Detection and characterization of *Clostridium difficile* in retail chicken. Lett Appl Microbiol 2010;50:362–5.
33. Harvey RB, Norman KN, Andrews K, et al. *Clostridium difficile* in poultry and poultry meat. Emerg Infect Dis 2011;8:1321–3.
34. Aleccia J. Tainted meats point to superbug C. diff in food. In: Health care @ 2012. Available at: http://www.msnbc.msn.com/id/27774614/print/1/displaymode/1098/. Accessed April 5, 2012.
35. Metcalf DS, Avery BP, Janecko N, et al. *Clostridium difficile* in seafood and fish. Anaerobe 2011;17:85–6.
36. Metcalf DS, Costa MC, Dew MW, et al. *Clostridium difficile* in vegetables, Canada. Lett Appl Microbiol 2010;51:600–2.
37. Warny M, Pepin J, Fang A, et al. Toxin production by an emerging strain of *Clostridium difficile* associated with outbreaks of severe disease in North America and Europe. Lancet 2005;366:1079–84.
38. Rodriguez-Palacios A, Staempfli HR, Duffield T, et al. *Clostridium difficile* PCR riboytpes in calves in Canada. Emerg Infect Dis 2006;12:1730–6.
39. Ackerlund T, Persson I, Unemo M, et al. Increased sporulation rate of epidemic *Clostridium difficile* Type 027/NAP1. J Clin Microbiol 2008;46:1530–3.
40. Truszczynski M, Pejsak Z. Pathogenicity of *Clostridium difficile* in humans and animals in the assessment of eventual connections. Med Weter 2012;68:451–5.
41. Koo H, Darkoh C, Koo C, et al. Potential foodborne transmission of *Clostridium difficile* infection in a hospital setting. In: IDSA press conferences @ 2010. Available at: https://idsa.confex.com/idsa/2010/webprogram/Paper5071.html. Accessed March 2, 2013.
42. Laino C, Martin LJ. Hospital food contaminated with *C. difficile*. In: WebMD @ 2012. Available at: http://www.webmd.com/healthy-aging/news/20121019/hospital-food-contaminated-c-diff. Accessed March 2, 2013.
43. Navaneethan U, Schauer D, Giannella R. Awareness about *Clostridium difficile* infection among internal medicine residents in the United States. Minerva Gastroenterol Dietol 2011;57(3):231–40.
44. Rodriguez-Palacios A, LeJeune JT, Hoover DG. *Clostridium difficile*: an emerging food safety risk. Food Technol 2012;66:40–9.

Foodborne Disease
The Global Movement of Food and People

Jennifer McEntire, PhD

KEYWORDS

• Foodborne illness • Parasites • Global • International

KEY POINTS

• Different types of foodborne illness are endemic to certain parts of the world.
• Food produced in other parts of the world may contain illness-causing pathogens that are not normally encountered in the United States.
• Global travel should be investigated when a patient presents with symptoms of foodborne illness.

THE CONTRIBUTION OF GLOBAL TRAVEL TO FOODBORNE ILLNESS

With the acceleration of international travel, clinicians will be treating foreign diseases on a more frequent basis. It is not only people who travel; the food that we eat also increasingly originates or makes a stop in another part of the world and therefore may be contaminated with pathogens that are not typically encountered in the United States.

Between 2011 and 2012, the number of trips overseas by US citizens increased by about 5.5%.[1] **Box 1** shows the number of trips taken to each part of the world, although certain areas may be more commonly associated with foodborne illness than others. One's risk of contracting a foodborne illness during travel may depend on how stringently food and water precautions are taken, as well as the duration of travel without access to safe food/water. How people may inadvertently become exposed during travel, such as brushing teeth, showering, freshwater swimming, drinking beverages on ice, eating of uncooked fresh salads and already peeled fruits, should also be considered.

In this article, the global burden of foodborne illness is discussed and the types of foodborne illness that are endemic in, or associated with, certain parts of the world are identified. Awareness of these patterns allows clinicians to better diagnose and treat patients who may have acquired a foodborne infection overseas, or who may

The Acheson Group, 1 Old Frankfort Way, Frankfort, IL 60423, USA
E-mail address: jennifer@achesongroup.com

Infect Dis Clin N Am 27 (2013) 687–693
http://dx.doi.org/10.1016/j.idc.2013.05.007
0891-5520/13/$ – see front matter © 2013 Elsevier Inc. All rights reserved.

id.theclinics.com

Box 1	
Foreign trips by US citizens	
Country/Region	**Number of Trips by US Citizens**
Europe	11,244,637
Caribbean	6,435,343
Asia	4,312,544
South America	1,702,867
Central America	2,394,332
Oceania	547,271
Middle East	1,500,282
Africa	364,867
Mexico	20,366,668
Canada	11,853,981

Data from ITA Office of Travel & Tourism Industries. US citizen traffic to overseas regions, Canada and Mexico, 2012. [Online]. 2013. Available at: http://tinet.ita.doc.gov/view/m-2012-O-001/index.html. Accessed March 22, 2013.

have eaten a food grown or processed outside the United States that was contaminated with a pathogen not commonly seen in the United States.

FOODBORNE ILLNESS ON A GLOBAL SCALE

As described by others, estimating the burden of foodborne illness worldwide is not possible, because many countries, especially developing countries, do not have systems in place that require clinicians to notify government health officials that foodborne illness has occurred. In 2006, the World Health Organization began an effort called the Initiative to Estimate the Global Burden of Foodborne Diseases to better understand the levels of foodborne illness around the world.[2]

Research reports and studies specific to certain parts of the world are described later, but it is often difficult to compare data because of the different public health monitoring systems in place in different regions, and the different methods used for analysis. However, there have been attempts to collect and analyze data from various regions to estimate and compare foodborne illness in those areas. A notable study by Majowicz and colleagues[3] reviewed cases of nontyphoidal *Salmonella* gastroenteritis and reported the estimates obtained by the model used. These estimates are provided in **Table 1**. Although the estimates are based on numerous assumptions and limited data, they do show that, at least for 1 pathogen, the rate of illness is related to region of the world. Determining why some areas have higher rates of salmonellosis requires additional study, but clearly individuals traveling to these areas have a greater chance of being exposed to *Salmonella*, and likely other pathogens, particularly those that are transmitted by the fecal-oral route.

FOODBORNE ILLNESS IN THE UNITED STATES

There are several causative agents of foodborne disease that are typically encountered in the United States. The US public health agencies work tirelessly to collect data related to foodborne illness, both outbreaks and sporadic cases, so that the burden of disease is understood and so that efforts can be put in place to prevent further illness.

For example, in the United States, the illnesses identified in **Table 2** are notifiable, meaning that clinicians need to inform their state or local public health officials that

Table 1
Estimated incidence of nontyphoidal *Salmonella* gastroenteritis worldwide

Region	Population (2006)	Estimated Number of Cases Nontyphoidal Salmonellosis Per Year	Incidence Rate Per 100,000 Population
Europe	738,071,000	5,065,000	686
Caribbean	40,525,000	42,000	104
Asia	3,707,089,000	86,425,000	2331
South America	300,623,000	235,000	78
Central America	215,172,000	229,000	106
Oceania	9,002,000	24,000	267
Middle East	410,800,000	563,000	137
Africa	767,239,000	2,458,000	320

Data from Majowicz SE, Musto J, Scallan E, et al. The global burden of nontyphoidal *Salmonella* gastroenteritis. Clin Infect Dis 2010;50(6):882–9.

Table 2
Select notifiable diseases that are potentially or likely related to food

Illness	Notes
Botulism	Foodborne disease is associated with unprocessed or underprocessed canned or jarred low acid foods
Brucellosis	Associated with consumption of unpasteurized milk or cheese, and wild game meat; virtually eradiated in animals in the United States but still problematic internationally
Cryptosporiasis	Generally caused by exposure to contaminated water; produce treated with contaminated water can transmit the parasite
Giardiasis	Generally caused by exposure to contaminated water; produce treated with contaminated water can transmit the parasite
Hepatitis (A)	Infected food handlers with poor personal hygiene can contaminate food
Listeriosis	Associated with ready-to-eat foods, and unpasteurized milk and cheese
Salmonellosis	Historically associated with poultry products, but increasingly associated with a diversity of products
Shiga toxin–producing *Escherichia coli*	Historically associated with ground beef products, but increasingly associated with a diversity of products, including produce
Shigellosis	Mostly associated with person-to-person contact, but food handlers with poor personal hygiene can contaminate food
Trichinellosis	Associated with pork products; generally controlled in the United States but still problematic internationally
Typhoid fever	Most cases are associated with international travel; the most recent US outbreak was associated with imported frozen fruit
Vibriosis	Associated with seafood, particularly shellfish harvested from contaminated water

a case has occurred. This information is shared with the Centers for Disease Control and Prevention, which looks at foodborne illness at a national level. **Table 2** shows a subset of notifiable diseases that can be transmitted via food[4]; there are other notifiable illnesses that could arguably also be food-related because they are related to water, and water is used heavily in the growth, manufacture, and preparation of food. Notes related to each illness are also included.

Several of the diseases listed in **Table 2** can be transmitted by contaminated water. In the United States, water is generally of high quality; however, sanitation and water treatment systems around the world may not meet the same standard. This situation means that the likelihood of acquiring some of these illnesses may increase in parts of the world with poor water quality, and food may serve as a transmission vehicle if the food was exposed to contaminated water during harvesting or washing; contaminated ice can also serve as a vehicle for water-associated pathogens. Food should be considered as a source of illness, especially if patients have recently traveled to parts of the world where water quality is an issue.

Some of the other illnesses in **Table 2** are associated with food animals. In some instances, these pathogens have been controlled or eradicated in animals in the United States. However, the association between the pathogens and their animal hosts may persist elsewhere in the world. Again, the recognition that international travel can serve as a risk factor for certain types of foodborne illness is important.

Each year, the cases of illness for select areas of the country are reported by Food-Net. This information can be extrapolated to the rest of the United States to gain a better picture of foodborne illness. **Table 3** shows the latest FoodNet data, based on reporting sites that cover 15.2% of the US population.[5] The table also shows the percentage of cases who had traveled before illness (and therefore could have acquired illness during their travel), in which travel status was known. The table shows that some illnesses are associated with travel, with the most striking example being illness associated with the parasite *Cyclospora*, which is a water-borne pathogen. More than half the patients infected with *Cyclospora* traveled before the onset of illness.

Although FoodNet data are invaluable in monitoring foodborne illness, these numbers sorely underestimate the total number of cases of foodborne illness

Table 3
Proportion of foodborne illness related to travel

	Total Number of Illnesses Reported Through FoodNet	Incidence Rate in the United States (Per 100,000 Population)	% Cases Who Traveled Before Illness (Among Cases with Known Travel Status)
Salmonella	7813	16.4	8.7
Campylobacter	6785	14.28	16
Shigella	1541	3.24	12.5
Cryptosporidium	1355	2.85	9
STEC non-O157:H7	521	1.1	13.7
STEC O157:H7	463	0.97	3.1
Yersinia	163	0.34	2.2
Vibrio	156	0.33	7.6
Listeria	145	0.31	1.6
Cyclospora	22	0.05	52.4

Abbreviation: STEC, Shiga toxin–producing *Escherichia coli.*

because most illness is self-limiting and ill consumers generally do not seek medical attention.

Compared with other countries, the United States is fortunate to have the resources to investigate foodborne illness in its citizenry. Foodborne illness is not so well documented or studied in other parts of the world, as described in the following sections.

FOODBORNE ILLNESS IN EUROPE

The European Food Safety Authority reports on foodborne illness in the European Union (EU). The report summarizing data from 2011[6] shows that the microbiological agents responsible for foodborne illness in the EU are similar to those in the United States; however, some of the proportions are different. For example, the EU detects higher levels of campylobacteriosis compared with salmonellosis (>220,000 confirmed cases of campylobacteriosis compared with <100,000 confirmed cases of salmonellosis), although more foodborne outbreaks are related to *Salmonella*. Compared with the United States, there are a high number of cases of yersiniosis, and a notable number of illnesses related to *Mycobacterium bovis*.

Although rates of salmonellosis are decreasing in the EU, unlike in the United States, animal husbandry practices are different and could account for the different types of zoonosis, and the relative proportion of each, in the EU compared with the United States. In addition, consumption of unpasteurized milk products, including unpasteurized cheese, is an accepted practice in some parts of the EU. Many of these products are deemed high risk in the United States (particularly for *Listeria monocytogenes*) and are generally not permitted. Thus, travelers to Europe may encounter different risks when eating in the EU compared with the United States.

FOODBORNE ILLNESS IN CHINA

Like in other parts of the world, it is difficult to estimate the total burden of foodborne illness in China. One analysis combed nearly 2500 Chinese articles reporting on illness between 1994 and 2005 and identified 1082 cases of bacterial foodborne illness (an extraordinarily low number given the number of Chinese citizens).[7] Unlike the EU and United States, the most common cause of illness was *Vibrio parahaemolyticus*, which is related to seafood, and was not surprisingly associated with provinces that border water. *Salmonella* was the second most common cause of illness and was associated with inland provinces. The greatest number of deaths were caused by the toxin produced by *Clostridium botulinum* (in the EU and United States, *L monocytogenes* is generally responsible for a high proportion of deaths).[7]

It is difficult to rely on numbers that likely severely underestimate foodborne illness in China. Alcorn and Ouyang note that it is rare for Chinese citizens to seek medical attention for foodborne illness.[8] In addition, China has started to use a system like PulseNet in-country to keep track of and relate foodborne pathogens. Between 2004 and 2011, most isolates submitted to PulseNet were *Salmonella*, followed by *Vibrio cholerae*, *Shigella*, *Yersinia enterocolitica*, *Vibrio parahaemolyticus*, *Listeria*, and *Escherichia coli*.[8]

FOODBORNE ILLNESS IN AUSTRALIA

In Australia, a country of roughly 20 million people, a 2008 report estimated that approximately 5.4 million cases of foodborne gastroenteritis occur annually. The leading cause of illness, *Campylobacter*, causes roughly 225,000 cases annually, with *Salmonella* causing less than 50,000. *L monoyctogenes* and Shiga toxin–producing *E coli* cause a few cases.[9] The use of a PulseNet-like system of foodborne illness tracking has helped the Australians identify several imported products that have resulted in illness, again showing that the global travel of food as well as people carries pathogens around the world.

FOODBORNE ILLNESS IN OTHER PARTS OF THE WORLD

Different factors make it difficult to collect data related to foodborne disease in different parts of the world and different methods in collecting data make it nearly impossible to score countries against each other. For example, in many African nations, the proportion of the population afflicted with human immunodeficiency virus and AIDS skews foodborne illness data, and the fact that a high percentage of food is imported also makes it difficult to analyze root causes of infection. However, the objective of this article is to point out that the risk of foodborne illness does vary in different parts of the world, and travelers to these regions may acquire illness more readily and may acquire illnesses that are less common in the United States.

IMPACT OF GLOBAL FOOD SUPPLY CHAIN

When patients present with suspected foodborne illness, clinicians are well served to inquire about recent international travel. As discussed, the profiles of foodborne disease vary around the world, based in part on the sophistication and regulation of food production systems, and more generally, the ability to control sanitation and hygiene. However, Americans are not only exposed to these conditions when they visit these countries; they may also be exposed when they consume food (anywhere in the world) that was handled in these countries.

The United States has access to one of the most diverse food supplies on the planet, but this is because the United States imports food from all over the world, year round. Imported food accounts for a growing percentage of food consumed annually, and between 1998 and 2007, the value of food imported into the United States nearly doubled.[10] Food import line items have increased at a rate of 10% annually throughout the last decade and show no sign of slowing down.

An analysis of outbreak data from 2005 to 2010 shows that 39 outbreaks and 2348 illnesses were linked to imported food from 15 countries.[10] This finding represents 1.5% of outbreaks associated with a reported food, up from 0.2% of outbreaks in the 1998 to 2004 time frame. Although this finding may seem like a small fraction of outbreaks, this could be because it is more difficult to trace food back to its origin if the origin is outside the United States. Nevertheless, the relative number of outbreaks associated with imported foods has increased, and nearly half of the outbreaks associated with imports occurred in 2009 and 2010, the most recent years analyzed. One-third of outbreaks were associated with *Salmonella* (13), followed by histamine in fish (10) and ciguatoxin (5). Nearly 45% of the outbreaks were associated with foods from Asia. The countries most often associated with outbreaks were Canada and Mexico, with 7 each. The food most commonly associated with illness was fish, with 17 outbreaks (11 of which were from Asia). Spices were the second most common; of the 6 outbreaks, 5 were associated with fresh or dried peppers.

Other parts of the world also struggle with ensuring the safety of imports. After Spain experienced 2 outbreaks of hepatitis A over the course of a decade associated with Peruvian clams, a study was undertaken to evaluate the levels of hepatitis A, norovirus, and astrovirus in mollusks from Peru, Morocco, Vietnam, and South Korea. Although the mollusks complied with current sanitary standards, 40% were positive for at least 1 virus.[11] This is but 1 example showing how practices in 1 part of the world can affect public health in other parts of the world.

IMPACT OF GLOBALIZATION ON FOODBORNE ILLNESS IN THE UNITED STATES

The public health community has a sense of the common foodborne pathogens in patients. With the increase in global travel, and the increasing consumption of foods from around the world, clinicians may need to broaden their thinking when it comes to diagnosing foodborne disease.

REFERENCES

1. ITA Office of Travel & Tourism Industries. US citizen traffic to overseas regions, Canada and Mexico, 2012 2013 [Online]. Available at: http://tinet.ita.doc.gov/view/m-2012-O-001/index.html. Accessed March 22, 2013.
2. World Health Organization. Food safety: initiative to estimate global burden of foodborne disease 2012 [Online]. Available at: http://www.who.int/foodsafety/foodborne_disease/ferg/en/index2.html. Accessed March 22, 2013.
3. Majowicz SE, Musto J, Scallan E, et al. The global burden of nontyphoidal *Salmonella* gastroenteritis. Clin Infect Dis 2010;50(6):882–9.
4. CDC. Summary of notifiable diseases–United States, 2010. MMWR Morb Mortal Wkly Rep 2012;59(53):1–116.
5. Centers for Disease Control and Prevention. Foodborne diseases active surveillance network (FoodNet): FoodNet surveillance report for 2001 (final report). Atlanta (GA): US Department of Health and Human Services CDC; 2012.
6. European Food Safety Authority. The European Union summary report on trends and sources of zoonoses, zoonotic agents and food-borne outbreaks in 2011. EFSA Journal 2013;11(4):3129–379.
7. Wang S, Duan H, Zhang W, et al. Analysis of bacterial foodborne disease outbreaks in China between 1994–2005. FEMS Immunol Med Microbiol 2007; 51(1):8–13.
8. Alcorn T, Ouyang Y. China's invisible burden of foodborne illness. Lancet 2012; 379(9818):789–90.
9. Kirk M, McKay I, Hall G, et al. Food safety: foodborne disease in Australia: the OzFoodNet experience. Clin Infect Dis 2008;47(3):392–400.
10. Centers for Disease Control and Prevention. CDC research shows outbreaks linked to imported foods increasing 2012 [Online]. Available at: http://www.cdc.gov/media/releases/2012/p0314_foodborne.html. Accessed May 12, 2013.
11. Polo D, Vilarino M, Manso C, et al. Imported mollusks and dissemination of human enteric viruses. Emerg Infect Dis 2010;16(6):1036–8.

Index

Note: Page numbers of article titles are in **boldface** type.

A

Acupuncture/acupressure
   in food-borne illness management, 564
AIDS
   food-borne diseases in patients with, 622–623
Antibiotic(s). *See* Antimicrobial agents
Antiemetics
   in food-borne illness management, 564
Antihistamines
   in food-borne illness management, 564
Antimicrobial agents
   Clostridium difficile associated with, 678
   in food-borne illness management, 565–570
      Campylobacter-related, 567
      Cryptosporidium-related, 570
      EHEC–related, 567, 570
      Entamoeba histolytica–related, 570
      enteroaggregative Shiga toxin–producing *E. coli* 0104:H4–related, 570
      Giardia-related, 570
      Salmonella-related, 565–567
      Shigella-related, 567
   in HUS patients, 590
   resistance to
      in emerging trends in food-borne diseases, 524
Antimotility agents
   in food-borne illness management, 562–563
Antispasmodics
   in food-borne illness management, 563
Arthritis
   reactive
      food-borne infections and, 606
Autoimmune disorders
   food-borne infections and, 606–607
Autoimmune thyroid disease
   food-borne infections and, 607

B

Bismuth salts
   in food-borne illness management, 563
Bowel dysfunction
   chronic
      food-borne infections and, 600–606

Infect Dis Clin N Am 27 (2013) 695–704
http://dx.doi.org/10.1016/S0891-5520(13)00060-3
0891-5520/13/$ – see front matter © 2013 Elsevier Inc. All rights reserved.

id.theclinics.com

Moving?

Make sure your subscription moves with you!

To notify us of your new address, find your **Clinics Account Number** (located on your mailing label above your name), and contact customer service at:

Email: **journalscustomerservice-usa@elsevier.com**

800-654-2452 (subscribers in the U.S. & Canada)
314-447-8871 (subscribers outside of the U.S. & Canada)

Fax number: **314-447-8029**

Elsevier Health Sciences Division
Subscription Customer Service
3251 Riverport Lane
Maryland Heights, MO 63043

*To ensure uninterrupted delivery of your subscription, please notify us at least 4 weeks in advance of move.

Printed and bound by CPI Group (UK) Ltd, Croydon, CR0 4YY

03/10/2024

01040390-0001